Handbook of Experimental Pharmacology

Volume 291

The *Handbook of Experimental Pharmacology* is one of the most authoritative and influential book series in pharmacology. It provides critical and comprehensive discussions of the most significant areas of pharmacological research, written by leading international authorities. Each volume in the series represents the most informative and contemporary account of its subject available, making it an unrivalled reference source.

HEP is indexed in Medline/PubMed and Scopus.

Elaine Gray • John Hogwood
Editors

Antithrombotic and Antiplatelet Agents

Springer

Editors
Elaine Gray
Institute of Pharmaceutical Sciences
King's College London
London, UK

John Hogwood
Therapeutic Reference Materials
Medicines and Healthcare Products
Regulatory Agency
South Mimms, Hertfordshire, UK

ISSN 0171-2004 ISSN 1865-0325 (electronic)
Handbook of Experimental Pharmacology
ISBN 978-3-032-22899-4 ISBN 978-3-032-22900-7 (eBook)
https://doi.org/10.1007/978-3-032-22900-7

This Springer imprint is published by the registered company Springer Nature Switzerland AG
The registered company address is: Gewerbestrasse 11, 6330 Cham, Switzerland

Preface

The knowledge of blood being vital for life was a concept dating back to ancient Greece, where the term haemostasis originated. It was known that loss of blood could lead to loss of life, and coagulating agents such as ash were used to try and stem haemorrhage. It was also known that the inverse, unexpected clotting termed thrombosis could give rise to loss of life. While there were some methods of preventing haemorrhage since ancient Greece, the prevention of thrombosis is a relatively more recent development. Over the last century, antithrombotics and anticoagulants have been developed to combat thrombosis for a range of indications and enabling trauma-related surgery. While an extract from leeches could be considered the first known clot preventer, it is heparin that was the first mainstream antithrombotic following its discovery in the 1910s. The chapter by Hogwood and Gray outlines a brief history of antithrombotic developments, their clinical uses, and some explanation of why antithrombotics are needed, especially given the rapid increase in cardiovascular diseases.

The first section on antithrombotics covers vitamin K antagonists, principally warfarin. This section was placed first, as arguably, the mechanism of action was understood for warfarin before any other anticoagulant. The role that warfarin has in a clinical setting is still complex, and despite the development of more targeted agents, warfarin is still an effective agent as a thrombosis prophylaxis (Pengo et al). However, the use of warfarin as an oral antithrombotic has one crucial requirement, in that there is a need for monitoring which ensures safety and efficacy in patients (Jennings and Kitchen).

Heparin has previously been covered in detail by this book series in 2012. Therefore, only a brief overview of the antithrombotic/anticoagulant properties, the mechanism of action coupled with the indications for heparin treatment/prophylaxis is given (Hogwood and Gray). One interesting development for heparin is the securing of the supply chain, and this may involve changing the main source of raw starting material from porcine origin, back to bovine or even ovine sources. The interchangeability of heparin from different sources is not guaranteed and requires consideration, especially if low molecular weight heparins are prepared from non-porcine sources (Jeske).

In the section on direct anticoagulants, we have focused on the oral direct anticoagulants as these are more widely used clinically over parental direct anticoagulants. Their rapid use from development, due to oral availability and precise mode of action and the ease of reversal, has led to broad replacement over warfarin despite their higher costs (Hassan and Lester). However, the monitoring of patients on these drugs is complex due to varying effects on coagulation assays, and furthermore in the laboratory setting the exact therapy may be unknown to the laboratory scientist investigating a patient sample (Reilly-Stitt).

In the last section, platelets, or perhaps using an older name, thrombocytes, are covered. These non-nucleated "cells" were early on known to be involved in thrombosis, and over the years, a huge array of signaling pathways that influence platelet activation have been determined (Pollitt et al). Aspirin had been the sole antiplatelet agent for decades, but now more specific drugs have been developed to target some of these platelet membrane proteins. Some of these antiplatelet agents are used not only as an antithrombotic but increasingly used as anti-inflammatory therapeutics as the role of platelets in inflammation is now better understood (Amison and Pitchford). With the variety of antiplatelet agents available, laboratory monitoring and the effect of these agents on platelet function tests, and indeed what tests should be used requires consideration (Davidson).

While there was recognition of thrombosis as harmful, undoubtedly for hundreds of years, it was not until the last century that treatment options became available. The initial options in use, heparin, warfarin and aspirin, could be thought of as broad-spectrum agents having multiple targets and effects, some of which are non-antithrombotic. The advent of targeted therapies has greatly increased the options available for treatment and prophylaxis of thrombosis with further therapies under development. Given that cardiovascular disease is on the rise across the world, antithrombotics, which have been in use for over a century, will continue to have a critical healthcare role.

London, UK Elaine Gray
South Mimms, UK John Hogwood

Contents

Haemostasis and the Need for Antithrombotics: An Introduction

John Hogwood and Elaine Gray

Contents

Abstract

Antithrombotic and antiplatelet agents have been in use for over 100 years, with many listed as WHO essential medicines. Mortality and morbidity caused by cardiovascular diseases and due to arterial and venous thrombosis are increasing globally. The old legacy products such as heparin and warfarin, and the newer generation of agents, such as DOACs and anti-platelet agents, are needed to protect public health and reduce the burden on global healthcare systems. With new technologies and an increased understanding of the underlining mechanisms of thrombotic diseases, new drugs/therapies will continue to be developed. In addition, these therapies require monitoring to ensure safety and efficacy. This chapter sets the framework for this book.

J. Hogwood (✉)
Therapeutic Reference Materials, Medicines and Healthcare Products Regulatory Agency, South Mimms, Hertfordshire, UK
e-mail: john.hogwood@mhra.gov.uk

E. Gray
Institute of Pharmaceutical Sciences, King's College London, London, UK

E. Gray, J. Hogwood (eds.), *Antithrombotic and Antiplatelet Agents*, Handbook of Experimental Pharmacology 291, https://doi.org/10.1007/164_2026_796

Keywords

Anticoagulant · Antithrombotics · Coagulation · Platelet · Thrombosis

The word haemostasis literally means halting (stasis) of blood (hema) from its Greek origins, and early manuscripts indicate that ancient Greek already had theories on the importance of blood and circulation (Meletis and Konstantopoulos, 2010). Our current knowledge of the interaction of blood vessel endothelium and various blood components such as soluble coagulation factors and platelets has enabled the understanding of the mechanism of the cardiovascular system and aids in the diagnosis of blood-related diseases. This has been well described in the 2002 book by Charles Owen 2002. While haemostasis that leads to generation of clots is an important defence for bleeding, overt formation of clots or thrombi is also detrimental. Both arterial and venous thromboses are significant causes of global mortality and morbidity (Weitz, 2024; Lozano et al., 2012). Antithrombotics are therefore crucial for prevention and treatment of thrombosis. This chapter gives a brief overview of thrombosis, its risk factors and the treatment options to give background to later chapters of this book.

1 What Is Thrombosis?

The maintenance of blood fluidity is a fine balance of the elements in the haemostatic system, which incorporates cellular and soluble components within the blood stream. This fine balance is required to ensure passage of nutrients around the body and to respond very rapidly to 'seal' any site of damage or leakage. The act of sealing a site of damage is a tightly orchestrated process which results in the formation of a blood clot, a thrombus. The process is well described elsewhere (Versteeg et al. 2013) but essentially can be separated into two steps – firstly a cellular response involving platelets followed by a cascade reaction that produces insoluble fibrin.

Thrombus formation is physiologically important to prevent blood loss but it can become unbalance and this can often occur without an underlining event. This will lead to thrombosis and can occur in any location within the cardiovascular system. Venous thrombosis (VT) occurs when clots form from coagulation factors in a vein and are frequently found in deep veins in the leg as deep vein thrombosis (DVT). One of the major complications of DVT is pulmonary embolism (PE) and this occurs when a venous clot breaks off and travels to the lung. Due to the involvement of the coagulation cascade, anticoagulants that target the cascade are the main treatment options for DVT and PE. Arterial thrombi (AT) usually form from activation of both platelets and the coagulation cascade and are the common cause of acute coronary syndrome (ACS) and strokes. Because of the involvement of platelets, anti-platelet agents are important treatment options for arterial thrombosis.

As mentioned above, the primary haemostatic drivers for venous and arterial thrombosis are slightly different. A venous thrombosis is primarily formed through secondary haemostasis with coagulation factors showing an imbalance perhaps due to restricted blood flow (Schulman et al. 2024), whilst arterial thrombosis is primarily driven via platelet activation, following adherence to the endothelium often at a location where an atherosclerotic plaque has formed (Prandoni 2009; Yamashita and Asada 2023). The treatment options for the two types of thrombosis can be different with VT treatment and prophylaxis focused on the clotting cascade, for which heparin, warfarin and the direct oral anticoagulants (DOACs) are the mainstay and AT treatment targeting platelets by use of anti-platelet agents such as aspirin or clopidogrel and are described below.

2 Risk Factors for Thrombosis

There are a range of risk factors associated with thrombosis which can be split into high, medium and low. The highest risk associated with thrombosis is severe trauma (Paffrath et al. 2010) and its treatment, alongside major surgical interventions (Previtali et al. 2011). A recent meta-analysis of major trauma with an Injury Severity Score (ISS) of $\geq$16 (Tran et al. 2024a) has shown that underlying factors such as age, obesity, location of injury, such as spinal or pelvic, will greatly increase the thrombotic risk. The use of anticoagulation in such circumstances is not without complications, as in seeking to treat or prevent thrombosis, there is an associated risk of haemorrhage (Ghafil et al. 2024). In the case of minor trauma, an ISS <9, thrombosis risk is more complex but generally considered medium, with a meta-analysis indicating that leg-related injury clearly increases VT risk, but more generally if hospitalization is required, thromboprophylaxis should be considered (Tran et al. 2024b) due to the possibility of thrombosis following discharge (Thomas et al. 2025). Further, medium-level risk factors include cancer, hormone replacement therapy, auto-immune diseases and thrombophilia, and the lower risk factors include pregnancy, age, obesity, diabetes and immobility (Lowe 2008; Grilz et al. 2018; Pastori et al. 2023).

3 Treatment/Prophylaxis of Thrombosis

As briefly outlined above, the treatment or prevention of thrombosis is complex due to the range of risk factors that a patient may have. For arterial thrombosis treatment, several guidelines have been published which outline indications and the treatment options for these (Kernan et al. 2014; Levine et al. 2016; Gerhard-Herman et al. 2017; Deng and Passam 2025) with a publication by May and Moll summarizing an approach to investigating unexplained arterial thrombosis (May and Moll 2020). Depending on the clinical setting, treatment options are the use of antiplatelet agents, anticoagulants (heparin, DOACs, warfarin) or thrombolytics, the latter of which are used to dissolve thrombi for immediate treatment (Margaglione et al. 1992; Ali et al.

2014). More extensive guidelines are available for VT, covering VT-related disease (Stevens et al. 2024; Wilkins et al. 2025), cancer-associated VT (Lyman et al. 2021; Farge et al. 2022), pregnancy (Kalaitzopoulos et al. 2022) and post-operative conditions (Anderson et al. 2019). Further, depending on the clinical setting, the treatment options can be heparin/low molecular weight heparin, DOACs and warfarin.

4 A Short History of the Use of Antithrombotic Agents

The first 'known' antithrombotic or anticoagulant agent was from leeches, which were used for medicinal purposes, although these purposes are highly dubious in today's glare ('The Medicinal Leech' 1826). It was known that the secretion from leeches contain an anticoagulant-like substance, which enabled the drawing of blood from animals. However, it was not until the 1980s that this material, now known as hirudin was produced for medical purposes (Markwardt 2002). Therefore, heparin which was developed clinically in the 1930s, can be considered as the first 'true' anticoagulant. The first reference material for the potency control of biologically extracted heparin was established in 1941 (Gray 2012). At the time of its initial use, the exact mechanism of how heparin worked as an anticoagulant was unknown, and through the decades, more information about the nature of heparin and its mechanism of action were determined (Barrowcliffe 2012). The primary mechanism of heparin is through interaction with inhibitors of the coagulation cascade (secondary haemostasis), which is briefly summarized in this book (Hogwood and Gray 2025). Low molecular weight heparins work in a similar manner and more broadly have a lower risk of off-target effects, such as causing heparin-induced thrombocytopenia (Arepally and Padmanabhan 2021). A further possible complication is the interest in diversifying the source of heparin from porcine to bovine and possibly ovine, and whether they can be classed as interchangeable (Jeske 2025).

Heparin as a class of biological medicine is widely used, being a WHO Essential Medicine, with interest now moving to a role beyond the haemostatic system. Interest in the non-anticoagulant role of heparin is quite broad, which some recent publications indicating anti-complement, anti-inflammatory and potential anti-cancer properties which could be harnessed for therapeutic use (Lever and Page 2012). Given the increasing accumulation of evidence linking haemostasis and inflammation (Margetic 2012; Foley and Conway 2016; Kuijpers et al. 2022), it may be that non-anticoagulant heparins developed for anti-inflammatory use may still have antithrombotic activity (Casu et al. 2008; Shastri et al. 2014).

The development of warfarin as an anticoagulant was through a series of linked observations. Firstly, it was determined that vitamin K was essential for maintaining haemostasis (Ferland 2012), with a lack of this vitamin leading to bleeding. A second observation was of increased bleeding in cows that had eaten clover coated in a fungus, this led to the finding of dicumarol as the compound which caused bleeding by disrupting vitamin K (Link 1959). Whilst this was being developed into an anticoagulant product, warfarin a similar compound was also being investigated in parallel. Warfarin was then developed into an anticoagulant for clinical use in 1954 (Ball and Featherstone 2025) and is still used today albeit (Pengo et al. 2026) with continuous monitoring being required, as described in a later chapter in this book (Jennings and Kitchen 2025).

Both heparin and warfarin could be viewed as 'broad-spectrum' anticoagulants as multiple elements within the coagulation cascade are targeted, with heparin having an advantage in being reversible and the advantage of warfarin being a minimal cost option. However, heparin and warfarin treatment requires intensive monitoring, and both heparin and low molecular weight heparins are parenteral preparations that are difficult for outpatient use. With the detailed understanding of the interaction of the elements of the coagulation cascade (Davie 2003; Palta et al. 2014), the possibility of developing more specific inhibitors arose. The first synthetic specific inhibitor used clinically is fondaparinux, the structure of which is based on the antithrombin binding pentasaccharide sequence found in heparin (Bauer 2001). Fondaparinux specifically potentiates antithrombin's ability to inhibit activated factor X (FXa), and unlike heparin and low molecular weight heparin, it has no activity against thrombin (FIIa). It also carries lower risk of bleeding and heparin-induced thrombocytopenia (HIT) than heparin. However, it is an injectable and therefore not easily used by patients post-hospitalization.

The development of direct oral anticoagulants (DOACs), a class of chemically synthesized specific inhibitors, heralded the next generation of antithrombotics. Dabigatran, a specific thrombin inhibitor, was licensed for clinical use firstly in the USA in 2010 and then in Europe in 2011 (Ageno et al. 2024; Galanaud et al. 2025). Globally, dabigatran is the only licensed oral direct thrombin inhibitor, but there are a number of marketed oral direct FXa inhibitors – rivaroxaban, apixaban, edoxaban ((CKS/NICE 2025) accessed Feb 2026) and Betrixaban (Skelley et al. 2018). With oral route of administration, short half-life and predictable pharmacokinetics, these new-generation DOACs have overtaken warfarin and other vitamin K antagonists (VKAs) for the majority of thrombotic indications (Hassan and Lester 2025). One major advantage of DOACs over VKAs is that there is no need for routine regular monitoring. However, post-administration monitoring is still required for some patient groups and can prove challenging (Reilly-Stitt 2025). In addition, DOACs are not superior to VKAs for certain indications; for example, anti-phospholipid syndrome and reversal of DOACs are also complicated and costly (Levy et al. 2014; Pengo et al. 2026).

The next generation of specific inhibitors is now being developed. Milvexian and asundexian are two small molecule oral FXIa inhibitors currently in clinical trials. Preliminary data suggest that both milvexian and asundexian could be promising therapeutics with less or equivalent bleeding side effects to current DOACs (Chan and Weitz 2023; Sammut et al. 2024). Other FXIa inhibitors in the pipelines are mostly intravenous monoclonal antibodies, where these candidates have a longer half-life. Another new target for thrombosis is FXIIa, with small molecules (Davoine et al. 2023; Dumas et al. 2024), peptides, siRNA and monoclonal antibodies (Kalinin 2021) being considered. Interestingly, garadacimab, a recombinant monoclonal antibody against FXIIa, has been licensed not for prevention or treatment of thrombotic-related disease, but for patients aged 12 years and older with hereditary angioedema (HAE) to prevent angioedema attacks (Fung 2025). Given the targets of these new inhibitors, it will be interesting to see if, when in clinical use, they are viewed as antithrombotic, anticoagulant or another class of medicine.

The use of agents which target the clotting cascade could be viewed as 'downstream' as invariably platelets form the basis upon which the cascade forms (Scridon 2022). Therefore, the inhibition of platelet activation is logical to reduce the possibility of secondary haemostasis. It was therefore with great interest in the 1960s, that aspirin, or more correctly acetylsalicylic acid as aspirin is technically a trade name, was found to have platelet-suppressing properties (Miner and Hoffhines 2007). Despite aspirin being in clinical use as a patented analgesic since establishment in 1900, it is now also used as an anti-platelet agent (Montinari et al. 2019). The mechanism of aspirin on platelets is well described (Schror 1997), with the suppression of platelet response giving rise to long-term use to prevent or reduce the risk of thrombosis, although this view is now changing (Cofer et al. 2022; Gaziano et al. 2018; Rothwell et al. 2018).

The success of platelet suppression in reducing thrombosis, coupled with an increased understanding of platelet function, led to interest in targeting other platelet activation pathways. The first of these drugs to be developed was ticlopidine, which irreversibly targets the ADP pathway in platelets (Saltiel and Ward 1987). The analogue of ticlopidine, clopidogrel, was then developed (Sangkuhl et al. 2010) and is now broadly used to treat patients with high risk of stroke or myocardia infraction (Patti et al. 2020; Dou et al. 2025) and thus used in the treatment of ACS. With many pathways for platelet activation, as described in a later chapter (Pollitt et al. 2025), there are numerous possible options for developing targeted inhibitors. The first such generated therapy is the monoclonal antibody abciximab, which targets a specific platelet activation pathway (Mascelli et al. 1998) reducing/dampening platelet activation. Other molecules which target platelet activation pathways in use and under development are described in a later chapter (Amison and Pitchford 2026). The continual interest in platelet-based therapies as antithrombotics and anti-inflammatory agents, and the complexity in patient indications, means that the monitoring of platelet response is an aspect that still requires good understanding by laboratory scientists and clinicians (Davidson 2025).

5 Summary

As described, albeit briefly within this chapter, antithrombotics and anticoagulants play a critical role in healthcare. From the first determination of the potential use of heparin over a century ago for treating thrombosis, the options now available have steadily increased. As described in the chapters of this book, there are still challenges associated with these therapeutics from the choice of therapeutic for different indications to the complexity in monitoring/measuring patient samples. However, given the proven benefit of antithrombotics, as evidenced by the development of new drugs, they will continue to have a critical role in global healthcare.

References

Ageno W, Caramelli B, Donadini MP, Girardi L, Riva N (2024) Changes in the landscape of anticoagulation: a focus on direct oral anticoagulants. Lancet Haematol 11:e938–e950

Ali MR, Salim Hossain M, Islam MA, Saiful Islam Arman M, Sarwar Raju G, Dasgupta P, Noshin TF (2014) Aspect of thrombolytic therapy: a review. ScientificWorldJournal 2014:586510

Amison RT, Pitchford SC (2026) Antiplatelet therapy. Handb Exp Pharmacol. https://doi.org/10.1007/164_2025_784

Anderson DR, Morgano GP, Bennett C, Dentali F, Francis CW, Garcia DA, Kahn SR, Rahman M, Rajasekhar A, Rogers FB, Smythe MA, Tikkinen KAO, Yates AJ, Baldeh T, Balduzzi S, Brozek JL, Ikobaltzeta IE, Johal H, Neumann I, Wiercioch W, Yepes-Nunez JJ, Schunemann HJ, Dahm P (2019) American Society of Hematology 2019 guidelines for management of venous thromboembolism: prevention of venous thromboembolism in surgical hospitalized patients. Blood Adv 3:3898–3944

Arepally GM, Padmanabhan A (2021) Heparin-induced thrombocytopenia: a focus on thrombosis. Arterioscler Thromb Vasc Biol 41:141–152

Ball CM, Featherstone PJ (2025) The history of warfarin. Anaesth Intensive Care 53:148–150

Barrowcliffe TW (2012) History of heparin. Handb Exp Pharmacol 207:3–22

Bauer KA (2001) Fondaparinux sodium: a selective inhibitor of factor Xa. Am J Health Syst Pharm 58(Suppl 2):S14–S17

Casu B, Vlodavsky I, Sanderson RD (2008) Non-anticoagulant heparins and inhibition of cancer. Pathophysiol Haemost Thromb 36:195–203

Chan NC, Weitz JI (2023) New therapeutic targets for the prevention and treatment of venous thromboembolism with a focus on factor XI inhibitors. Arterioscler Thromb Vasc Biol 43:1755–1763

CKS/NICE (2025) Anticoagulation – oral : Licensed indications. https://cks.nice.org.uk/topics/anticoagulation-oral/background-information/licensed-indications/

Cofer LB, Barrett TJ, Berger JS (2022) Aspirin for the primary prevention of cardiovascular disease: time for a platelet-guided approach. Arterioscler Thromb Vasc Biol 42:1207–1216

Davidson S (2025) Platelet function tests and monitoring antiplatelet therapies. Handb Exp Pharmacol. https://doi.org/10.1007/164_2025_788

Davie EW (2003) A brief historical review of the waterfall/cascade of blood coagulation. J Biol Chem 278:50819–50832

Davoine C, Traina A, Evrard J, Lanners S, Fillet M, Pochet L (2023) Coumarins as factor XIIa inhibitors: potency and selectivity improvements using a fragment-based strategy. Eur J Med Chem 259:115636

Deng E, Passam FH (2025) Managing patients with a history of arterial disease and new venous thromboembolism. Hematology Am Soc Hematol Educ Program 2025:22–33

Dou N, Ma H, Zhang P, Lu R, Hang J, Sun J (2025) Advances in the clinical use of Clopidogrel: a review of individualized treatment strategies and monitoring optimization based on genetic polymorphisms. Pharmgenomics Pers Med 18:163–177

Dumas A, Goyal N, Mottamal M, Afosah DK, Al-Horani RA (2024) Discovery of a new lead molecule to develop a novel class of human factor XIIa inhibitors. J Thromb Thrombolysis 57:1308–1314

Farge D, Frere C, Connors JM, Khorana AA, Kakkar A, Ay C, Munoz A, Brenner B, Prata PH, Brilhante D, Antic D, Casais P, Esposito MCG, Ikezoe T, Abutalib SA, Meillon-Garcia LA, Bounameaux H, Pabinger I, Douketis J, Thrombosis International Initiative on, and panel Cancer advisory (2022) 2022 international clinical practice guidelines for the treatment and prophylaxis of venous thromboembolism in patients with cancer, including patients with COVID-19. Lancet Oncol 23:e334–ee47

Ferland G (2012) The discovery of vitamin K and its clinical applications. Ann Nutr Metab 61:213–218

Foley JH, Conway EM (2016) Cross talk pathways between coagulation and inflammation. Circ Res 118:1392–1408

Fung S (2025) Garadacimab: first approval. Drugs 85:827–832
Galanaud JP, Laroche JP, Righini M (2025) The history and historical treatments of deep vein thrombosis: toward the era of new anticoagulants. J Thromb Haemost 23:3654–3664
Gaziano JM, Brotons C, Coppolecchia R, Cricelli C, Darius H, Gorelick PB, Howard G, Pearson TA, Rothwell PM, Ruilope LM, Tendera M, Tognoni G, Arrive Executive Committee (2018) Use of aspirin to reduce risk of initial vascular events in patients at moderate risk of cardiovascular disease (ARRIVE): a randomised, double-blind, placebo-controlled trial. Lancet 392: 1036–1046
Gerhard-Herman MD, Gornik HL, Barrett C, Barshes NR, Corriere MA, Drachman DE, Fleisher LA, Fowkes FG, Hamburg NM, Kinlay S, Lookstein R, Misra S, Mureebe L, Olin JW, Patel RA, Regensteiner JG, Schanzer A, Shishehbor MH, Stewart KJ, Treat-Jacobson D, Walsh ME (2017) 2016 AHA/ACC guideline on the management of patients with lower extremity peripheral artery disease: a report of the American College of Cardiology/American Heart Association task force on clinical practice guidelines. Circulation 135:e726–ee79
Ghafil C, Park C, Yu J, Drake A, Sundaram S, Thiele L, Graham C, Inaba K, Matsushima K (2024) The risk of hemorrhagic complications after anticoagulation therapy in trauma patients: a multicenter evaluation. J Trauma Acute Care Surg 96:757–762
Gray E (2012) Standardisation of unfractionated and low-molecular-weight heparin. Handb Exp Pharmacol 207:65–76
Grilz E, Konigsbrugge O, Posch F, Schmidinger M, Pirker R, Lang IM, Pabinger I, Ay C (2018) Frequency, risk factors, and impact on mortality of arterial thromboembolism in patients with cancer. Haematologica 103:1549–1556
Hassan E, Lester W (2025) Direct oral anticoagulant inhibitors: mode of action, clinical aspects. Handb Exp Pharmacol. https://doi.org/10.1007/164_2025_786
Hogwood J, Gray E (2025) Heparin: over 100 years of anticoagulation. Handb Exp Pharmacol. https://doi.org/10.1007/164_2025_780
Jennings I, Kitchen D (2025) Laboratory and point of care monitoring of vitamin K antagonist treatment. Handb Exp Pharmacol. https://doi.org/10.1007/164_2025_782
Jeske W (2025) Comparison of the biologic activity of different species of heparin. Handb Exp Pharmacol. https://doi.org/10.1007/164_2025_781
Kalaitzopoulos DR, Panagopoulos A, Samant S, Ghalib N, Kadillari J, Daniilidis A, Samartzis N, Makadia J, Palaiodimos L, Kokkinidis DG, Spyrou N (2022) Management of venous thromboembolism in pregnancy. Thromb Res 211:106–113
Kalinin DV (2021) Factor XII(a) inhibitors: a review of the patent literature. Expert Opin Ther Pat 31:1155–1176
Kernan WN, Ovbiagele B, Black HR, Bravata DM, Chimowitz MI, Ezekowitz MD, Fang MC, Fisher M, Furie KL, Heck DV, Johnston SC, Kasner SE, Kittner SJ, Mitchell PH, Rich MW, Richardson D, Schwamm LH, Wilson JA, Council on Cardiovascular American Heart Association Stroke Council, Council on Clinical Cardiology Stroke Nursing, and Disease Council on Peripheral Vascular (2014) Guidelines for the prevention of stroke in patients with stroke and transient ischemic attack: a guideline for healthcare professionals from the American Heart Association/American Stroke Association. Stroke 45:2160–2236
Kuijpers MJE, Heemskerk JWM, Jurk K (2022) Molecular mechanisms of hemostasis, thrombosis and thrombo-inflammation. Int J Mol Sci 23:5825
Lever R, Page CP (2012) Non-anticoagulant effects of heparin: an overview. Handb Exp Pharmacol 207:281–305
Levine GN, Bates ER, Bittl JA, Brindis RG, Fihn SD, Fleisher LA, Granger CB, Lange RA, Mack MJ, Mauri L, Mehran R, Mukherjee D, Newby LK, O'Gara PT, Sabatine MS, Smith PK, Smith SC Jr, Halperin JL, Levine GN, Al-Khatib SM, Birtcher KK, Bozkurt B, Brindis RG, Cigarroa JE, Curtis LH, Fleisher LA, Gentile F, Gidding S, Hlatky MA, Ikonomidis JS, Joglar JA, Pressler SJ, Wijeysundera DN (2016) 2016 ACC/AHA guideline focused update on duration of dual antiplatelet therapy in patients with coronary artery disease: a report of the American

College of Cardiology/American Heart Association task force on clinical practice guidelines. J Thorac Cardiovasc Surg 152:1243–1275
Levy JH, Spyropoulos AC, Samama CM, Douketis J (2014) Direct oral anticoagulants: new drugs and new concepts. JACC Cardiovasc Interv 7:1333–1351
Link KP (1959) The discovery of dicumarol and its sequels. Circulation 19:97–107
Lowe GD (2008) Common risk factors for both arterial and venous thrombosis. Br J Haematol 140: 488–495
Lozano R, Naghavi M, Foreman K, Lim S, Shibuya K, Aboyans V, Abraham J, Adair T, Aggarwal R, Ahn SY, Alvarado M, Anderson HR, Anderson LM, Andrews KG, Atkinson C, Baddour LM, Barker-Collo S, Bartels DH, Bell ML, Benjamin EJ, Bennett D, Bhalla K, Bikbov B, Bin Abdulhak A, Birbeck G, Blyth F, Bolliger I, Boufous S, Bucello C, Burch M, Burney P, Carapetis J, Chen H, Chou D, Chugh SS, Coffeng LE, Colan SD, Colquhoun S, Colson KE, Condon J, Connor MD, Cooper LT, Corriere M, Cortinovis M, de Vaccaro KC, Couser W, Cowie BC, Criqui MH, Cross M, Dabhadkar KC, Dahodwala N, De Leo D, Degenhardt L, Delossantos A, Denenberg J, Des Jarlais DC, Dharmaratne SD, Dorsey ER, Driscoll T, Duber H, Ebel B, Erwin PJ, Espindola P, Ezzati M, Feigin V, Flaxman AD, Forouzanfar MH, Fowkes FG, Franklin R, Fransen M, Freeman MK, Gabriel SE, Gakidou E, Gaspari F, Gillum RF, Gonzalez-Medina D, Halasa YA, Haring D, Harrison JE, Havmoeller R, Hay RJ, Hoen B, Hotez PJ, Hoy D, Jacobsen KH, James SL, Jasrasaria R, Jayaraman S, Johns N, Karthikeyan G, Kassebaum N, Keren A, Khoo JP, Knowlton LM, Kobusingye O, Koranteng A, Krishnamurthi R, Lipnick M, Lipshultz SE, Ohno SL, Mabweijano J, MacIntyre MF, Mallinger L, March L, Marks GB, Marks R, Matsumori A, Matzopoulos R, Mayosi BM, McAnulty JH, McDermott MM, McGrath J, Mensah GA, Merriman TR, Michaud C, Miller M, Miller TR, Mock C, Mocumbi AO, Mokdad AA, Moran A, Mulholland K, Nair MN, Naldi L, Narayan KM, Nasseri K, Norman P, O'Donnell M, Omer SB, Ortblad K, Osborne R, Ozgediz D, Pahari B, Pandian JD, Rivero AP, Padilla RP, Perez-Ruiz F, Perico N, Phillips D, Pierce K, Pope CA 3rd, Porrini E, Pourmalek F, Raju M, Ranganathan D, Rehm JT, Rein DB, Remuzzi G, Rivara FP, Roberts T, De Leon FR, Rosenfeld LC, Rushton L, Sacco RL, Salomon JA, Sampson U, Sanman E, Schwebel DC, Segui-Gomez M, Shepard DS, Singh D, Singleton J, Sliwa K, Smith E, Steer A, Taylor JA, Thomas B, Tleyjeh IM, Towbin JA, Truelsen T, Undurraga EA, Venketasubramanian N, Vijayakumar L, Vos T, Wagner GR, Wang M, Wang W, Watt K, Weinstock MA, Weintraub R, Wilkinson JD, Woolf AD, Wulf S, Yeh PH, Yip P, Zabetian A, Zheng ZJ, Lopez AD, Murray CJ, AlMazroa MA, Memish ZA (2012) Global and regional mortality from 235 causes of death for 20 age groups in 1990 and 2010: a systematic analysis for the Global Burden of Disease Study 2010. Lancet 380:2095–2128
Lyman GH, Carrier M, Ay C, Di Nisio M, Hicks LK, Khorana AA, Leavitt AD, Lee AYY, Macbeth F, Morgan RL, Noble S, Sexton EA, Stenehjem D, Wiercioch W, Kahale LA, Alonso-Coello P (2021) American Society of Hematology 2021 guidelines for management of venous thromboembolism: prevention and treatment in patients with cancer. Blood Adv 5: 927–974
Margaglione M, Grandone E, Di Minno G (1992) Mechanisms of fibrinolysis and clinical use of thrombolytic agents. Prog Drug Res 39:197–217
Margetic S (2012) Inflammation and haemostasis. Biochem Med (Zagreb) 22:49–62
Markwardt F (2002) Hirudin as alternative anticoagulant – a historical review. Semin Thromb Hemost 28:405–414
Mascelli MA, Lance ET, Damaraju L, Wagner CL, Weisman HF, Jordan RE (1998) Pharmacodynamic profile of short-term abciximab treatment demonstrates prolonged platelet inhibition with gradual recovery from GP IIb/IIIa receptor blockade. Circulation 97:1680–1688
May JE, Moll S (2020) How I treat unexplained arterial thrombosis. Blood 136:1487–1498
Meletis J, Konstantopoulos K (2010) The beliefs, myths, and reality surrounding the word hema (blood) from homer to the present. Anemia 2010:857657
Miner J, Hoffhines A (2007) The discovery of aspirin's antithrombotic effects. Tex Heart Inst J 34: 179–186

Montinari MR, Minelli S, De Caterina R (2019) The first 3500 years of aspirin history from its roots – a concise summary. Vasc Pharmacol 113:1–8
Owen C (2002) Coagulation: a history of blood coagulation. JAMA 287:1051–1052
Paffrath T, Wafaisade A, Lefering R, Simanski C, Bouillon B, Spanholtz T, Wutzler S, Maegele M, D. G. U. Trauma Registry of (2010) Venous thromboembolism after severe trauma: incidence, risk factors and outcome. Injury 41:97–101
Palta S, Saroa R, Palta A (2014) Overview of the coagulation system. Indian J Anaesth 58:515–523
Pastori D, Cormaci VM, Marucci S, Franchino G, Del Sole F, Capozza A, Fallarino A, Corso C, Valeriani E, Menichelli D, Pignatelli P (2023) A comprehensive review of risk factors for venous thromboembolism: from epidemiology to pathophysiology. Int J Mol Sci 24:3169
Patti G, Micieli G, Cimminiello C, Bolognese L (2020) The role of Clopidogrel in 2020: a reappraisal. Cardiovasc Ther 2020:8703627
Pengo V, Marongiu F, Barcellona D (2026) Are the direct oral anticoagulants better than warfarin for the prevention and treatment of stroke and atrial fibrillation? Handb Exp Pharmacol
Pollitt AY, Hughes CE, Jones CI (2025) Platelet membrane receptors and signalling pathways. Handb Exp Pharmacol. https://doi.org/10.1007/164_2025_787
Prandoni P (2009) Venous and arterial thrombosis: two aspects of the same disease? Clin Epidemiol 1:1–6
Previtali E, Bucciarelli P, Passamonti SM, Martinelli I (2011) Risk factors for venous and arterial thrombosis. Blood Transfus 9:120–138
Reilly-Stitt C (2025) Laboratory testing of direct oral anticoagulants. Handb Exp Pharmacol. https://doi.org/10.1007/164_2025_783
Rothwell PM, Cook NR, Gaziano JM, Price JF, Belch JFF, Roncaglioni MC, Morimoto T, Mehta Z (2018) Effects of aspirin on risks of vascular events and cancer according to bodyweight and dose: analysis of individual patient data from randomised trials. Lancet 392:387–399
Saltiel E, Ward A (1987) Ticlopidine. A review of its pharmacodynamic and pharmacokinetic properties, and therapeutic efficacy in platelet-dependent disease states. Drugs 34:222–262
Sammut MA, Elamin N, Storey RF (2024) Factor XI and XIa inhibition: a new approach to anticoagulant therapy. Br J Cardiol 31:018
Sangkuhl K, Klein TE, Altman RB (2010) Clopidogrel pathway. Pharmacogenet Genomics 20: 463–465
Schror K (1997) Aspirin and platelets: the antiplatelet action of aspirin and its role in thrombosis treatment and prophylaxis. Semin Thromb Hemost 23:349–356
Schulman S, Makatsariya A, Khizroeva J, Bitsadze V, Kapanadze D (2024) The basic principles of pathophysiology of venous thrombosis. Int J Mol Sci 25:11447
Scridon A (2022) Platelets and their role in hemostasis and thrombosis-from physiology to pathophysiology and therapeutic implications. Int J Mol Sci 23:12772
Shastri MD, Peterson GM, Stewart N, Sohal SS, Patel RP (2014) Non-anticoagulant derivatives of heparin for the management of asthma: distant dream or close reality? Expert Opin Investig Drugs 23:357–373
Skelley JW, Thomason AR, Nolen JC, Candidate P (2018) Betrixaban (Bevyxxa): a direct-acting oral anticoagulant factor Xa inhibitor. P T 43:85–120
Stevens SM, Woller SC, Baumann Kreuziger L, Doerschug K, Geersing GJ, Klok FA, King CS, Murin S, Vintch JRE, Wells PS, Wasan S, Moores LK (2024) Antithrombotic therapy for VTE disease: compendium and review of CHEST guidelines 2012-2021. Chest 166:388–404
The Medicinal Leech (1826) Med Chir Rev 5:52–72
Thomas RM, Sparks AD, Wilkinson K, Gergi M, Repp AB, Roetker NS, Smith NL, Muthukrishnan P, Martin K, Zakai NA (2025) Risk factors for venous thrombosis after discharge from medical hospitalizations: the Medical Inpatient Thrombosis and Hemostasis study. J Thromb Haemost 23:2190–2197
Tran A, Fernando SM, Rochwerg B, Hameed MS, Dawe P, Hawes H, Haut E, Inaba K, Engels PT, Zarychanski R, Siegal DM, Carrier M (2024a) Prognostic factors associated with venous

thromboembolism following traumatic injury: a systematic review and meta-analysis. J Trauma Acute Care Surg 97:471–477

Tran A, Lutsey PL, Carrier M (2024b) Minor trauma and venous thromboembolism: the threshold for antithrombotic prophylaxis. Haematologica 109:3860–3867

Versteeg HH, Heemskerk JW, Levi M, Reitsma PH (2013) New fundamentals in hemostasis. Physiol Rev 93:327–358

Weitz JI (2024) Arterial thrombosis: present and future. Circulation 150:905–907

Wilkins CR, Chiu AM, Kishore SA (2025) Medical management of acute venous thromboembolism. Semin Intervent Radiol 42:558–562

Yamashita A, Asada Y (2023) Underlying mechanisms of thrombus formation/growth in atherothrombosis and deep vein thrombosis. Pathol Int 73:65–80

Part I

Vitamin K Antagonist (Warfarin)

Are the Direct Oral Anticoagulants Better Than Warfarin for the Prevention and Treatment of Stroke and Atrial Fibrillation?

Vittorio Pengo, Francesco Marongiu, and Doris Barcellona

Contents

V. Pengo (✉)
University of Padova, Padova, Italy

Arianna Foundation on Anticoagulation, Bologna, Italy

F. Marongiu
Arianna Foundation on Anticoagulation, Bologna, Italy

University of Cagliari, Cagliari, Italy

D. Barcellona
Arianna Foundation on Anticoagulation, Bologna, Italy

Hemostasis and Thrombosis Unit, University of Cagliari, Cagliari, Italy

E. Gray, J. Hogwood (eds.), *Antithrombotic and Antiplatelet Agents*, Handbook of Experimental Pharmacology 291, https://doi.org/10.1007/164_2025_785

Abstract

Atrial fibrillation is the most common cardiac arrhythmia in adults, affecting approximately 59.7 million people worldwide as of 2019—a 111% increase since 1990. Over the past 20 years, the prevalence of AF has risen by 33%, and it is projected to increase by more than 60% by 2050. Age plays a critical role in the factors that contribute to AF. Its prevalence is low (0.1%) in adults under 55 years old but rises to 5.9% in individuals aged 65 and older and 9.0% in those aged 80 and older. In this chapter, we provide a brief history of vitamin K antagonists and direct oral anticoagulants, both of which play a paramount role in atrial fibrillation. We also review the main differences between these two classes of anticoagulants. Furthermore, we aim to address the most common issues associated with DOACs use, particularly concerning patients with renal failure, obesity, and elderly or frail individuals. Lastly, we will discuss some remarks on randomized controlled trials and their limitations. The pivotal role of anticoagulation clinics is also highlighted here, underscoring the need for regular follow-up of both VKAs and DOACs.

1 Introduction

Atrial fibrillation (AF) is the most common sustained cardiac arrhythmia in adults, affecting 59.7 million adults worldwide as of 2019, an increase of 111% since 1990 (Martin et al. 2024; Roth et al. 2020). AF has increased its rates by 33% in the past 20 years, but is expected to increase further by more than 60% in 2050 (Lippi et al. 2021). Atrial fibrosis induces AF, which in turn causes dysfunction of the left atrium and its appendage with the consequence of a fivefold increase in the risk of ischemic stroke (Kamel et al. 2018). Unfortunately, AF is often asymptomatic and the risk of stroke may be underestimated (Bernstein et al. 2021). The prevalence of AF is low (0.1%) in adults younger than 55 years but ranges from 5.9% in those older than 65 years and peaks to 9.0% in those older than 80 years of age (Feinberg et al. 1995). The purpose of this chapter is to answer the question posed to the authors: are direct oral anticoagulants better than Warfarin for stroke prevention in atrial fibrillation? We will try to retrace the steps that have shaped the new era of oral anticoagulation in the prevention of cardio-embolism due to AF along with such dramatic changes in the anticoagulant approach to this topic.

2 A Brief History of Warfarin, AF, and Cardio-embolism

In the 1960s and based on autopsy finding in 1969 (Aberg 1969), it was known that AF was associated with an increased risk of cardio-embolic stroke. This evidence was confirmed in 1977 by Hinton et al. who studied 333 autopsies of patients with AF who had shown embolic episodes. Their findings indicated a high risk of embolism in AF of any origin, particularly due to ischemic heart disease and mitral valvulopathy (Hinton et al. 1977). Results of the Framingham study published by Wolf et al. revealed a close relationship between chronic AF and stroke over a 24-year follow-up (Wolf et al. 1978). They stated that people with chronic AF, with or without rheumatic heart disease (RHD), had a significant risk of stroke "probably due to embolism." Specifically, chronic AF, without RHD, was associated with a five-fold increase in stroke incidence. They concluded that controlled trials of anticoagulants were needed to demonstrate whether stroke could be prevented in people with chronic AF. In 1980, Eaton and Sherman reported that anticoagulation had proven very useful in preventing cerebral embolism in patients with "a cardiac source of embolism" (Easton and Sherman 1980). This statement referred specifically to patients with RHD in whom anticoagulation had been shown to be effective in preventing cardio-embolism. However, while stating that the effect of anticoagulation in patients with nonrheumatic AF was not yet known, they cited the study by Darling et al. in which 40% of patients with AF and systemic embolism had atrial thrombi at autopsy (Darling et al. 1967). These findings clearly suggested that anticoagulation could be an important therapeutic strategy even in patients with AF without RHD. The answer to this question required a randomized controlled trial to demonstrate the efficacy of warfarin versus placebo in patients with AF. Finally, Petersen et al. published the results of a placebo-controlled clinical trial of warfarin and aspirin for the prevention of thromboembolism in chronic AF (Petersen et al. 1989). A total of 1007 patients were randomized to receive warfarin, aspirin (75 mg), or placebo for 2 years. Only 5 patients treated with Warfarin had thromboembolic complications compared with 20 patients treated with aspirin and 21 with placebo. The authors concluded that warfarin could be recommended to prevent thromboembolism in patients with AF. Five additional randomized trials were subsequently conducted and incorporated into a meta-analysis (Hart et al. 1999). Overall, Warfarin reduced stroke by 62% with an absolute risk reduction of 2.7% (number need to treat: 37) per year in primary prevention and 8.4% per year in secondary prevention (number need to treat: 12) at the cost of 0.3% per year increase in major extracranial bleeding.

3 The New Era of Direct Oral Anticoagulants

After many years when the only available anticoagulants were vitamin K antagonists (VKAs), several molecules were developed to replace warfarin as an oral antithrombotic drug in AF. The primary goal was to discover new drugs inducing direct inhibition of coagulation factors without the burden of INR monitoring.

Secondary goals were to reduce bleeding (particularly intracerebral hemorrhage), drug interference, and dietary restrictions. To address all these challenges, a new direct thrombin inhibitor was developed: Ximelagatran (Eriksson et al. 2003).

This new drug opened a revolutionary road in the prevention of cardio-embolism in AF. Ximelagatran was challenged against warfarin in two phase 3 non-inferiority randomized controlled trial (RCT): an open-label one performed in Europe (SPORTIF III) and a double-blind trial conducted in the United States (SPORTIF V). Compared to warfarin, the primary outcome rate (cardio-embolic events) was lower with Ximelagatran in SPORTIF III but higher in SPORTIF V in which non-inferiority goal was not reached. Consequently, results of the trial were deemed invalid by the Food and Drug Administration (FDA) and the development of Ximelagatran was discontinued (Albers and Investigators S 2004).

From 2009 to 2013, four new anticoagulants have been challenged against warfarin in non-inferiority trials: Dabigatran, Rivaroxaban, Apixaban, and Edoxaban (Connolly et al. 2009; Patel et al. 2011; Granger et al. 2011; Giugliano et al. 2013). These new anticoagulants were thought to have a reduced toxicity and a more predictable pharmacokinetics and pharmacodynamics by inhibiting directly the single coagulation factor thrombin (FIIa) or factor Xa (FXa) and were collectively referred to as direct-acting oral anticoagulants (DOACs) or non-vitamin K antagonist oral anticoagulants (NOACs).

Approved by the European Medicines Agency (EMA) in 2008 and by the Food and Drug Administration (FDA) in 2010, the FIIa inhibitor Dabigatran was the first DOAC to be introduced in clinical practice for prevention and treatment of thrombosis and cardio-embolic events. Ensuing the FXa inhibitors Rivaroxaban, Apixaban and Edoxaban were approved.

In comparison with VKAs, DOACs offered a number of clinical advantages: no routine laboratory monitoring or frequent dose adjustments because of a more predictable anticoagulant effect (Denas and Pengo 2011). In all these RCTs, the inferiority margin was taken at 1.46. Main results of registration trials are reported in Table 1. Dabigatran 150 mg BID and Apixaban 5 mg BID were superior while Rivaroxaban (20/15 mg OD) and Edoxaban (60/30 mg QD) were non-inferior to warfarin in stroke/systemic embolism prevention in patients with non-valvular AF. Only Edoxaban 30/15 mg OD resulted inferior to warfarin when only ischemic stroke was considered (HR: 1.41, 95% CI: 1.19–1.67). All-cause mortality was similar or reduced in patients with AF receiving DOACs as compared with warfarin therapy.

As far as major bleeding is concerned, all the DOACs were superior to warfarin. In particular, the number of intracranial hemorrhages (ICH) was halved compared to warfarin. How can this striking result be explained? Tissue Factor-Factor VIIa (TF-FVIIa) complex plays a key role in *idling* (keeping *a* motor running at a very low speed) the clotting cascade. Factor VII is crucial to ensure everyday local hemostasis. In other words, even a very small vascular injury in the brain is counterbalanced by the TF-FVIIa hemostatic complex. Hemostasis may not take place in case of VKAs treatment when the vitamin K-dependent factor VII is reduced thereby not allowing a rapid vascular repair (Mackman 2009) (Fig. 1).

Table 1 Main outcomes in the 4 RCT versus warfarin

Anticoagulant	Stroke/SE	RR vs. warfarin	Major bleeding	RR vs. warfarin	ICH	RR vs. warfarin
Dabigatran 150	1.11	0.66 (0.53–0.82)	3.11	0.93 (0.81–1.07)	0.30	0.40 (0.27–0.60)
Dabigatran 110	1.53	0.91 (0.74–1.11)	2.71	0.80 (0.69–0.93)	0.23	0.31 (0.20–0.47)
Warfarin	1.69		3.36		0.74	
Rivaroxaban	2.1	0.88 (0.75–1.03)	3.6	1.04 (0.90–1.20)	0.5	0.67 (0.47–0.93)
Warfarin	2.4		3.4		0.7	
Apixaban	1.27	0.79 (0.66–0.95)	2.13	0.69 (0.60–0.80)	0.33	0.42 (0.30–0.58)
Warfarin	1.60		3.09		0.80	
Edoxaban 60	1.57	0.79 (0.63–0.99)	2.75	0.80 (0.71–0.91)	0.39	0.47 (0.34–0.63)
Edoxaban 30	2.04	1.07 (0.87–1.31)	1.61	0.47 (0.41–0.55)	0.26	0.30 (0.21–0.43)
Warfarin	1.80		3.43		0.85	

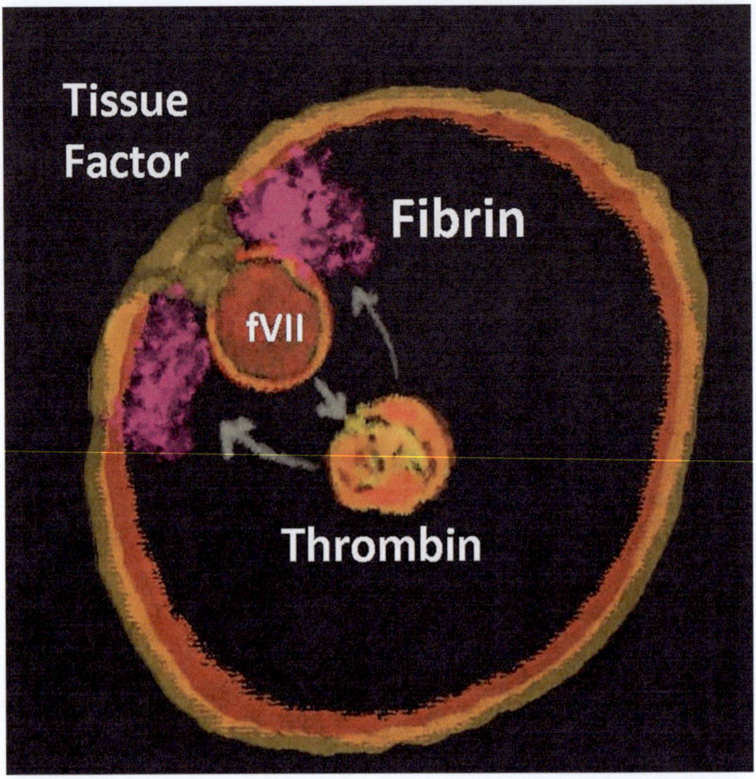

Fig. 1 TF-FVIIa complex plays a key role in idling (a motor running at a very low speed) of the clotting cascade. Factor VII is crucial to ensure everyday local hemostasis which may be lost if factor VII is reduced by VKAs

In 2014, Ruff et al. published a meta-analysis which included 42,411 patients treated with DOACs and 29,272 who received Warfarin. In comparison with warfarin, DOACs reduced cardio-embolic events (RR 0·81, 95% CI 0·73–0·91), all-cause mortality (RR 0.90, 95% CI: 0.85–0.95), and intracranial hemorrhage (RR 0.48, 95% CI: 0.39–0.59) (Ruff et al. 2014). These data were confirmed in a systematic review and network meta-analysis (Lopez-Lopez et al. 2017) and by using administrative data and propensity score methodology (Denas et al. 2017). Nevertheless, despite a reduced rate of major bleeding by 14%, post-authorization data showed that the risk of hemorrhagic complications during DOACs treatment remains worrying. With these agents, major bleedings have been reported at an annual rate of 2.1–3.5%, along with 0.25–0.51% of intracranial bleeding (ICH) and an increased rate of gastrointestinal bleeding (GIB) (HR = 1.25, 95% CI: 1.01–1.55) (Zoppellaro et al. 2018). The latter figure was confirmed later by a systematic review and network meta-analysis which found higher rates of GIB (+47%, +40% and +22% versus warfarin) induced by Rivaroxaban 20 mg, Dabigatran 300 mg, and Edoxaban 60 mg daily, respectively. Apixaban 5 mg twice daily showed lower major GIB in

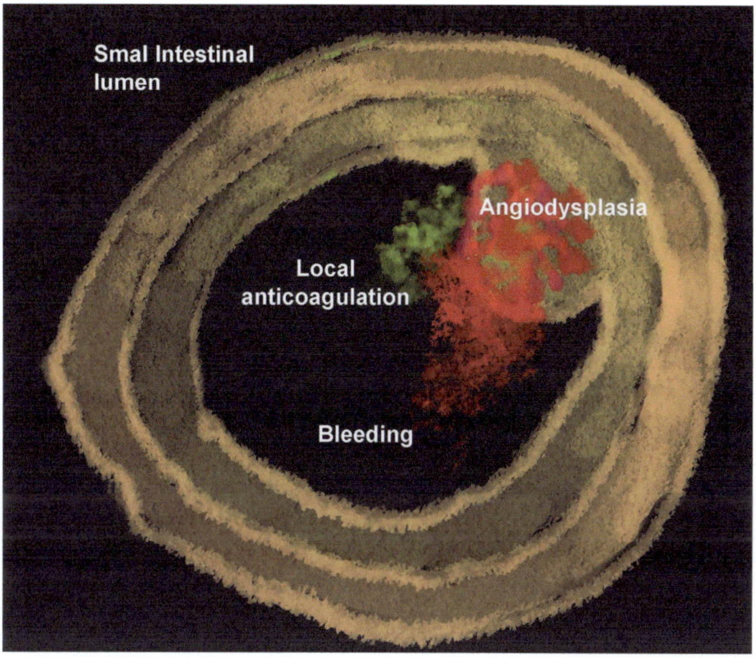

Fig. 2 Non-adsorbed DOACs along the intestinal tract are still active thus promoting bleeding if peptic ulcer, gastritis, angiodysplasia, diverticulosis, polyps, cancer, or hemorrhoids are present

comparison with dabigatran 300 mg (OR, 0.63; 95% CI, 0.44–0.88) and Rivaroxaban 20 mg (OR, 0.60; 95% CI, 0.43–0.83) daily (Radadiya et al. 2021). Accordingly, Ingason reported that the use of Rivaroxaban was associated with a higher risk of GIB when compared with other DOACs (Ingason et al. 2022). Why do most of the DOACs increase the risk of GIB? A possible explanation is that amounts of non-adsorbed still active DOACs promote bleeding in the presence of unknown lesions of the intestinal tract such as peptic ulcer, gastritis, angiodysplasia, diverticulosis, polyps, cancer, or hemorrhoids (Desai et al. 2013; Coleman et al. 2012). Despite a careful collection of patient's personal history, this was found to be neither a predictor for GIB bleeding nor a guide to the choice of the oral anticoagulant to be offered. Nevertheless, a good clinical choice is to check the hemoglobin level and search of occult blood in the stool before starting and during the follow-up of DOAC-treated patients (Barcellona et al. 2021a) (Fig. 2).

3.1 Real-World Evidence and Guidelines

In 2018, Potpara reported that the real-world evidence substantially confirms the results of registration RCTs (Potpara 2018) despite several limitations of post-approval observational studies (Potpara and Lip 2017). Indeed, DOACs are today

Table 2 ICH in AF patients treated with warfarin[a]

Study	ICH %/year
Palareti et al. Prospective study (28.1% >80 years)	0.43
Poli D et al. Prospective study (80–104 years)	0.55
Connolly SJ et al. RE-LY (Dabigatran)	1.0
Patel MR et al. ROCKET-AF (Rivaroxaban)	0.83
Granger CB et al. ARISTOTLE (Apixaban)	1.29
Giugliano RP et al. ENGAGE.AF (Edoxaban)	1.20

[a]Prospective observational studies and RCT in patients >75 years of age

recommended over warfarin for the prevention of cardio-embolic stroke in patients with AF (Joglar et al. 2024).

3.2 Remarks on the Registration Trials

Some points deserve attention on the four DOACs registration RCT. In 2017, Palareti et al. reported the rate of major bleeding and ICH of 5707 patients treated with VKAs and monitored during a follow-up of 8906 patient-years by the Italian Anticoagulation Clinics (FCSA) (Palareti et al. 2017). Mean age was 73.0 years (28.1% >80 years) and 61.6% were treated for AF. The rate of major bleeding and ICH in the AF group was 1.4%/year and 0.43%/year respectively. Previously, Poli et al. published a prospective study on the bleeding risk in very old patients (80–104 years old) treated with VKAs and followed by FCSA during a period of 7,560 person/years in the AF population (Poli et al. 2011). The rate of major bleeding and ICH in the AF patients were 1.73% pts/years and 0.55% pts/years respectively. Taken together, these figures appear to be significantly lower than those reported in the four RCTs. The difference between these data collected in real life was even greater in patients ≥75 years of age in the four RCT in comparison with Warfarin as reported by Schäfer et al. (2020) (Table 2). The striking reduction seen in the Italian Anticoagulation Clinics could account for better surveillance than that of the world centers involved in the four RCTs as reported by Wallentin et al. (2010).

4 Comparison of DOACs vs. Warfarin in Special Situations

4.1 DOAC vs. Warfarin in Obese Patients

A systematic review analyzed the efficacy and safety of DOACs versus warfarin in obese patients (BMI >30Kg/m^2) with AF. As compared to warfarin, DOACs use showed a significant reduction in stroke (RR = 0.80, 95% CI: 0.65–0.90), hemorrhagic stroke (RR = 0.58, 95% CI: 0.38, 0.88), major bleeding (RR = 0.76, 95% CI: 0.63, 0.92), GIB (RR = 0.59, 95% CI: 0.49, 0.72), and ICH (RR = 0.45, 95% CI 0.34, 0.60) (Karakasis et al. 2024). The same results were obtained in patients with

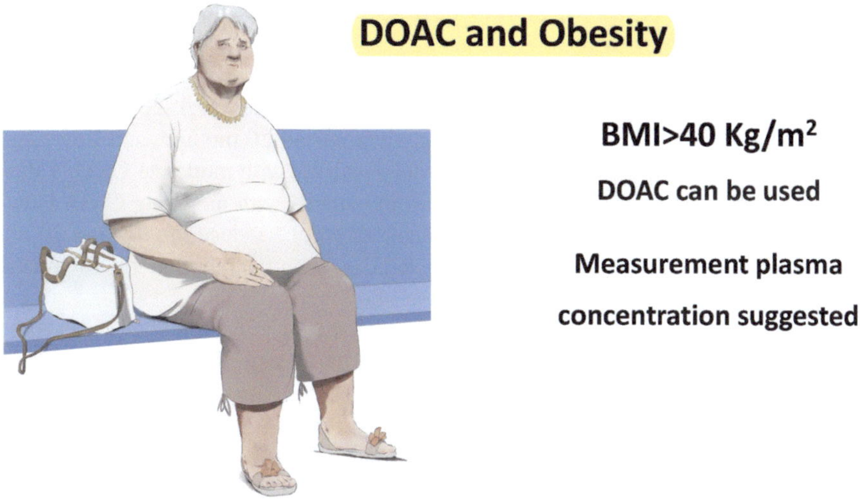

Fig. 3 In the obesity patients with AF, DOACs can be offered but the measurement at through and peak of plasma concentration at steady-state is suggested

BMI >40 kg/m^2 although the composite endpoint (stroke and systemic embolism) was not statistically different between warfarin and DOACs use (Sagris et al. 2025). Measuring trough and peak plasma DOACs concentration in 160 patients with a median BMI of 32.3 kg/m^2, Menichelli et al. found a significant percentage of patients with below optimal range drug concentration. The authors suggested that measuring DOACs plasma concentration in obesity class ≥ II (BMI 35–39.9 Kg/m^2) may be important. This may be another wise indication that the assessment of plasma DOAC concentration may be needed other than those recognized to be crucial; such as before surgical or invasive procedures (Tripodi et al. 2018) (Fig. 3).

4.2 DOACs and Chronic Kidney Disease

All DOACs are excreted by the kidneys and treatment dosage varies according to the glomerular filtration rate (Elenjickal et al. 2024). Dabigatran, a strong thrombin inhibitor, is mainly excreted by kidneys (80%) and the binding to plasma protein is low (26–28%) thus allowing its removal by hemodialysis (Ganetsky et al. 2011). Apixaban metabolism involves both kidneys (27%) and oxidative pathways via P450, biliary and direct intestinal excretion (Byon et al. 2019). The percentage of Rivaroxaban excreted by the kidneys is 35% of the administered dose while two-thirds are metabolized by the liver via cytochrome P450 enzymes (CYP3A4, CYP2J2) (Kreutz 2012). Edoxaban metabolism includes both kidneys (50%) and extra-kidneys (50%) pathways (cytochrome CYP3A4) (Parasrampuria and Truitt 2016). All factor Xa inhibitors bind plasma protein and are only marginally removed by hemodialysis (Mavrakanas et al. 2015).

4.2.1 DOACs Versus VKAs in Patients with AF and Moderate CKD (CrCl 30–50 mL/min)

Dabigatran 150 mg and Apixaban 5 mg BID showed lower rates of stroke/SE in patients with moderate CKD (Hijazi et al. 2014; Hohnloser et al. 2012) while the rates of stroke/SE with dabigatran 110 mg, rivaroxaban 20 mg OD, and Edoxaban 60 mg OD were not different from warfarin in patients with moderate CKD. Taken together, DOACs are preferable to warfarin in patients with moderate CKD. However, the dose of Rivaroxaban and Edoxaban should be reduced to 15 and 30 mg daily and that of Dabigatran to 110 mg BID as recently reported by Elenjickal et al. (2024).

4.2.2 DOACs Versus VKAs in Patients with AF and Severe CKD (CrCl <30 mL/min)

Patients with creatinine clearance (CrCl) below 30 mL/min were excluded from registration in RCTs. Lack of good-quality evidence in CKD has led to differences in recommendations by various guidelines (Mavrakanas et al. 2020). In a "post hoc" analysis from the ARISTOTLE trial, 269 patients with CrCl of 25–30 mL/min received either apixaban (2.5/5 mg) or warfarin. Apixaban was associated with lower rate of stroke/SE (HR 0.55, 95% CI: 0.20–1.51) and major bleeding (HR 0.34, 95% CI: 0.14–0.80) and this dosage is recommended in patients with severe CKD (Stanifer et al. 2020). However, a more recent report stated that 5 mg BID was associated with higher rates of major bleeding in comparison with that of 2.5 mg BID. Accordingly, the dose recommended in patients with severe CKD is 2.5 mg/BID (Xu et al. 2023). Only retrospective data suggest a reduced dose of Rivaroxban and Edoxaban in these patients. Specifically, in patients with CKD stage 4 (eGFR 15–29 ml/min), DOACs (but not dabigatran) should be used with caution because of lack of clear evidence. DOACs plasma concentration may be a useful tool in severe CKD, as recommended by the International Society of Thrombosis and Hemostasis (ISTH) (Baglin et al. 2013), although a great interpatient variability was noted (Testa et al. 2016) and plasma levels poorly correlate with GFR (Testa et al. 2019). Concerning the estimate of renal function, the Cockcroft-Gault equation was used in registration RCTs but more precise formulas as the Modification of Diet in Renal Disease Study (MDRD) and Chronic Kidney Disease Epidemiology Collaboration (CKD-EPI) are now recommended (Schaeffner et al. 2012; Michels et al. 2010). MDRD or CKD-EPI do not consider body weight and are more suitable in the clinical wards, where the measurement of weight in bedridden patients is often impossible to obtain. Both equations, however, may overestimate GFR in elderly patients (Dowling et al. 2013).

4.2.3 Oral Anticoagulants in Patients with Atrial Fibrillation and End-Stage Kidney Disease (ESKD)

There is no robust study to recommend the use of DOAC in patients with CKD Stage 5 (<15 ml/min) or on long-term dialysis. Hence, the use of DOACs in this setting is not recommended (Grandone et al. 2021). Warfarin should be used with caution since bleeding risk increases with the severity of CKD (Mavrakanas et al. 2015) and

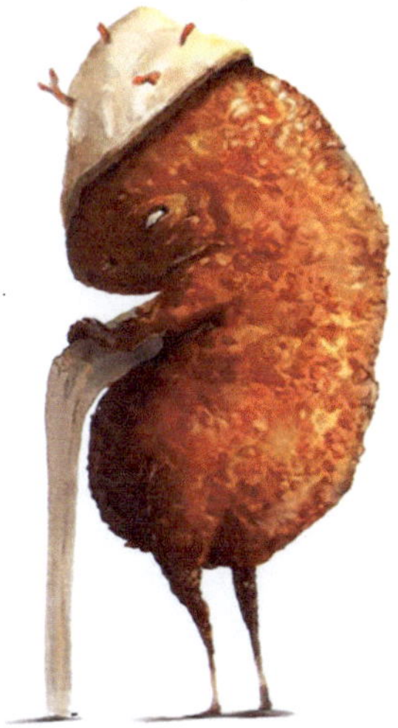

Fig. 4 In chronic kidney disease DOACs are *recommended, **suggested, *** limited data, use with caution, consider risks and benefits. ****Warfarin is to be used with caution

stage 4 patients require a 20% dose reduction to maintain INR in the therapeutic range (De Vriese et al. 2021) with 5.8-fold higher risk of bleeding at supratherapeutic INRs (Limdi et al. 2015). This is why Nephrologists spur the use of oral anticoagulants in ESKD unless the thrombosis risk is very high (Fig. 4).

5 DOACs vs. VKAs in AF and Acute Coronary Syndrome

Until the advent of DOACs, patients with AF undergoing percutaneous coronary intervention (PCI) with stent placement were treated with VKAs combined with dual antiplatelet therapy (DAPT) consisting of a $P2Y_{12}$ receptor inhibitor and aspirin to reduce the risk of coronary thrombosis and cardio-embolic stroke. To reduce the risk of bleeding, DOACs have been tested in this clinical setting where the sample size calculation was targeted for safety and not for efficacy. In the PIONEER AF-PCI (Gibson et al. 2016) and RE-DUAL PCI studies (Cannon et al. 2017), rivaroxaban and dabigatran combined with a $P2Y_{12}$ inhibitor (Clopidogrel in about 90% of cases) were compared with the classic triple therapy (Warfarin plus ASA plus a $P2Y_{12}$ inhibitor).

In the PIONEER AF-PCI study, 2124 patients were randomly assigned to low-dose Rivaroxaban (15 mg) OD plus a $P2Y_{12}$ inhibitor in one arm, very low-dose rivaroxaban (2.5 mg) BD plus DAPT in the second arm vs. classical triple therapy. Clinically significant bleeding was lower in the two arms receiving rivaroxaban than in the group receiving standard therapy (HR 0.63, 95% CI: 0.50–0.80 and HR 0.59, 95% CI: 0.47–0.76, respectively). The rates of death from cardiovascular events, myocardial infarction, or stroke were similar in the three groups.

In the RE-DUAL PCI study, 2725 patients were randomly assigned to the Dabigatran (110 mg or 150 mg BD) plus a $P2Y_{12}$ inhibitor (Clopidogrel or Ticagrelor) and no Aspirin versus triple therapy with Warfarin plus a $P2Y_{12}$ inhibitor (Clopidogrel or Ticagrelor) and Aspirin for 1–3 months.

The incidence of major and clinically relevant bleeding was similar to that of triple therapy using dabigatran 150 mg (HR 0.72, 96% CI: 0.58–0.88, $p < 0.001$ for non-inferiority) while it was significantly lower using Dabigatran 110 mg (HR 0.52, 96% CI: 0.42–0.63, $p < 0.001$ for superiority).

The AUGUSTUS study randomized assigned patients to apixaban at a dose of 5 mg or 2.5 mg BID plus a $P2Y_{12}$ inhibitor versus warfarin combined with ASA and a $P2Y_{12}$ inhibitor or warfarin combined with a $P2Y_{12}$ inhibitor, for 6 months (Lopes et al. 2019). Results showed that major and clinically relevant non-major bleeding were significantly lower in the group treated with Apixaban and a $P2Y_{12}$ inhibitor compared to the other treatment arms. Moreover, patients in the Apixaban group had a lower incidence of death or hospitalization than those in the VKAs group (HR 0.83, 95% CI: 0.74–0.93) and a similar incidence of ischemic events. In the ENTRAST study, Edoxaban at a dose of 60 mg or 30 mg OD in association with a $P2Y_{12}$ inhibitor was tested versus the classic triple therapy with VKAs. Edoxaban compared to VKAs showed non-inferiority in terms of safety (HR 0.83, 95%: 0.65–1.05, p non-inferiority $= 0.001$) (Vranckx et al. 2019). A recent meta-analysis of registration studies on almost 11,000 patients confirmed that DOACs associated with a $P2Y_{12}$ inhibitor reduce the overall risk of bleeding (OR 0.59, 95% CI: 0.41–0.86) with similar efficacy (OR 1.03, 95% CI: 0.86–1.24) in terms of cardiovascular events (Zoppellaro et al. 2020).

Yet, it is not clear whether the reduction in bleeding events is attributable to the early suspension of ASA (on average after 7 days in all the studies) or is a specific effect related to the use of DOACs. Summing up, results showed that dual therapy (DOACs associated with a $P2Y_{12}$ inhibitor) is as effective as triple therapy in reducing major cardiovascular events and reducing the risk of bleeding. However, a trend toward an increase in stent thrombosis and cardiovascular events in patients with ACS with this strategy was noted. DOACs associated with antiplatelet therapy are in the new AF guidelines as the first choice in patients undergoing PCI and stent placement.

6 Safety of VKA and DOAC in Elderly Patients

Elderly patients with AF are burdened with a combination of a higher risk of both stroke and bleeding (Hanon et al. 2013). Despite the net clinical benefit in favor of oral anticoagulation use (Karamichalakis et al. 2016; Ng et al. 2016; Patti et al. 2017), elderly patients are undertreated due to safety concern (Steffel et al. 2021).

Overall, women pay more for this inappropriate behavior (Marongiu et al. 2024). Indeed, the risk of bleeding during anticoagulant therapy with VKAs is amplified by age, thus requiring frequent monitoring and management. Sensitivity to warfarin, polypharmacy, and comorbidities make it difficult to maintain stable anticoagulation (Bungard et al. 2000). A suboptimal Time in the Therapeutic Range (TTR <70%) was often evident in patients treated with Warfarin with consequent increase in bleeding risk particularly in the elderly (Zulkifly et al. 2022). The better safety profile boosted an increased use of DOACs in elderly AF patients (Ko et al. 2022). A recent meta-analysis showed a lower risk of intracranial bleeding, hemorrhagic stroke, and fatal bleeding using DOACs vs. VKAs in the elderly patients (Silverio et al. 2021). In a timely nationwide study in patients 75 years of age and older a better safety profile for DOACs was found. In comparison with warfarin, major bleeding was reduced using dabigatran (HR 0.75 95% CI: 0.52 to 1.08), rivaroxaban (HR 0.96, 95% CI 0.78–1.16), and significantly for Apixaban (HR 0.74, 95% CI 0.60–0.91) (Rutherford et al. 2022). As already mentioned, an increased risk of GIB in the older patients (over 75 years old) was observed with DOACs as compared to warfarin.

7 Safety of Oral Anticoagulants in Frail and Other Frailty-Related Conditions

Frailty is defined as a clinical condition characterized by a decline in reserve and function classified as low grip strength, low energy, slow walking speed, low level of physical activity, and weight loss (Fried et al. 2001). One of the most common reasons to underprescribe oral anticoagulation is frailty (Volgman et al. 2022). This condition has not been specifically evaluated in DOACs registration trials and post-marketing observational cohorts. One prospective, multicenter cohort study that enrolled consecutive very elderly (≥80 years) anticoagulation-naïve patients starting recommended doses of Edoxaban found that anticoagulation is feasible in very elderly patients with AF even if frail (Denas et al. 2023).

The incidence rate ratio for major bleeding and clinically relevant nonmajor (CRNM) bleeding did not statistically differ between frail and fitter patients (RR 0.7, 95% CI: 0.1–2.7 and 0.7, 95% CI: 0.2–2.2, respectively). The strengths of the study included the enrollment of consecutive very elderly patients, a significant number of elderly women (often underrepresented in clinical trials), and a standardized and reproducible pre-enrollment frailty score rather than a simple evaluation of the phenotype. A post hoc analysis of the ENGAGE TIMI 48 trial (Wilkinson et al. 2020) showed that Edoxaban was similarly efficacious to Warfarin across the frailty spectrum and was associated with lower rates of bleeding. Overall, available data highlight that frailty is not a contraindication to offset the benefit of anticoagulation.

8 DOACs Drug-Drug Interaction and Rare Adverse Events

Potential limitations of DOACs use derive from pharmacokinetic and pharmacodynamic drug interactions (Vranckx et al. 2018). Although less common than with VKAs, evidence regarding interactions of DOACs with co-administered drugs is accumulating (Steffel et al. 2021). All DOACs are substrates of P-glycoprotein and may interact with strong inducers or inhibitors of this transporter. Rivaroxaban and, to a lesser extent, Apixaban are also substrates of cytochrome P450 (Harskamp et al. 2019). Rarer non-bleeding adverse events are reported by pharmacovigilance and case reports. Hepatic impairment, gastrointestinal disorders, and rare renal complications have been described (Raschi et al. 2016; Maura et al. 2018). From a practical point of view, dyspepsia has been found to be one of the main reasons for DOACs discontinuation (Beyer-Westendorf et al. 2016; Hecker et al. 2016). Other rare adverse events as increased liver enzymes, hyperbilirubinemia (Caldeira et al. 2014), acute hepatitis treated with venovenous hemodiafiltration (Porru et al. 2017), and severe skin adverse events with dabigatran, rivaroxaban, and apixaban (An et al. 2017; Barrett et al. 2015; Pansuriya et al. 2021) have been described.

9 DOAC Adherence and Persistence

Although DOACs are now the recommended oral anticoagulants to be offered to patients with AF, adherence is suboptimal. In a retrospective study of a large number of patients in Israel, Arbel et al. calculated adherence by means of the proportion of days adequately covered (PDC) in the first year of treatment (Arbel et al. 2022). Good adherence was defined as PDC $\geq$80%. The proportion of good adherent patients treated with DOACs was unsatisfactory being approximately 75%. Importantly, the risk of stroke was lower among adherent patients in comparison with patients with PDC $<$80% indicating that good adherence halves the risk of stroke (HR 0.56, 95% CI: 0.45–0.71). The figures of adherence and persistence were even worse in a recent meta-analysis where adherence and persistence were 66% (95% CI, 63%–70%) and 69% (95% CI, 65%–72%), respectively (Ozaki et al. 2020). Specifically, adherence was 71% (95% CI, 64%–78%) for Apixaban, 60% (95% CI, 52%–68%) for Dabigatran, and 70% (95% CI, 64%–75%) for Rivaroxaban. As expected, DOACs nonadherence was associated with an increased risk of stroke (HR 1.39, 95% CI: 1.06–1.81). The authors concluded stating that clinical monitoring of patients could increase their adherence and persistence. Recently, a meta-analysis explored whether a single dose of DOACs could impact better in terms of adherence and persistence (Quiros Lopez et al. 2025). The authors analyzed thirty-nine studies, for a total of 976,494 patients. The single-dose regimen (OD) was associated with a significantly higher adherence and persistence ($P < 0.05$) than the double regimen (BID) in most studies. Similarly, persistence was higher with the OD in 67.7% of cases in comparison with 14.9% of the BID regimen. However, another systematic review did not find any difference between BID and OD DOACs' dosages in terms of safety and efficacy (Mainbourg et al. 2021). Poor compliance and the OD regimen have been identified as the major flaws for explaining the failure of DOAC in favor of Warfarin in the INVICTUS trial where patients with AF and a severe mitral stenosis were treated with Rivaroxaban versus Warfarin (Connolly et al. 2022). The OD approach is also subjected to poor adherence if patients are left alone without strict clinical monitoring. Gregory Lip, in an accompanying editorial (Lip 2022), acutely expressed the need for a "*holistic treatment of patients with rheumatic heart disease–associated atrial fibrillation, beyond the anticoagulation per se*." In other words, periodical follow-up of patients treated with DOACs is important for a complete approach in terms of personalized care, especially if other comorbidities are present as is frequently the case in anticoagulated patients. One can also speculate that rivaroxaban weakness in counterbalancing a hypercoagulable state derives from an important inflammatory milieu typical of severe mitral stenosis (Sharma et al. 2020). Moreover, the OD regimen probably does not properly cover high thrombotic risk conditions since the half-life of those drugs is about 12 h suggesting that a BID regimen may be more appropriate (Marongiu and Barcellona 2024). To reinforce the need of a regular follow-up of anticoagulated patients comes from the study of Barcellona et al. (2021b) who assessed the patients' adherence by the Morisky Medication Adherence Scale 8-items. The study included 785 consecutive outpatients, of whom 384 were on VKAs and 401 on DOACs. All the patients constantly attended the Haemostasis and Thrombosis Departmental Unit of the University of Cagliari in Italy. The Morisky Medication Adherence Scale 8-items score was 8 in both groups thus showing a high degree of adherence. The intentional non-adherence reached the lowest score while the unintentional non-adherence is the most frequent drawback in patients treated with either VKAS or DOACs. The high adherence to the therapy obtained in both groups of patients was probably due to the educational course administered to each patient at the beginning of their anticoagulant treatment and during all the follow-up period.

10 The Role of the Anticoagulation Clinics

When DOACs became available on the market, most physicians sang the *de profundis* for Warfarin along with the anticoagulation clinics and this assumption was greatly boosted by the aggressive behavior of Industries' marketing policy. However, the role of the Anticoagulation Clinics has been slowly reevaluated over time when healthcare professional and patients realized that the Anticoagulation Clinics were a reference point for all anticoagulated patients not only those treated with VKAs. It is worth noting that the Anticoagulation Clinics first appeared in the Netherlands many years ago (*Federatie van Nederlandse Trombosediensten*) and greatly contributed to optimization of VKAs management (van den Besselaar et al. 1988). In 1989 in Italy was founded the *Federazione Centri per la Sorveglianza della terapia Anticoagulante* (FCSA) which created a great number of Thrombosis Centers widespread in the Country with the aim of improving the management of VKAs in terms of diagnosis, laboratory monitoring, and preparing the patients to surgery or invasive procedures (Berrettini 1997). A lot of seminars, annual

Congresses, debates, and several clinical research studies were organized further contributing to disseminate a culture not only dedicated to the anticoagulant management but also to the knowledge of the Hemostasis and Thrombosis principles. In 2005, when new anticoagulants started to be challenged against warfarin, the role of the Anticoagulation Clinics was projected into the future hoping that they would have been a reference organization to be dedicated to both VKAs and DOACs (Marongiu and Barcellona 2005). Over the time, the Anticoagulation Clinics have not been officially recognized by most Italian regions despite the approval in 2010 of a formal document (so-called *Stato-Regioni*). It described very well the characteristics and functions of the Thrombosis Centers. Recently, it became clear that patients with AF treated with DOACs could not be left alone after the drug prescription, usually done by cardiologists. A regular follow-up to obtain a good adherence and persistence to the anticoagulant drugs and surveillance of patient's rapidly changing clinical conditions especially in elderly and frail patients is mandatory (Ten Cate 2024). Finally, it is worth noting that some conditions still require VKAs treatment such as the anti-phospholipid syndrome, the mechanical heart valves, and the severe mitral stenosis with atrial fibrillation (Pengo 2024). In addition, a recent study in Thrombosis Centers in the Netherlands showed that bleeding occurs more frequently in patients switched from VKAs to DOACs, thus indicating that if a frail patient is well managed with VKAs it is perhaps not appropriate to change that route (Joosten et al. 2024).

11 Conclusions

The answer to the question proposed by the title of this chapter is certainly positive (Table 3). DOACs are better than warfarin in the management of AF in terms of efficacy and safety. However, DOACs have limitations that should be known by physicians (Table 4). Overall, a follow-up should be always performed for these patients in order to assure good adherence and to protect them from serious bleeding episodes along with preparation to surgery and invasive procedures. To reach all these goals the Anticoagulation Clinics or, better, the Thrombosis Centers, should be the checkpoints which deserve much more attention by the politicians and the administrative personnel recognizing them an important social role in the community (Box 1).

Table 3 General pros and cons of DOAC versus warfarin

DOAC vs. warfarin	
Pros	Cons
Rapid onset	Increased GI bleeding (except Apixaban)
Fixed dose	Poor compliance
Superior or non-inferior (stroke, ICH, and major bleeding)	Renal dependent excretion
No monitoring tests (INR)	Great patients' variability
No food interaction (except rivaroxaban)	Not indicated in some conditions

Table 4 DOACs in patients with atrial fibrillation

DOACs contraindicated	DOACs not preferred	DOACs considered (thrombosis in uncommon sites)
Mechanical heart valves (any type) Antiphospholipid syndrome (triple-positivity) AF in mitral stenosis Switch from warfarin in well-managed elderly patients (to be confirmed)	High-risk GI bleeding Obesity (BMI >30) ESRD (CrCl <15 mL/min)[a]	Cardiac chambers Cerebral venous thrombosis Splanchnic thrombosis Catheter-related thrombosis

[a]Only apixaban may be considered

Box 1: Warfarin: An Old Drug but Still Used in Some Conditions

Many years ago, the first anticoagulant drugs to be employed in the primary and secondary prevention of thromboembolic events in patients with AF were the vitamin K antagonists (VKAs), such as Warfarin and Acenocoumarol. The discovery of Warfarin is a fascinating history (Marongiu and Barcellona 2015). All started from the observation that the hemorrhages in cows were due to the ingestion of spoiled sweet clover because a substance (coumarin) was oxidized in moldy clover (catalyzed by Aspergillus hay mold) to form dicumarol 4-idrossi¬coumarin. Its structure was first described by Cambell in 1941 (Campbell et al. 1940). The employment of Warfarin in humans was first published by Bingham et al. in 1941 (Bingham 1941). Coumarins block the enzyme epoxide reductase that brings back the vitamin K epoxide (coming from having driven carboxylation) to its reduced form which is able to induce carboxylation of the Gla-protein residues which bind Ca ions, essential for the coagulability of four factors of the coagulation cascade of four vitamin K-dependent coagulative factors (II, VII, IX, and X) (Stenflo et al. 1974) and the function of Protein C, Protein S and Protein Z, the so-called natural anticoagulants. The final result is to reduce the function of all these proteins in a dose-dependent effect (De Caterina et al. 2013). Warfarin is a racemic mixture of two isomers: the enantiomers R and S. Warfarin is soluble in water and is adsorbed by the gastrointestinal tract. It binds to albumin, and its half-life is about 36 h (Ageno et al. 2012). It goes through an oxidative metabolism in the liver by the enzyme CYP2C9 of the cytochrome P450 system (Miners and Birkett 1998). Acenocoumarol and Phenprocoumon are other available VKAs. The former is believed to have a half-life of about 10 h while the second has a half-life of about 120 h. The power of the different VKAs differs in that the Acenocoumarol is about twice as potent as Warfarin (Barcellona et al. 1998) while the relationship between Warfarin and Phenprocoumon dosages is 0.40 (van Leeuwen et al. 2008). Because VKAs inhibit the function of four vitamin K-dependent factors, a monitoring test

(continued)

Box 1 (continued)
such as prothrombin time (PT) is required. This test, developed by Quick (1935), has been expressed for many years, and sometimes also nowadays, as a percentage of activity, but the results differed greatly among laboratories because of the diversity of the reagent used. Kirkwood (1983) developed a system called INR (international normalized ratio), which had the aim to harmonize the results among the different reagents. This method provides the calibration of a working reagent against an international thromboplastin reference through the measurement of pairs of log-transformed PTs in 60 stable patients treated with VKAs and in 20 normal subjects. Monitoring PT INR is also available today by means of portable coagulometers (van den Besselaar et al. 2015; Barcellona et al. 2017).

Aknowledgment The authors would like to thank Marzia Barcellona for drawing the figures in this chapter.

References

Aberg H (1969) Atrial fibrillation. I. A study of atrial thrombosis and systemic embolism in a necropsy material. Acta Med Scand 185(5):373–379

Ageno W, Gallus AS, Wittkowsky A et al (2012) Oral anticoagulant therapy, antithrombotic therapy and prevention of thrombosis. In: American College of Chest Physicians evidence-based clinical practice guidelines, ninth ed. Chest 141(Suppl):e44S–e88S

Albers GW, Investigators S (2004) Stroke prevention in atrial fibrillation: pooled analysis of SPORTIF III and V trials. Am J Manag Care 10(14 Suppl):S462–S469; discussion S9–73

An J, Garje R, Wanat KA, Leone JP (2017) Dabigatran-related leukocytoclastic vasculitis. BMJ Case Rep 2017

Arbel A, Abu-Ful Z, Preis M, Cohen S, Saliba W (2022) Adherence with direct oral anticoagulants in patients with atrial fibrillation: trends, risk factors, and outcomes. J Arrhythm 38(1):67–76

Baglin T, Hillarp A, Tripodi A, Elalamy I, Buller H, Ageno W (2013) Measuring Oral Direct Inhibitors (ODIs) of thrombin and factor Xa: a recommendation from the Subcommittee on Control of Anticoagulation of the Scientific and Standardisation Committee of the International Society on Thrombosis and Haemostasis. J Thromb Haemost 11:756

Barcellona D, Vannini ML, Fenu L et al (1998) Warfarin or Acenocoumarol: which is better in the management of oral anticoagulants? Thromb Haemost 80:899–902

Barcellona D, Fenu L, Marongiu F (2017) Point-of-care testing INR: an overview. Clin Chem Lab Med 55(6):800–805

Barcellona D, Fenu L, Marongiu F (2021a) Clinical history and gastrointestinal bleeding in patients taking oral anticoagulants. Int J Cardiol 339:134–137

Barcellona D, Mameli A, Cornacchini S, Perra F, Diovaldi M, Farci N et al (2021b) Patients' adherence to oral anticoagulants therapy: comparison between vitamin K antagonists and direct oral anticoagulants. Int J Cardiol 333:162–166

Barrett P, Vuppalanchi R, Masuoka H, Chalasani N (2015) Severe drug-induced skin and liver injury from rivaroxaban. Dig Dis Sci 60(6):1856–1858

Bernstein RA, Kamel H, Granger CB, Piccini JP, Sethi PP, Katz JM et al (2021) Effect of long-term continuous cardiac monitoring vs usual care on detection of Atrial fibrillation in patients with

stroke attributed to large- or small-vessel disease: the STROKE-AF randomized clinical trial. JAMA 325(21):2169–2177
Berrettini M (1997) Anticoagulation clinics: the Italian experience. Haematologica 82(6):713–717
Beyer-Westendorf J, Ehlken B, Evers T (2016) Real-world persistence and adherence to oral anticoagulation for stroke risk reduction in patients with atrial fibrillation. Europace 18(8): 1150–1157
Bingham JB, Meyer OO, Pohle FJ (1941) Studies on the hemorrhagic agent 3,3′-methylene-bis-(4-hydroxycoumarin): its effect on the prothrombin and coagulation time of the blood of dogs and humans. Am J Med Sci 202:563–578
Bungard TJ, Ghali WA, Teo KK, McAlister FA, Tsuyuki RT (2000) Why do patients with atrial fibrillation not receive warfarin? Arch Intern Med 160(1):41–46
Byon W, Garonzik S, Boyd RA, Frost CE (2019) Apixaban: a clinical pharmacokinetic and pharmacodynamic review. Clin Pharmacokinet 58(10):1265–1279
Caldeira D, Barra M, Santos AT, de Abreu D, Pinto FJ, Ferreira JJ et al (2014) Risk of drug-induced liver injury with the new oral anticoagulants: systematic review and meta-analysis. Heart 100(7):550–556
Campbell HA, Roberts WL, Smith WK et al (1940) Studies of the hemorrhagic sweet clover disease: the preparation of hemorrhagic concentrates. J Biol Chem 1940136:47–55
Cannon CP, Bhatt DL, Oldgren J, Lip GYH, Ellis SG, Kimura T et al (2017) Dual antithrombotic therapy with dabigatran after PCI in atrial fibrillation. N Engl J Med 377(16):1513–1524
Coleman CI, Sobieraj DM, Winkler S, Cutting P, Mediouni M, Alikhanov S et al (2012) Effect of pharmacological therapies for stroke prevention on major gastrointestinal bleeding in patients with atrial fibrillation. Int J Clin Pract 66(1):53–63
Connolly SJ, Ezekowitz MD, Yusuf S, Eikelboom J, Oldgren J, Parekh A et al (2009) Dabigatran versus warfarin in patients with atrial fibrillation. N Engl J Med 361(12):1139–1151
Connolly SJ, Karthikeyan G, Ntsekhe M, Haileamlak A, El Sayed A, El Ghamrawy A et al (2022) Rivaroxaban in rheumatic heart disease-associated atrial fibrillation. N Engl J Med 387(11): 978–988
Darling RC, Austen WG, Linton RR (1967) Arterial embolism. Surg Gynecol Obstet 124(1): 106–114
De Caterina R, Husted S, Wallentin L et al (2013) Vitamin K antagonists in heart disease: current status and perspectives (section III). Position paper of the ESC Working Group on Thrombosis – Task Force on Anticoagulants in Heart Disease. Thromb Haemost 110(6):1087–1107
De Vriese AS, Caluwe R, Van Der Meersch H, De Boeck K, De Bacquer D (2021) Safety and efficacy of vitamin K antagonists versus rivaroxaban in hemodialysis patients with atrial fibrillation: a multicenter randomized controlled trial. J Am Soc Nephrol 32(6):1474–1483
Denas G, Pengo V (2011) Emerging anticoagulants. Expert Opin Emerg Drugs 16(1):31–44
Denas G, Gennaro N, Ferroni E, Fedeli U, Saugo M, Zoppellaro G et al (2017) Effectiveness and safety of oral anticoagulation with non-vitamin K antagonists compared to well-managed vitamin K antagonists in naive patients with non-valvular atrial fibrillation: propensity score matched cohort study. Int J Cardiol 249:198–203
Denas G, Zoppellaro G, Granziera S, Pagliani L, Noventa F, Iliceto S et al (2023) Very elderly patients with atrial fibrillation treated with edoxaban: impact of frailty on outcomes. JACC Adv 2(7):100569
Desai J, Kolb JM, Weitz JI, Aisenberg J (2013) Gastrointestinal bleeding with the new oral anticoagulants – defining the issues and the management strategies. Thromb Haemost 110(2): 205–212
Dowling TC, Wang ES, Ferrucci L, Sorkin JD (2013) Glomerular filtration rate equations overestimate creatinine clearance in older individuals enrolled in the Baltimore Longitudinal Study on Aging: impact on renal drug dosing. Pharmacotherapy 33(9):912–921
Easton JD, Sherman DG (1980) Management of cerebral embolism of cardiac origin. Stroke 11(5): 433–442

Elenjickal EJ, Travlos CK, Marques P, Mavrakanas TA (2024) Anticoagulation in patients with chronic kidney disease. Am J Nephrol 55(2):146–164

Eriksson UG, Bredberg U, Hoffmann KJ, Thuresson A, Gabrielsson M, Ericsson H et al (2003) Absorption, distribution, metabolism, and excretion of ximelagatran, an oral direct thrombin inhibitor, in rats, dogs, and humans. Drug Metab Dispos 31(3):294–305

Feinberg WM, Blackshear JL, Laupacis A, Kronmal R, Hart RG (1995) Prevalence, age distribution, and gender of patients with atrial fibrillation. Analysis and implications. Arch Intern Med 155(5):469–473

Fried LP, Tangen CM, Walston J, Newman AB, Hirsch C, Gottdiener J et al (2001) Frailty in older adults: evidence for a phenotype. J Gerontol A Biol Sci Med Sci 56(3):M146–M156

Ganetsky M, Babu KM, Salhanick SD, Brown RS, Boyer EW (2011) Dabigatran: review of pharmacology and management of bleeding complications of this novel oral anticoagulant. J Med Toxicol 7(4):281–287

Gibson CM, Mehran R, Bode C, Halperin J, Verheugt FW, Wildgoose P et al (2016) Prevention of bleeding in patients with atrial fibrillation undergoing PCI. N Engl J Med 375(25):2423–2434

Giugliano RP, Ruff CT, Braunwald E, Murphy SA, Wiviott SD, Halperin JL et al (2013) Edoxaban versus warfarin in patients with atrial fibrillation. N Engl J Med 369(22):2093–2104

Grandone E, Aucella F, Barcellona D, Brunori G, Forneris G, Gresele P et al (2021) Position paper on the safety/efficacy profile of direct oral anticoagulants in patients with chronic kidney disease: consensus document of Societa Italiana di Nefrologia (SIN), Federazione Centri per la diagnosi della trombosi e la Sorveglianza delle terapie Antitrombotiche (FCSA) and Societa Italiana per lo Studio dell'Emostasi e della Trombosi (SISET). J Nephrol 34(1):31–38

Granger CB, Alexander JH, McMurray JJ, Lopes RD, Hylek EM, Hanna M et al (2011) Apixaban versus warfarin in patients with atrial fibrillation. N Engl J Med 365(11):981–992

Hanon O, Assayag P, Belmin J, Collet JP, Emeriau JP, Fauchier L et al (2013) Expert consensus of the French Society of Geriatrics and Gerontology and the French Society of Cardiology on the management of atrial fibrillation in elderly people. Arch Cardiovasc Dis 106(5):303–323

Harskamp RE, Teichert M, Lucassen WAM, van Weert H, Lopes RD (2019) Impact of polypharmacy and P-glycoprotein- and CYP3A4-modulating drugs on safety and efficacy of oral anticoagulation therapy in patients with atrial fibrillation. Cardiovasc Drugs Ther 33(5): 615–623

Hart RG, Benavente O, McBride R, Pearce LA (1999) Antithrombotic therapy to prevent stroke in patients with atrial fibrillation: a meta-analysis. Ann Intern Med 131(7):492–501

Hecker J, Marten S, Keller L, Helmert S, Michalski F, Werth S et al (2016) Effectiveness and safety of rivaroxaban therapy in daily-care patients with atrial fibrillation. Results from the Dresden NOAC Registry. Thromb Haemost 115(5):939–949

Hijazi Z, Hohnloser SH, Oldgren J, Andersson U, Connolly SJ, Eikelboom JW et al (2014) Efficacy and safety of dabigatran compared with warfarin in relation to baseline renal function in patients with atrial fibrillation: a RE-LY (Randomized Evaluation of Long-term Anticoagulation Therapy) trial analysis. Circulation 129(9):961–970

Hinton RC, Kistler JP, Fallon JT, Friedlich AL, Fisher CM (1977) Influence of etiology of atrial fibrillation on incidence of systemic embolism. Am J Cardiol 40(4):509–513

Hohnloser SH, Hijazi Z, Thomas L, Alexander JH, Amerena J, Hanna M et al (2012) Efficacy of apixaban when compared with warfarin in relation to renal function in patients with atrial fibrillation: insights from the ARISTOTLE trial. Eur Heart J 33(22):2821–2830

Ingason AB, Hreinsson JP, Bjornsson ES (2022) Gastrointestinal bleeding on oral anticoagulation: what is currently known. Drug Saf 45(12):1449–1456

Joglar JA, Chung MK, Armbruster AL, Benjamin EJ, Chyou JY, Cronin EM et al (2024) 2023 ACC/AHA/ACCP/HRS guideline for the diagnosis and management of atrial fibrillation: a report of the American College of Cardiology/American Heart Association Joint Committee on Clinical Practice Guidelines. Circulation 149(1):e1–e156

Joosten LPT, van Doorn S, van de Ven PM, Kohlen BTG, Nierman MC, Koek HL et al (2024) Safety of switching from a vitamin K antagonist to a non-vitamin K antagonist oral anticoagulant in frail older patients with atrial fibrillation: results of the FRAIL-AF randomized controlled trial. Circulation 149(4):279–289

Kamel H, Bartz TM, Elkind MSV, Okin PM, Thacker EL, Patton KK et al (2018) Atrial cardiopathy and the risk of ischemic stroke in the CHS (cardiovascular health study). Stroke 49(4):980–986

Karakasis P, Ktenopoulos N, Pamporis K, Sagris M, Soulaidopoulos S, Gerogianni M et al (2024) Efficacy and safety of direct oral anticoagulants versus warfarin in obese patients (BMI >/= 30 kg/m(2)) with atrial fibrillation or venous thromboembolism: an updated systematic review and meta-analysis. J Clin Med 13(13)

Karamichalakis N, Georgopoulos S, Vlachos K, Liatakis I, Efremidis M, Sideris A et al (2016) Efficacy and safety of novel anticoagulants in the elderly. J Geriatr Cardiol 13(8):718–723

Kirkwood TB (1983) Calibration of reference thromboplastins and standardisation of the prothrombin time ratio. Thromb Haemost 49(3):238–244

Ko D, Lin KJ, Bessette LG, Lee SB, Walkey AJ, Cheng S et al (2022) Trends in use of oral anticoagulants in older adults with newly diagnosed atrial fibrillation, 2010–2020. JAMA Netw Open 5(11):e2242964

Kreutz R (2012) Pharmacodynamic and pharmacokinetic basics of rivaroxaban. Fundam Clin Pharmacol 26(1):27–32

Limdi NA, Nolin TD, Booth SL, Centi A, Marques MB, Crowley MR et al (2015) Influence of kidney function on risk of supratherapeutic international normalized ratio related hemorrhage in warfarin users: a prospective cohort study. Am J Kidney Dis 65(5):701–709

Lip GYH (2022) Anticoagulation in atrial fibrillation and rheumatic heart disease. N Engl J Med 387(11):1036–1038

Lippi G, Sanchis-Gomar F, Cervellin G (2021) Global epidemiology of atrial fibrillation: an increasing epidemic and public health challenge. Int J Stroke 16(2):217–221

Lopes RD, Heizer G, Aronson R, Vora AN, Massaro T, Mehran R et al (2019) Antithrombotic therapy after acute coronary syndrome or PCI in atrial fibrillation. N Engl J Med 380(16): 1509–1524

Lopez-Lopez JA, Sterne JAC, Thom HHZ, Higgins JPT, Hingorani AD, Okoli GN et al (2017) Oral anticoagulants for prevention of stroke in atrial fibrillation: systematic review, network meta-analysis, and cost effectiveness analysis. BMJ 359:j5058

Mackman N (2009) The role of tissue factor and factor VIIa in hemostasis. Anesth Analg 108(5): 1447–1452

Mainbourg S, Cucherat M, Provencher S, Bertoletti L, Nony P, Gueyffier F et al (2021) Twice- or once-daily dosing of direct oral anticoagulants, a systematic review and meta-analysis. Thromb Res 197:24–32

Marongiu F, Barcellona D (2005) The future of anticoagulation clinics: a journey to thrombosis centers? Haematologica 90(3):298

Marongiu F, Barcellona D (2015) Vitamin K antagonists (Coumarins), drugs used in the prevention and treatment of cardioembolism, deep vein thrombosis, and pulmonary embolism. In: Watson R, Preedy V (eds) Bioactive nutraceuticals and dietary supplements in neurological and brain disease. Prevention and therapy. Chapter 40. Academic (Elsevier), London, pp 395–398

Marongiu F, Barcellona D (2024) Why does rivaroxaban not work in severe mitral stenosis? Semin Thromb Hemost 50(2):303–306

Marongiu F, Grandone E, Marongiu S, Mameli A, Barcellona D (2024) Stroke in women: anticoagulation in a complicated puzzle. Bleed Thromb Vasc Biol 3:137

Martin SS, Aday AW, Almarzooq ZI, Anderson CAM, Arora P, Avery CL et al (2024) 2024 heart disease and stroke statistics: a report of US and global data from the American Heart Association. Circulation 149(8):e347–e913

Maura G, Billionnet C, Coste J, Weill A, Neumann A, Pariente A (2018) Non-bleeding adverse events with the use of direct oral anticoagulants: a sequence symmetry analysis. Drug Saf 41(9): 881–897

Mavrakanas TA, Samer C, Fontana P, Perrier A (2015) Direct oral anticoagulants: efficacy and safety in patient subgroups. Swiss Med Wkly 145:w14081
Mavrakanas TA, Charytan DM, Winkelmayer WC (2020) Direct oral anticoagulants in chronic kidney disease: an update. Curr Opin Nephrol Hypertens 29(5):489–496
Michels WM, Grootendorst DC, Verduijn M, Elliott EG, Dekker FW, Krediet RT (2010) Performance of the Cockcroft-Gault, MDRD, and new CKD-EPI formulas in relation to GFR, age, and body size. Clin J Am Soc Nephrol 5(6):1003–1009
Miners JO, Birkett DJ (1998) Cytochrome P4502C9: an enzyme of major importance in human drug metabolism. Br J Clin Pharmacol 45:525–538
Ng KH, Shestakovska O, Connolly SJ, Eikelboom JW, Avezum A, Diaz R et al (2016) Efficacy and safety of apixaban compared with aspirin in the elderly: a subgroup analysis from the AVERROES trial. Age Ageing 45(1):77–83
Ozaki AF, Choi AS, Le QT, Ko DT, Han JK, Park SS et al (2020) Real-world adherence and persistence to direct oral anticoagulants in patients with atrial fibrillation: a systematic review and meta-analysis. Circ Cardiovasc Qual Outcomes 13(3):e005969
Palareti G, Antonucci E, Migliaccio L, Erba N, Marongiu F, Pengo V et al (2017) Vitamin K antagonist therapy: changes in the treated populations and in management results in Italian anticoagulation clinics compared with those recorded 20 years ago. Intern Emerg Med 12(8): 1109–1119
Pansuriya T, Nguyen T, Sadat MA, Raza SA, Sarva ST (2021) A 78-year-old man with a pulmonary embolism who developed skin necrosis 7 days after treatment with the direct oral anticoagulant factor Xa inhibitor apixaban. Am J Case Rep 22:e929002
Parasrampuria DA, Truitt KE (2016) Pharmacokinetics and pharmacodynamics of edoxaban, a non-vitamin K antagonist oral anticoagulant that inhibits clotting factor Xa. Clin Pharmacokinet 55(6):641–655
Patel MR, Mahaffey KW, Garg J, Pan G, Singer DE, Hacke W et al (2011) Rivaroxaban versus warfarin in nonvalvular atrial fibrillation. N Engl J Med 365(10):883–891
Patti G, Lucerna M, Pecen L, Siller-Matula JM, Cavallari I, Kirchhof P et al (2017) Thromboembolic risk, bleeding outcomes and effect of different antithrombotic strategies in very elderly patients with Atrial fibrillation: a sub-analysis from the PREFER in AF (PREvention oF Thromboembolic Events-European Registry in Atrial Fibrillation). J Am Heart Assoc 6(7)
Pengo V (2024) The warfarin renaissance. Intern Emerg Med 19(4):1177–1179
Petersen P, Boysen G, Godtfredsen J, Andersen ED, Andersen B (1989) Placebo-controlled, randomised trial of warfarin and aspirin for prevention of thromboembolic complications in chronic atrial fibrillation. The Copenhagen AFASAK study. Lancet 1(8631):175–179
Poli D, Antonucci E, Testa S, Tosetto A, Ageno W, Palareti G, et al (2011) Bleeding risk in very old patients on vitamin K antagonist treatment: results of a prospective collaborative study on elderly patients followed by Italian Centres for Anticoagulation. Circulation 124(7):824–829
Porru M, Mameli A, Cianchetti ME, Musu M, Schirru P, Ruberto MF et al (2017) Dabigatran overdose: a case report of acute hepatitis. Extracorporeal treatment. Int J Hematol 105(4): 532–535
Potpara TS (2018) Comparing non-vitamin K antagonist oral anticoagulants (NOACs) to different Coumadins: the win-win scenarios. Thromb Haemost 118(5):803–805
Potpara TS, Lip GY (2017) Postapproval observational studies of non-vitamin K antagonist oral anticoagulants in atrial fibrillation. JAMA 317(11):1115–1116
Quick AJ (1935) The prothrombin in hemophilia and in obstructive jaundice. J Biol Chem 109:73–74
Quiros Lopez R, Formiga Perez F, Beyer-Westendorf J (2025) Adherence and persistence with direct oral anticoagulants by dose regimen: a systematic review. Br J Clin Pharmacol 91(4): 1096–1113
Radadiya D, Devani K, Brahmbhatt B, Reddy C (2021) Major gastrointestinal bleeding risk with direct oral anticoagulants: does type and dose matter? – a systematic review and network meta-analysis. Eur J Gastroenterol Hepatol 33(1S Suppl 1):e50–ee8

Raschi E, Bianchin M, Ageno W, De Ponti R, De Ponti F (2016) Adverse events associated with the use of direct-acting oral anticoagulants in clinical practice: beyond bleeding complications. Pol Arch Med Wewn 126(7–8):552–561
Roth GA, Mensah GA, Johnson CO, Addolorato G, Ammirati E, Baddour LM et al (2020) Global burden of cardiovascular diseases and risk factors, 1990-2019: update from the GBD 2019 study. J Am Coll Cardiol 76(25):2982–3021
Ruff CT, Giugliano RP, Braunwald E, Hoffman EB, Deenadayalu N, Ezekowitz MD et al (2014) Comparison of the efficacy and safety of new oral anticoagulants with warfarin in patients with atrial fibrillation: a meta-analysis of randomised trials. Lancet 383(9921):955–962
Rutherford OW, Jonasson C, Ghanima W, Soderdahl F, Halvorsen S (2022) Effectiveness and safety of oral anticoagulants in elderly patients with atrial fibrillation. Heart 108(5):345–352
Sagris M, Ktenopoulos N, Pamporis K, Gerogianni M, Karakasis P, Theofilis P et al (2025) The efficacy and safety of direct oral anticoagulants compared to warfarin in morbidly obese patients on anticoagulation: a systematic review and meta-analysis. Curr Vasc Pharmacol 23:404
Schaeffner ES, Ebert N, Delanaye P, Frei U, Gaedeke J, Jakob O et al (2012) Two novel equations to estimate kidney function in persons aged 70 years or older. Ann Intern Med 157(7):471–481
Schafer A, Flierl U, Berliner D, Bauersachs J (2020) Anticoagulants for stroke prevention in atrial fibrillation in elderly patients. Cardiovasc Drugs Ther 34(4):555–568
Sharma G, Ghati N, Sharique M, Sharma S, Shetkar S, Karmakar S et al (2020) Role of inflammation in initiation and maintenance of atrial fibrillation in rheumatic mitral stenosis – an analytical cross-sectional study. J Arrhythm 36(6):1007–1015
Silverio A, Di Maio M, Prota C, De Angelis E, Radano I, Citro R et al (2021) Safety and efficacy of non-vitamin K antagonist oral anticoagulants in elderly patients with atrial fibrillation: systematic review and meta-analysis of 22 studies and 440 281 patients. Eur Heart J Cardiovasc Pharmacother 7(FI1):f20–ff9
Stanifer JW, Pokorney SD, Chertow GM, Hohnloser SH, Wojdyla DM, Garonzik S et al (2020) Apixaban versus warfarin in patients with atrial fibrillation and advanced chronic kidney disease. Circulation 141(17):1384–1392
Steffel J, Collins R, Antz M, Cornu P, Desteghe L, Haeusler KG et al (2021) 2021 European Heart Rhythm Association practical guide on the use of non-vitamin K antagonist oral anticoagulants in patients with atrial fibrillation. Europace 23(10):1612–1676
Stenflo J, Fernlund P, Egan W et al (1974) Vitamin K dependent modifications of glutamic acid residues in prothrombin. Proc Natl Acad Sci USA 71:2730–2733
Ten Cate H (2024) The wonders of anticoagulation. Front Cardiovasc Med 11:1517109
Testa S, Tripodi A, Legnani C, Pengo V, Abbate R, Dellanoce C et al (2016) Plasma levels of direct oral anticoagulants in real life patients with atrial fibrillation: results observed in four anticoagulation clinics. Thromb Res 137:178–183
Testa S, Legnani C, Antonucci E, Paoletti O, Dellanoce C, Cosmi B et al (2019) Drug levels and bleeding complications in atrial fibrillation patients treated with direct oral anticoagulants. J Thromb Haemost 17(7):1064–1072
Tripodi A, Marongiu F, Moia M, Palareti G, Pengo V, Poli D et al (2018) The vexed question of whether or not to measure levels of direct oral anticoagulants before surgery or invasive procedures. Intern Emerg Med 13(7):1029–1036
van den Besselaar AM, van der Meer FJ, Gerrits-Drabbe CW (1988) Therapeutic control of oral anticoagulant treatment in The Netherlands. Am J Clin Pathol 90(6):685–690
van den Besselaar AM, Biedermann JS, Kruip MJ et al (2015) Point-of-care testing and INR within-subject variation in patients receiving a constant dose of vitamin K antagonist. Thromb Haemost 114(6):1260–1267
van Leeuwen Y, Rosendaal FR, van der Meer FJ et al (2008) The relationship between maintenance dosages of three vitamin K antagonists: acenocoumarol, warfarin and phenprocoumon. Thromb Res 123:225–230

Volgman AS, Nair G, Lyubarova R, Merchant FM, Mason P, Curtis AB et al (2022) Management of atrial fibrillation in patients 75 years and older: JACC state-of-the-art review. J Am Coll Cardiol 79(2):166–179

Vranckx P, Valgimigli M, Heidbuchel H (2018) The significance of drug-drug and drug-food interactions of Oral anticoagulation. Arrhythm Electrophysiol Rev 7(1):55–61

Vranckx P, Valgimigli M, Eckardt L, Tijssen J, Lewalter T, Gargiulo G et al (2019) Edoxaban-based versus vitamin K antagonist-based antithrombotic regimen after successful coronary stenting in patients with atrial fibrillation (ENTRUST-AF PCI): a randomised, open-label, phase 3b trial. Lancet 394(10206):1335–1343

Wallentin L, Yusuf S, Ezekowitz MD, Alings M, Flather M, Franzosi MG et al (2010) Efficacy and safety of dabigatran compared with warfarin at different levels of international normalised ratio control for stroke prevention in atrial fibrillation: an analysis of the RE-LY trial. Lancet 376(9745):975–983

Wilkinson C, Wu J, Searle SD, Todd O, Hall M, Kunadian V et al (2020) Clinical outcomes in patients with atrial fibrillation and frailty: insights from the ENGAGE AF-TIMI 48 trial. BMC Med 18(1):401

Wolf PA, Dawber TR, Thomas HE Jr, Kannel WB (1978) Epidemiologic assessment of chronic atrial fibrillation and risk of stroke: the Framingham study. Neurology 28(10):973–977

Xu Y, Chang AR, Inker LA, McAdams-DeMarco M, Grams ME, Shin JI (2023) Associations of apixaban dose with safety and effectiveness outcomes in patients with atrial fibrillation and severe chronic kidney disease. Circulation 148(19):1445–1454

Zoppellaro G, Zanella L, Denas G, Gennaro N, Ferroni E, Fedeli U et al (2018) Different safety profiles of oral anticoagulants in very elderly non-valvular atrial fibrillation patients. A retrospective propensity score matched cohort study. Int J Cardiol 265:103–107

Zoppellaro G, Marchese GM, Squizzato A, Denas G, Patti G, De Caterina R et al (2020) Benefit of dual antithrombotic therapy with direct oral anticoagulants in patients with atrial fibrillation undergoing percutaneous coronary intervention: a systematic review and metaanalysis of randomized clinical trials. Intern Emerg Med 15(6):1093–1104

Zulkifly H, Lip GYH, Lane DA (2022) Anticoagulation control in older atrial fibrillation patients receiving vitamin K antagonist therapy for stroke prevention. Int J Clin Pract 2022:5951262

Laboratory and Point of Care Monitoring of Vitamin K Antagonist Treatment

Ian Jennings and Dianne Kitchen

Contents

Abstract

Vitamin K antagonist (VKA) therapy is given to patients either after a thrombosis or prophylactically to prevent a thrombotic event. VKAs block the action of vitamin K reductase which converts inactive forms of Factors II, FVII, FIX, FX, protein C, S and Z to their functional enzyme zymogens. In this way the levels of functional clotting factors in the circulation are reduced and thus the potential of the blood to clot is lowered. VKA therapy requires careful monitoring as pharmacological responses vary significantly between individuals; too much anticoagulation can increase bleeding risks, but too little increases the risk of a new or extended thrombosis. The effects of VKA therapy are monitored using the International Normalised Ratio (INR). This is a standardised test based on the prothrombin time (PT), developed in the 1980s to allow comparability between all different methods and reagents. This then means that a patient can be tested anywhere in the world and the same INR results would be obtained. The INR tests

I. Jennings (✉) · D. Kitchen (✉)
UK NEQAS (Blood Coagulation), Sheffield, UK
e-mail: ian.jennings@nhs.net; dianne.kitchen@nhs.net

E. Gray, J. Hogwood (eds.), *Antithrombotic and Antiplatelet Agents*, Handbook of Experimental Pharmacology 291, https://doi.org/10.1007/164_2025_782

can be performed in a laboratory setting but also since the late 1990s as a Point of Care test (POCt). Although this test has been standardised, there is still potential to see differences between methods in particular samples or in certain patient conditions. An understanding of the factors affecting this straightforward test, and constant quality control, is required to ensure results are valid and reliable, and patient treatment is optimised. Comparability between different test systems for INR monitoring is greatest in over-anticoagulated patients, and strategies for treatment of these patients, for example, with reversal agents such as Vitamin K either orally or by injection need to be in place.

Keywords

INR · Laboratory tests · Monitoring · Point of care tests · Warfarin

1 Anticoagulant Therapy with Vitamin K Antagonists

Anticoagulant therapy using Vitamin K antagonists (VKA) was first introduced in the 1950s, following discovery of the ability of 4-hydroxy coumarin to prolong clotting times in humans (Townsend and Mills 1942; Wolff et al. 1953; Nicholson 1957; Shapiro et al. 1958; Baer et al. 1958). Of the VKAs, warfarin is the most commonly used worldwide, with acenocoumarol and phenindione also prescribed. The action of VKA is to disrupt the carboxylation of vitamin K cycle within the liver which affects the production of vitamin K-dependent clotting factors (Ageno et al. 2012) (Fig. 1).

Several clotting factors essential for balanced haemostasis are synthesised in the liver. These include factors II, VII, IX and X (plus proteins C, S and Z), termed vitamin K-dependent clotting factors. These factors are fully functional once the proteins have been modified by a process of post-translational carboxylation. This process involves oxidation of vitamin K, and so-called vitamin K antagonists (VKA) interfere with vitamin K oxide reductase, thus preventing the carboxylation of the vitamin K K-dependent clotting factors. An absence of dietary vitamin K also interferes with this carboxylation step, and instead of functional clotting factors, non-functional protein is released into the circulation –known as PIVKA (protein induced by vitamin K absence or antagonists) proteins. When a patient is undergoing VKA therapy, they will therefore have some circulating functional FII, FVII, FIX and FX and also PIVKA FII, PIVKA FVII, PIVKA FIX and PIVKA FX. These PIVKA proteins are important if reversal of the therapy is required using vitamin K and we shall briefly explore reversal therapy later in the chapter.

Vitamin K antagonists therefore reduce the level of functional clotting factors in the circulation, altering the haemostatic balance in a patient. They can be used therapeutically following a thrombotic event, or prophylactically where the risk of thrombosis is increased. However, the haemostatic balance following VKA therapy is important, as over-anticoagulation can lead to a bleeding event but too little can increase the risk of thrombosis (Hylek et al. 2003; Hylek 2003). There is a

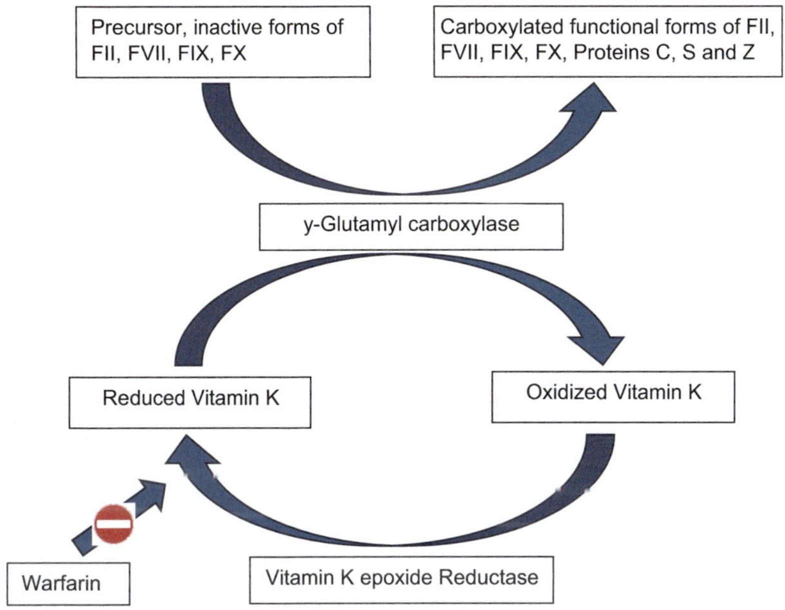

Fig. 1 Role of warfarin in disrupting the carboxylation of vitamin K-dependent clotting factors

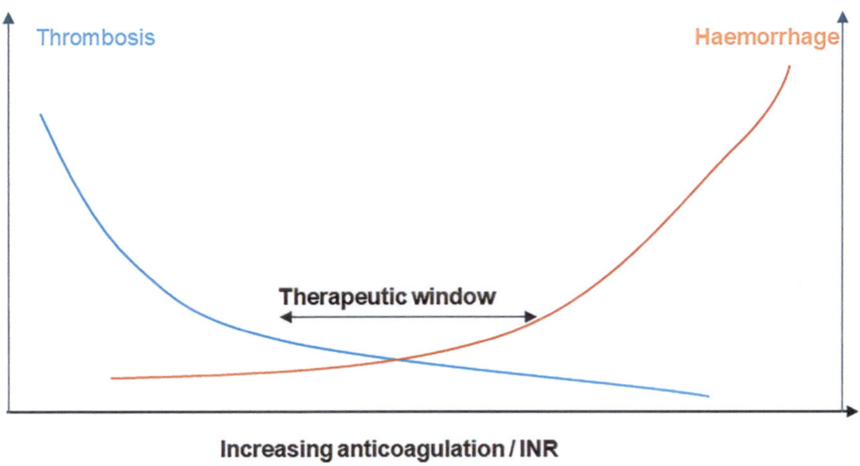

Fig. 2 Haemostatic balance in VKA therapy

therapeutic window whereby the advantage of therapy outweighs the bleeding risk as illustrated in Fig. 2. The therapeutic window varies depending on clinical indication for anticoagulation.

When VKA therapy is commenced, the level of functional vitamin K-dependent clotting factors starts to fall. The rate of reduction of clotting factors is dependent upon the half-life of each factor – as they are all different, the levels of FII, VII, IX and X fall at different rates. The half-life of FVII is the shortest at 6 h, FIX is 24 h, FX is 48 h and FII is 60 h. So, when VKA is commenced (induction phase) functional FVII levels fall rapidly, followed by FIX, FX and lastly FII. Typically, patients are given a 'loading dose' of VKA over 3 days followed by a maintenance dose. With this regime, at around day 5 the levels of all the vitamin K factors should have fallen to new 'steady state' below the levels seen in unanticoagulated individuals (Kumar et al. 1990). Therefore, it can take several days after commencement of therapy for these factors to stabilise at on-treatment levels.

Guidelines recommend specific target levels of anticoagulation, dependent on the indication for treatment (Keeling et al. 2011). However, individual responses to warfarin therapy are highly variable, with genetic variation (particularly in the *CYP2C9* and *VKORC1* genes), drug interactions and dietary effects all contributing to unpredictable dosage requirements (Ageno et al. 2012). Fixed dose regimes are therefore not possible, and to ensure optimal therapy, the level of anticoagulation therefore needs to be monitored closely and dosage adjustments made to maintain a patient's haemostatic balance within the therapeutic window.

2 Monitoring Anticoagulant Therapy – The INR System

The prothrombin time (PT), measuring the clotting activity of the extrinsic pathway (see Fig. 3), is sensitive to levels of 3 of the 4 vitamin K-dependent procoagulant factors (FII, FV, and FVII) and when VKA therapy was first introduced patients were monitored by the PT. However, marked variation in the sensitivity of different thromboplastins to the same level of anticoagulation hampered attempts to standardise treatment. In an attempt to improve this, a PT ratio was introduced to monitor treatment, by dividing the clotting time of the patient sample by a control value. This still failed to standardise results, with therapeutic ranges from 1.25 to 3.0 times normal quoted for different reagents (Bailey et al. 1971). Therefore, in the early 1980s, a system was introduced with the aim that all reagents used for VKA monitoring would give the same result and this would enable patients to expect the same assessment of their anticoagulant status regardless of where in the world they were tested.

The International Normalised Ratio (INR) was introduced in 1983 (Hermans et al. 1983; van den Besselaar 1985) with the premise that all candidate thromboplastins could be calibrated for sensitivity to VKAs against an international reference preparation (IRP), such that they would then give agreement between different methods. The first IRP was IRP67/40 and this was designated to have an International Sensitivity Index (ISI) of 1.0. The sensitivity of commercially available thromboplastins could then be compared to this reference preparation. The process of calibration involves performing PTs on 20 healthy normal control samples and at least 60 samples from anticoagulated patients. PTs are measured with the IRP using a manual (water bath) method, and the candidate thromboplastin using the routine method for this material. The log values of the PTs are plotted, and the slope of the

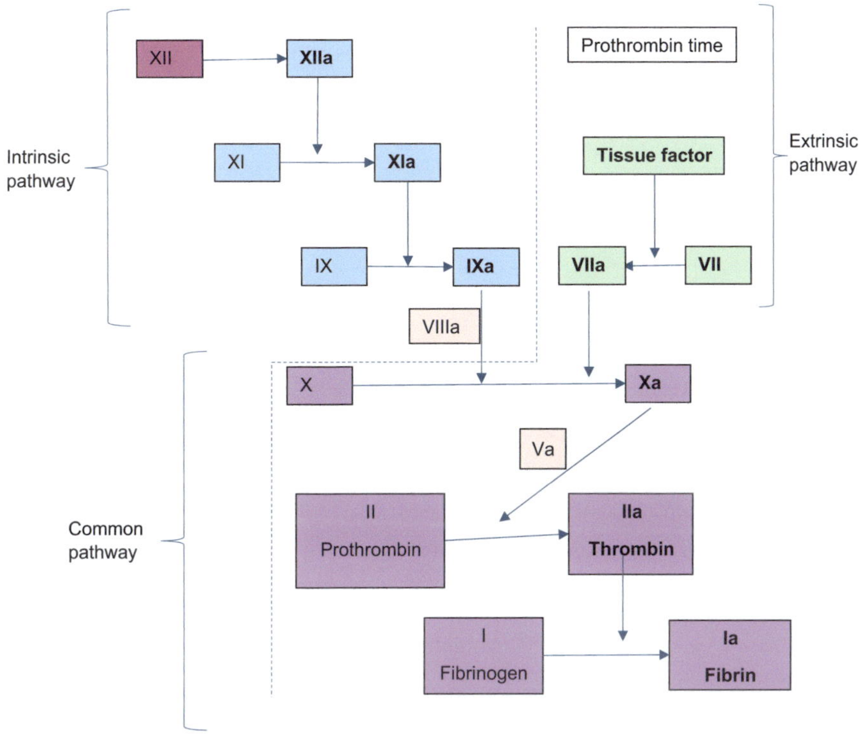

Fig. 3 The coagulation cascade (Macfarlane 1964)

line gives the ISI for the candidate thromboplastin (see Fig. 4). The INR can then be determined as:

$$\text{INR} = (\text{PT}/\text{MNPT})^{\text{ISI}}$$

where PT is the prothrombin time of the test sample, the MNPT is a geometric mean PT for 20 or more samples obtained from healthy normal subjects not on VKA therapy, and the ISI is the international sensitivity index for the thromboplastin in use.

It is important that the anticoagulated samples used are from individuals that have been on VKA for more than 6 weeks with stable levels of treatment – fluctuation in levels, or levels outside of the INR range 1.5–4.0 indicate a lack of stability, and the varying half-lives of the VK dependent clotting factors and the variable sensitivity of different thromboplastin preparations to clotting factor levels can affect the validity of any ISI calibration process. It is also important therefore to avoid samples from patients in the induction phase, or patients with any new medications as these can affect the action of VKA.

When diagnostic reagent manufacturer produces a new thromboplastin they are required to set an ISI for it using methods ultimately traceable to an IRP. Given the

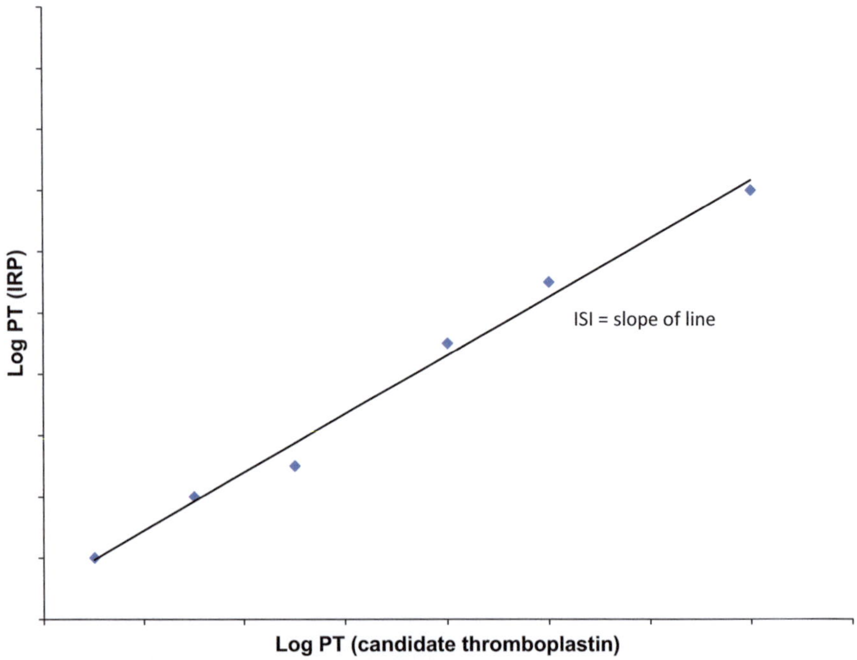

Fig. 4 Assignment of ISI values of thromboplastins against an IRP

restrictive volume of IRP available, this is usually achieved by use of an in-house standard which is compared directly to an IRP. The new thromboplastins have an ISI set by using the in-house standards. Over the years since the INR and ISI system was introduced, there has been a series of IRPs assigned, with each new product calibrated back to the original IRP 67/40 (Fig. 5) (van den Besselaar et al. 2018, 2024).

This method of assigning an ISI applies to both thromboplastin reagents used in laboratory settings, and Point of Care (POC) test strips which contain thromboplastin ensuring that laboratory and POC testing should agree within the INR system limits which we will discuss later.

An example of how the INR system works is shown in Table 1 showing results from the same patient tested with 5 different methods (labelled A-E). These data show quite different PT times for the same sample, and even when the PT ratio is calculated there is still some difference between reagents, but once the ISI is applied the results agree.

If the ISI is not set correctly in the calibration process this will affect all results to some extent with the higher INR values being more affected than the lower values as shown in Table 2.

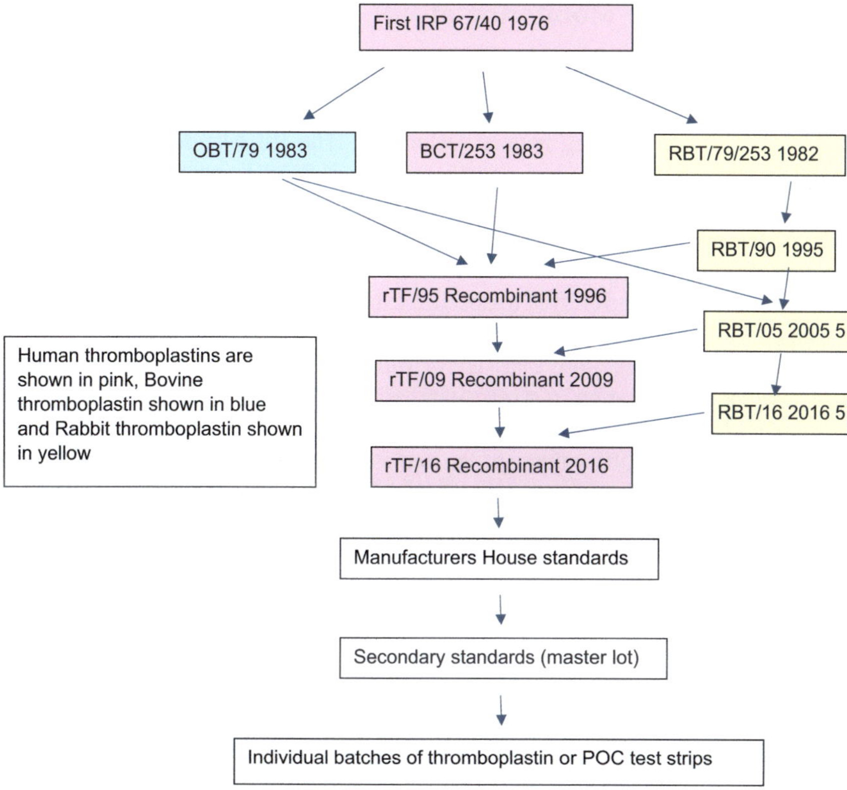

Fig. 5 Calibration of thromboplastin process

Table 1 ISI effect in standardising methods

Reagent	PT sec	MNPT	PT ratio	ISI	INR
A	23	14.5	1.6	1.5	2.1
B	30	14	2.1	1.0	2.1
C	28	16.5	1.7	1.4	2.1
D	33	17	1.9	1.1	2.1
E	19	13	1.5	1.9	2.1

Table 2 Effect of an inaccurate ISI in use on differing levels of INR (MNPT = 12.8 s)

Sample	PT (seconds)	ISI = 1.0	ISI = 1.1	ISI = 1.25	ISI = 1.4
	PT	INR	INR	INR	INR
A	15	1.2	1.2	1.2	1.2
B	25	2.0	2.1	2.3	2.6
C	35	2.7	3.0	3.5	4.1
D	45	3.5	4.0	4.8	5.8
E	55	4.3	5.0	6.2	7.7

3 Laboratory Monitoring of INR

With few automated systems in use in 1983, the process for determining INR values as described above generally comprised of PTs from IRP and candidate thromboplastin both measured using manual techniques. The ISI was determined for the candidate thromboplastin, and locally prepared MNPT values would allow laboratories to determine INRs for their reagent.

Since the introduction of the INR, automation has replaced manual techniques, and increasingly diagnostic manufacturers market analyser and reagent combinations, allowing for system-specific ISIs. Laboratories now have the option of using an ISI assigned by the manufacturer to their reagent/instrument system, or performing a local calibration to assign or validate ISIs for their reagent. Commercially available calibration plasmas with assigned INR values can be used to determine a local ISI by using the slope obtained when plotting the clotting times against the assigned INR values, in the same way as assignment of ISI values to commercial thromboplastins (see Fig. 4), or can even provide a calibration curve against which patient clotting times can be directly converted to an INR (Fig. 6). Guidelines are available with respect to approaches to INR determination with local calibration approaches (van den Besselaar et al. 2004; CLSI 2005).

The INR system allows for adjustment of patients' VKA dosing to aim for target anticoagulation levels dependent on the clinical indications (Keeling et al. 2011).

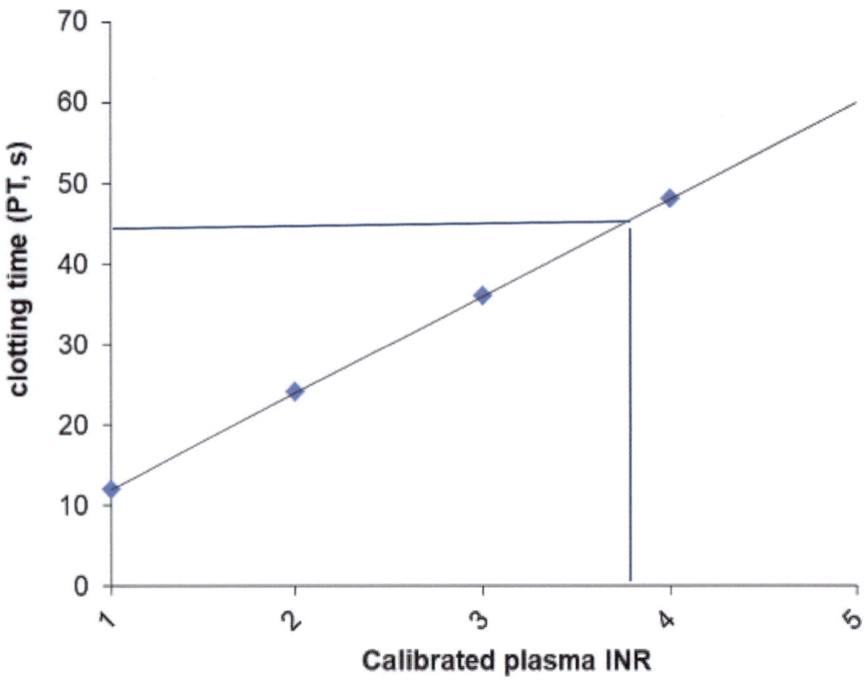

Fig. 6 Calibration curve demonstrating a direct calculation of clotting times with a local system against calibration plasmas with assigned INR values

Dosing algorithms and clinical decision support systems (CDSS) aid in dose adjustment and recall/retesting intervals. However, despite a system designed to ensure commutability of INR results between different methods (with a commonly quoted variation of up to 0.5 INR units being deemed acceptable), differences in results are still observed. Differing anticoagulant preparations (e.g., 3.2% or 3.8% citrate concentration) for venous blood samples have contributed to variability in the past (Chantarangkul et al. 1998), and manufacturers do not always successfully assign an accurate ISI value to their reagent. High ISI values for some reagents have in the past affected the sensitivity of the method to INR changes, but the majority of commercially available reagents now have assigned ISI values very close to 1.0.

4 Quality Control for INR Testing in the Laboratory

It is important therefore that laboratories perform regular Internal Quality Control (IQC) to detect any issues with precision of their testing, including during reagent lot changes. IQC should be performed at frequent intervals, determined by the volume and frequency of testing of clinical samples. Laboratories will have assigned target values or ranges for their IQC material, so these are known before the samples are tested. Centres should maintain records of IQC along with acceptance criteria (target ranges), and logs of any actions in the event of an IQC result outside of the target range. External Quality Assessment can help determine test accuracy by comparison with other centres using the same or different methodology. Plasma from patients receiving anticoagulant therapy is collected through plasmapheresis, following informed donor consent. The plasma is then buffered and aliquoted prior to freeze drying for stability, and subsequent distribution of samples to participating laboratories. Results are returned to the EQA provider for analysis, with target values assigned for performance assessment. Participants in the EQA programme do not therefore know the result of their sample when testing – assessment is retrospective, and IQC is necessary to compliment EQA participation. It is reasonable to expect INRs obtained in different centres and with different reagents to be within 0.5 units of each other – although at elevated INR levels, or in patients with unstable treatment and fluctuating INRs, agreement is not necessarily seen. External Quality Assessment programmes typically see a range of results reported for a homogenous sample tested in different laboratories; EQA data from the UK NEQAS Blood Coagulation programme shows over 900 centres using 14 different thromboplastins on 27 different analyser platforms. In general, between laboratories within method-specific groups, precision is very good with average between-lab CVs around 5% However, precision between different reagent peer groups is not always good, despite the theoretical standardisation introduced by the INR system – Fig. 7 shows the distribution of reported results for the same sample tested in an EQA exercise, with the total variation in this sample between 2.3 and 4.2.

Laboratories obtaining outlying results in an EQA exercise are required to investigate the cause, which may include checking the MNPT and ISI in local use.

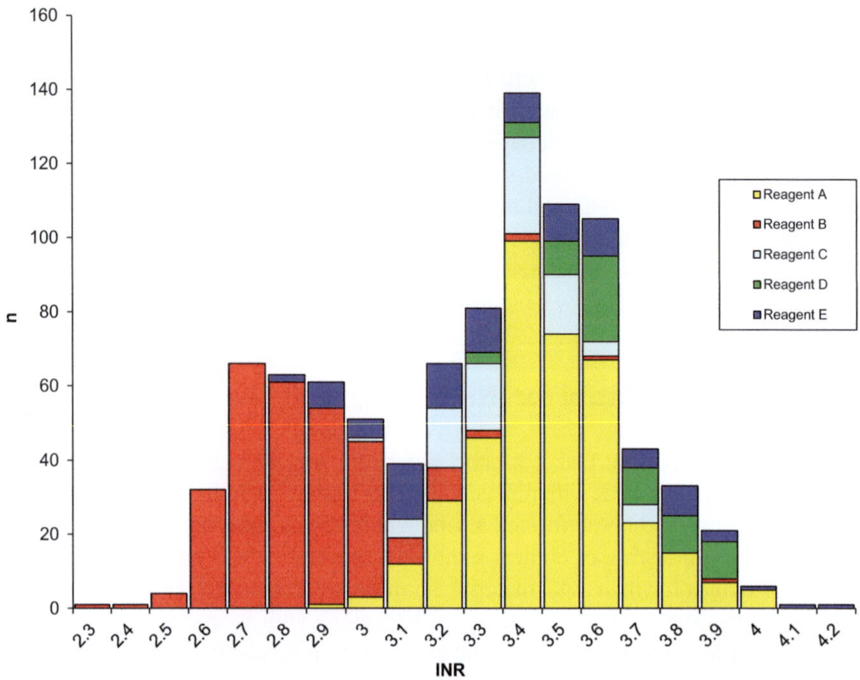

Fig. 7 Histogram showing INR values measured with different methods for the same external quality assessment sample

5 Point of Care Monitoring of INR

Point of care or near patient testing for INR monitoring was introduced in the late 1990s (Leaning and Ansell 1996; Fitzmaurice et al. 1998; Koerner and Fuller 1998; Murray et al. 1999). The POC devices were originally shoe-box-sized pieces of equipment which could be operated by non-laboratory-trained staff. They were designed to be easy to use and to give a result in a few minutes resulting in a much-reduced turnaround time when compared to laboratory testing which meant that the VKA dosage can be adjusted instantly. Now some 20 plus years later there are many POC INR devices available and they tend to be smaller handheld devices which have features such as quality control lockout, operator lockout, keypad identification which allows patients' ID to be linked to the result and a sizable memory for results. Test strips are now generally stored at room temperature (most state between 2° and 30°) and have liquid internal quality control (IQC) available (this usually needs reconstitution and refrigeration). As well as liquid IQC, many devices have built in 'electronic' QC in the test strips which checks that the test strip is suitable to use and has not been exposed to high heat or humidity. Many have a system check which activates when the device is turned on and checks the electric circuitry of the devices. The POC test strips (sometimes also called cartridges or cuvettes depending on the manufacturers) are calibrated in the same way as the laboratory thromboplastins so they are all traceable to an IRP. The endpoint detection system is the process by which the device measures clot formation and determines the eventual PT of the sample. This varies between methods and has evolved over the years such that the original methods are no longer in use. Devices vary in the endpoint detection system and also in the volume of the blood sample required. The cost of the device, test strips and quality control package (both IQC and EQA) should be considered when purchasing a POC device.

When POC INR testing was introduced, many publications showed how patients could be monitored using these new-style devices. There have also been many publications comparing a POC INR testing system to a laboratory test system. However, one issue with these studies is the assumption by the authors that the laboratory system is the truth. Very few have actually used an IRP to establish how accurate the POC devices actually were, one exception being a study by van den Besselaar et al. (2012) who concluded that the device and test strips studies were within 8% of the international standard. Early POC devices were often purchased and implanted without any comparison testing and very little training with the requirement of IQC and external quality control (EQA) not taken into account. This has improved over time and now training and requirement of IQC and EQA is a requirement of centres wishing to use POC INR testing. In the same way that IQC and EQA is required for laboratory methods, the POC devices also need this to ensure results are reliable and reproducible to enable VKA therapy to be as safe as possible.

Operators should have suitable training in the use of the device (Fitzmaurice et al. 2023), have understanding of the action of VKA, be able to operate the dosing software which is very frequently used and be able to perform IQC and EQA testing. They should be trained in obtaining a fingerstick sample and should be deemed to be competent in all of these areas and should maintain competency with regular checks. There should also be a process to follow should the IQC or EQA be out of range and written Standard Operating Procedures (SOP) which are regularly updated and reviewed. If POC INR testing is undertaken in a secondary care setting then this is usually overseen by the POC committee and the POC team and this gives vital support and laboratory assistance to operators who may not be familiar with laboratory processes. Unfortunately, in primary care in some countries there is often very little support available for POC testing. One area that is sometimes still not taken into account when costing and implementing a POC service is the provision of both IQC and EQA. In a survey undertaken by UK National external quality assurance service for blood coagulation (UK NEQAS BC) they asked participants enrolled in the EQA programme for POC INR testing how often IQC was performed. These were users who were already taking part in EQA so it is surprising that 2% of users did not perform IQC testing and just 15% perform IQC with each clinic as recommended by the then current UK guidelines (Kitchen et al. 2005, 2015). This shows a lack of understanding for the requirement of IQC to work in conjunction with EQA to ensure precise and accurate results. It is highly likely that there are many users that are not taking part in any EQA or performing any IQC whilst testing patients' samples.

6 Quality Control for POC Testing

Quality control for POC INR testing is an essential part of ensuring reliable results. A robust quality control requires both IQC and EQA at regular intervals (Kitchen et al. 2008). The IQC is an ongoing event that users determine when to perform and what to do if the IQC fails. IQC for POC INR testing is purchased from the manufacturer of the device and comes with preset acceptable ranges. The devices can often be set with a QC lockout so that if a QC test is due, the device cannot be used until a QC is performed. IQC results should be recorded and stored. This can be either as an online system, in a log book, or as part of the Computer decision software system (CDSS). SOPs should detail how to test, where to record and how to troubleshoot.

EQA is provided by an external organisation to test the device at regular intervals, often 4 or 6 times per year. It provides a test sample with an unknown result which the operator tests and submits their result. There are many international EQA providers for POC INR testing but one of the largest programmes is operated by UK NEQAS BC. Once results are received from the users, a median value is calculated and results are scored against this median value. An acceptable range is set around this median value and users who are outside of this range have failed the test. The principle behind this method of EQA is that if all the users test the same sample then they should all get very similar results. Devices/tests trips that are outside the acceptable range are performing differently and this may be affecting patient results and should be investigated.

UK NEQAS BC POC INR EQA programme was introduced in 1996 with just 30 devices and peaked in 2018 with 4718 devices registered (Kitchen et al. 2012). The introduction of direct oral anticoagulants (DOACs) has reduced the use of VKA therapy in many countries including the UK, and the Covid-19 pandemic has hastened many patients transitioning to DOACs. However, there are still patient groups that are not yet suitable for DOACs such as mechanic heart valve patients and antiphospholipid syndrome. VKA therapy is still much cheaper than DOACs and many resource-poor areas of the world will continue to use VKA for anticoagulation therapy.

UK NEQAS BC provides citrated samples from genuine patients on VKA therapy. The samples are lyophilised and provided to users with are measured diluent and a small disposable pipette to transfer the diluent into the lyophilised sample. Full instructions are supplied, and the test should only take around 5 min. It is important to provide a sample as near as possible to the genuine sample and this is difficult in the POC testing arena because the devices are designed to be used with fresh native whole blood (not containing any anticoagulant). However, it is not possible to produce a non-anticoagulated sample as this would clot within minutes of acquiring.

It is also not feasible to provide a whole blood sample because the red blood cells deteriorate rapidly and this would make the sample unstable, giving different results when tested on different days. EQA samples need to comply with the UKAS standards ISO 17043 such that all the samples provided for a test are homogeneous and stable over the period of the test. Commutability and stability are both very important aspects of EQA sample provision whereby samples that are commutable reflect accurately what would happen with fresh patient samples (Jennings et al. 2019). Stability is required so that samples do not deteriorate and give different results if tested at different times (Jennings et al. 2015; Kitchen et al. 2022). Various international EQA programmes provide EQA for POC INR devices although not all devices are covered. UK NEQAS BC currently provides EQA programmes for the Coagucheck INRange, Coaguchek Xs, Coaguchek XS Plus, Coaguchek XS Pro, Coaguchek Pro II, i-STAT1 and LumiraDX.

Each device type is peer reviewed so they are not cross-compared with a different device type. Table 3 shows data from the UK NEQAS BC point of care INR programmes during 2023.

As can be seen from the data, the CVs are good with all below 14% and some as low as 2.4% which is comparable to laboratory reagents. Percentage of users that were outside the acceptable range was also low in some devices with one survey or the LumiraDX having no devices out of range. The i-STAT device has the highest % CVs and also the highest % out of range results. However, this is the smallest group and if only one of the 20 devices is out of range this equates to a percentage of 5%.

We can compare the uncertainty of measurement (UoM) across these devices in the UK NEQAS BC POC INR programmes. For the year 2023, the average UoM for I-STAT was 0.113, for LumiraDX = 0.025, for Coaguchek XS Plus =0.0045 and for Coaguchek Pro II =0.006. For comparison, the average UoM over the same period in the EQA programme for hospital laboratory measurement of INRs (for the 3 most widely used thromboplastins, n > 90 users) were Werfen Recombiplastin 2G = 0.0112, Siemens Innovin = 0.0120, Stago Neoplastin R = 0.0217.

Table 3 Participation and EQA exercise results for UK NEQAS BC Point of Care INR progammes in 2023

POC INR EQA in 2023	Number of participants in programme	Medians ranged between	CV% ranged between	% outside of acceptable range was between
Coaguchek XS series	1749	1.8–3.1	4.1–8.4	0.3–1.4
Coaguchek Pro II	1780	1.9–3.3	5.1–9.6	0.8–2.0
i-STAT	21	3.25–4.6	9.2–11.7	11.1–22.2
LumiraDx	62	1.6–2.7	5.2–7.4	0.0–6.1

7 Comparison Between Laboratory and POC Device Results

In routine practice, it should not be necessary to send a venous comparison sample to the laboratory for testing when using POC INR measurement. If a patient's INR result is above 5.0, the guidelines state that a repeat test should be conducted using the POC device and the patient treated as clinically relevant. However, if a result of >8.0 is registered on the POC device, a venous sample should be taken for laboratory testing (Jennings et al. 2014). The reasoning behind this is that knowing the INR level may affect the treatment of the patient. For example if a POC reading is >8.0 and a venous sample is tested in the laboratory and that result is 8.2 and the patient is well and not bleeding then a pause in VKA therapy maybe the appropriate course of action. Whereas a laboratory INR reading of 15.0 in a patient that is not bleeding may need reversal using vitamin K therapy. It must be remembered that in patients who are over-anticoagulated, we cannot expect the INR system to work as well to give agreement and the expectation of the results being within 0.5 INR units is not possible. This is because when establishing the ISI, the samples used are in the range of 1.5–4.5 and samples over this are excluded from the process. It is also because as a patient is changing from being in a stable state to being over-anticoagulated their factor levels are falling yet further and they will fall in order of their half-lives with FVII falling first. Reagents/methods that are sensitive to the level of FVII will be more effected by the initial fall that reagents/methods that are not. Table 4 shows examples of 10 different patients comparing a laboratory system and a POC system.

It can be seen that the results do not show a particular trend; sometimes the POC is reading higher and sometimes the laboratory is reading higher and some samples show good agreement.

If there is a concern that there is a difference between 2 INR methods then we can perform some comparison studies to investigate but it is important to rule out over-anticoagulated patients. Other patient-related issues that may show difference between methods are patients with antiphospholipid antibodies, patients with very low or very high haematocrits, and any pre-analytical issues in either the laboratory or the POC system.

Table 4 Comparison of INR values on two different systems for over-anticoagulated samples

POC coaguchek XS	Laboratory innovin on sysmex CA 1500
5.0	4.6
5.5	4.6
6.5	4.8
6.1	6.1
5.6	6.9
5.5	5.4
6.7	5.7
5.5	5.8
7.8	6.4
>8.0	7.2

Once these have been ruled out, it is essential to establish if a genuine difference is seen across many samples so that all samples are affected to some degree. To perform such an investigation would require around 20 samples performed on the POC and then having a venous sample taken on the same day, preferably within around 2 h of the POC sample. We can plot this data on a Bland-Altman plot of the mean of the 2 results and the difference of the 2 results. Table 5 shows an example of such a set of results.

Once the results are plotted and a trend line is added (Fig. 8), a trend to higher INR results with the POC device can be identified. It can also be seen that as the INR increases, the difference between the 2 methods is more marked and this is typical of calibration errors in one or both systems. This is because if the ISI is miscalculated the affect will be seen in all the tests but the higher the INR the more marked the effect and thus a greater absolute difference between methods will occur (see Table 2). Of note it is not immediately possible to determine which of the 2 systems

Table 5 Series of INR results obtained with laboratory and Point of Care methods for comparison

Laboratory result	POC result	Average	Difference
2.3	2.2	2.25	0.1
2.9	3.6	3.25	−0.7
3.4	4.2	3.8	−0.8
2.2	2.6	2.4	−0.4
3.8	3.6	3.7	0.2
2.1	2.6	2.35	−0.5
4.2	4.9	4.55	−0.7
3.9	4.5	4.2	−0.6
2.7	2.9	2.8	−0.2

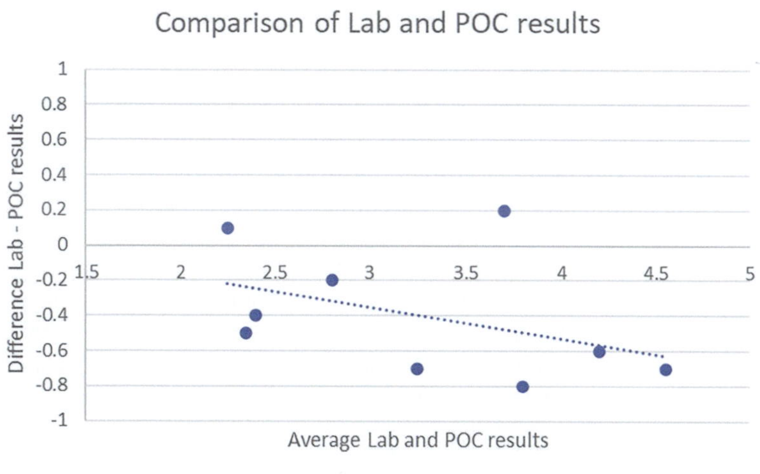

Fig. 8 Bland-Altman plot comparing laboratory and POC results

is giving a true result from the above we can only say that they are definitely giving different results and that it appears to be due to a calibration issue. To establish which is giving a correct result would require a comparison with an IRP and from this we could calculate the ISI of each method and compare this to the manufacturer's stated ISI.

8 VKA Reversal

If a patient has an INR above the therapeutic range (>4.5), the cause of action will depend on whether the patient has bleeding occurring. If there is no bleeding present, then it may be sufficient to pause the warfarin therapy for a day or so and then restart with regular monitoring of the INR. It is worth noting here that a bleeding event can occur at therapeutic levels of therapy (i.e., 2.0–4.5) although it is more likely if a patient is over-anticoagulated.

If VKA reversal is required due to a patient having a bleeding event, becoming over-anticoagulated with bleeding or in order to undergo a procedure this can be achieved by giving either vitamin K or in life-threatening bleeding the use of prothrombin complex (Keeling et al. 2011; Ansell et al. 2008). The reversal of VKA can be achieved in approximately 24 h by use of oral vitamin K or if required the use of IV vitamin K can reverse the VKA therapy in between 6–8 h. For an even quicker reversal, the use of prothrombin complex can correct the effect within 15 min. The choice of reversal agent is therefore dependent on the reason for reversal. If a patient is over-anticoagulated but with no bleeding present then it may be suitable to omit a VKA therapy and monitor before restarting VKA. The use of vitamin K to reverse the effect is achieved by the PIVKA proteins that are already circulating in the blood to be converted to active proteins using the carboxylation cycle that is no longer blocked by VKA.

Following reversal, if applicable warfarin therapy can be restarted and a baseline level of INR should be established together with regular monitoring of the INR until the patient has reached stabilisation of their INR.

To conclude although VKA therapy in the developed world has been superseded by the use of direct oral anticoagulants (DOACs), there is still a role for this treatment. In certain conditions, warfarin is still the recommended treatment – for antiphospholipid syndrome, mechanical heart valve replacement and for children requiring long-term anticoagulation. This treatment required careful monitoring, and this can be achieved with the use of the INR either in the laboratory or POC testing. The INR test should be performed by a precise and accurate method supported by a robust quality control system. This system needs both IQC and EQA in place to ensure good quality, reliable results to monitor treatment. Warfarin therapy can be easily reversed using vitamin K (oral or injections) or prothrombin complex concentrate depending on how quickly the reversal is required.

References

Ageno W, Gallus AS, Wittkowsky A, Crowther M, Hylek EM, Palareti G (2012) Oral anticoagulant therapy: Antithrombotic Therapy and Prevention of Thrombosis, 9th ed: American College of Chest Physicians Evidence-Based Clinical Practice Guidelines. Chest 141(2 Suppl):e44S–e88S

Ansell J, Hirsh J, Hylek E, Jacobson A, Crowther M, Palareti G (2008) Pharmacology and management of the vitamin K antagonists: American College of Chest Physicians Evidence-Based Clinical Practice Guidelines (8th Edition). Chest 133(6 Suppl):160S–198S

Baer S, Yarrow MW, Kravitz C, Markson V (1958) Clinical experiences with warfarin (coumadin) sodium as an anticoagulant. JAMA J Am Med Assoc 167(6):704–708

Bailey e, Harper A, Pinkerton PH (1971) The "therapeutic range" of the one-stage prothrombin time in the control of anticoagulant therapy: the effect of different thromboplastin preparations. CMAJ 105:1041

Chantarangkul V, Tripodi A, Clerici M, Negri B, Mannucci PM (1998) Assessment of the influence of citrate concentration on the International Normalized Ratio (INR) determined with twelve reagent-instrument combinations. Thromb Haemost 80(2):258–262

CLSI (2005) Procedures for validation of INR and local calibration, 1st edn. CLSI H54-A

Fitzmaurice DA, Hobbs FD, Murray ET (1998) Primary care anticoagulant clinic management using computerized decision support and near patient International Normalized Ratio (INR) testing: routine data from a practice nurse-led clinic. Fam Pract 15(2):144–146

Fitzmaurice DA, Geersing GJ, Armoiry X, Machin S, Kitchen S, Mackie I (2023) ICSH guidance for INR and D-dimer testing using point of care testing in primary care. Int J Lab Hematol 45(3): 276–281

Hermans J, van den Besselaar AM, Loeliger EA, van der Velde EA (1983) A collaborative calibration study of reference materials for thromboplastins. Thromb Haemost 50(3):712–717

Hylek EM (2003) Complications of oral anticoagulant therapy: bleeding and nonbleeding, rates and risk factors. Semin Vasc Med 3(3):271–278

Hylek EM, Go AS, Chang Y, Jensvold NG, Henault LE, Selby JV, Singer DE (2003) Effect of intensity of oral anticoagulation on stroke severity and mortality in atrial fibrillation. N Engl J Med 349(11):1019–1026

Jennings I, Kitchen D, Keeling D, Fitzmaurice D, Heneghan C, BCSH Committee (2014) Patient self-testing and self-management of oral anticoagulation with vitamin K antagonists: guidance from the British Committee for Standards in Haematology. Br J Haematol 167(5):600–607

Jennings I, Kitchen DP, Woods TA, Kitchen S, Preston FE, Walker ID (2015) Stability of coagulation proteins in lyophilized plasma. Int J Lab Hematol 37(4):495–502

Jennings I, Kitchen D, Kitchen S, Woods T, Walker I (2019) The importance of commutability in material used for quality control purposes. Int J Lab Hematol 41(1):39–45

Keeling D, Baglin T, Tait C, Watson H, Perry D, Baglin C, Kitchen S, Makris M, British Committee for Standards in Haematology (2011) Guidelines on oral anticoagulation with warfarin – fourth edition. Br J Haematol 154:311–324

Kitchen DP, Kitchen S, Jennings I, Woods TA, Walker ID, Preston FE (2005) Point of care testing by health care professionals: current practice amongst the UK National External Quality Assessment Scheme Participants. Br J Haematol 130(2):320–321

Kitchen DP, Kitchen S, Jennings I, Woods T, Walker I (2008) Quality assessment in point-of-care coagulation testing. Semin Thromb Hemost 34(7):647–653

Kitchen DP, Kitchen S, Jennings I, Woods TA, Fitzmaurice DA, Murray ET, Walker ID (2012) Point of Care INR testing devices: performance of the Roche CoaguChek XS and XS Plus in the UK NEQAS BC external quality assessment programme for healthcare professionals: four years' experience. J Clin Pathol 65(12):1119–1123

Kitchen DP, Jennings I, Kitchen S, Woods TA, Walker ID (2015) Bridging the gap between point-of-care testing and laboratory testing in hemostasis. Semin Thromb Hemost 41(3):272–278

Kitchen S, Bowyer A, Lowe A, Jennings I, Walker ID (2022) External quality assessment for one-stage and chromogenic factor IX assays in samples containing Alprolix (rFIXFc) or

Idelvion (rIX-FP) and evidence that UK National External Quality Assessment Scheme for blood coagulation samples are commutable with patient samples. Int J Lab Hematol 44(3): 619–625

Koerner SD, Fuller RE (1998) Comparison of a portable capillary whole blood coagulation monitor and standard laboratory methods for determining international normalized ratio. Mil Med 163(12):820–825

Kumar S, Haigh JR, Tate G, Boothby M, Joanes DN, Davies JA, Roberts BE, Feely MP (1990) Effect of warfarin on plasma concentrations of vitamin K dependent coagulation factors in patients with stable control and monitored compliance. Br J Haematol 74(1):82–85

Leaning KE, Ansell JE (1996) Advances in the monitoring of oral anticoagulation: point-of-care testing, patient self-monitoring, and patient self-management. J Thromb Thrombolysis 3(4): 377–383

Macfarlane RG (1964) An enzyme cascade in the blood clotting mechanism, and its function as a biochemical amplifier. Nature 202:498–499

Murray ET, Fitzmaurice DA, Allan TF, Hobbs FD (1999) A primary care evaluation of three near patient coagulometers. J Clin Pathol 52(11):842–845

Nicholson JH (1957) Clinical experiences with anticoagulants; a comparison of coumadin (warfarin) sodium and dicumarol (bishydroxycoumarin). Angiology 8(5):456–465

Shapiro CM, Lisker R, Lichtman AM, Josephson AM (1958) Comparative clinical study of coumadin sodium and dicumarol in patients with thromboembolic diseases. Am Heart J 55(1):66–72

Townsend SR, Mills ES (1942) Effect of synthetic haemorrhagic agent 3,3′-methylene-bis (4-hydroxycoumarin) in prolonging coagulation and prothrombin time in human subject. Canad MAJ 46:214

van den Besselaar AM (1985) Standardization of the prothrombin time in oral anticoagulant control. Haemostasis 15(4):271–277

van den Besselaar AM, Barrowcliffe TW, Houbouyan-Réveillard LL, Jespersen J, Johnston M, Poller L, Tripodi A, Subcommittee on Control of Anticoagulation of the Scientific and Standardization Committee of the ISTH (2004) Guidelines on preparation, certification, and use of certified plasmas for ISI calibration and INR determination. J Thromb Haemost 2(11): 1946–1953

van den Besselaar AM, Péquériaux NC, Ebben M, van der Feest J, de Jong K, Ganzeboom MB, van Ooijen J, Postema F, Witteveen E, van der Meer FJ (2012) Point-of-care monitoring of vitamin K-antagonists: validation of CoaguChek XS test strips with International Standard thromboplastin. J Clin Pathol 65(11):1031–1035

van den Besselaar AMHP, Chantarangkul V, Angeloni F, Binder NB, Byrne M, Dauer R, Gudmundsdottir BR, Jespersen J, Kitchen S, Legnani C, Lindahl TL, Manning RA, Martinuzzo M, Panes O, Pengo V, Riddell A, Subramanian S, Szederjesi A, Tantanate C, Herbel P, Tripodi A (2018) International collaborative study for the calibration of proposed international standards for thromboplastin, rabbit, plain, and for thromboplastin, recombinant, human, plain. J Thromb Haemost 16(1):142–149

van den Besselaar AMHP, Stavelin A, Kitchen S, Bryant M, Tripodi A, Scalambrino E, Clerici M, Herbel P, Jünschke A, Meyer Dos Santos S, Meijer P, Niessen RWLM, Meijers JCM, Thelwell C, Cuker A, Kung C, Cao Z, Zander N, Iwasaki Y, Depasse F, van Rijn C, Baktawar S, Abdoel C, Cobbaert CM (2024) Defining a metrologically traceable and sustainable calibration hierarchy of international normalized ratio for monitoring of vitamin K antagonist treatment in accordance with International Organization for Standardization (ISO) 17511:2020 standard: communication from the International Federation of Clinical Chemistry and Laboratory Medicine-SSC/ISTH working group on prothrombin time/international normalized ratio standardization. J Thromb Haemost. 22(4):1236–1248

Wolff JM, Barker NW, Gifford RW Jr, Mann FD (1953) Experience with a new intravenous coumarin anticoagulant (warfarin, sodium derivative). Proc Staff Meet Mayo Clin 28(18): 489–497

Part II

Heparin and Low Molecular Weight Heparin

Heparin: Over 100 Years of Anticoagulation

John Hogwood and Elaine Gray

Contents

Abstract

This chapter provides an overview of heparin, including discovery, structure, mechanism of action, and principal use for anticoagulation. For over 100 years, heparin has a central role in prophylaxis and treatment of prothrombotic states, be it used in the event of pulmonary embolism or maintaining blood fluidity during dialysis. Indeed, heparin had a role in enabling the development of

J. Hogwood (✉)
Therapeutic Reference Materials, Medicines and Healthcare Products Regulator Agency, South Mimms, UK
e-mail: john.hogwood@mhra.gov.uk

E. Gray
Institute of Pharmaceutical Sciences, King's College London, London, UK

E. Gray, J. Hogwood (eds.), *Antithrombotic and Antiplatelet Agents*, Handbook of Experimental Pharmacology 291, https://doi.org/10.1007/164_2025_780

cardiopulmonary bypass for the surgical treatment of cardiopulmonary diseases. The development of heparin depolymerization which produced low molecular weight heparin further enhanced the usefulness of this anticoagulant, where this type of heparin can be self-administered. There has been much written about heparin over the last century, and this chapter provides a concise overview.

Keywords

Anticoagulant · Heparin · Low Molecular Weight Heparin · Venous Thromboembolism

1 Discovery of Heparin

Numerous articles have been published on the discovery and history of heparin (Barrowcliffe 2012; Wardrop and Keeling 2008; Caen 1984; Paschoa 2016; Hemker 2016; Ong et al. 2019). The majority of these publications attributed the discovery of heparin to Jay McLean who was working in William Howell's Baltimore laboratory. In 1916, he accidentally isolated an anticoagulant while extracting a "thromboplastin" material from a dog's liver (McLean 1916). There is however some controversy as to whether McLean did discover heparin. Howell and Holt continued with McLean's work and in 1918 described the isolation of an anticoagulant which they claimed not to be similar to the substance described by McLean. Nonetheless, they acknowledged McLean's contribution and named this material heparin (Howell and Holt 1918). However, there is evidence that this anticoagulant from the liver has been described by other scientists even in the late 1880s. Jorpes in his 1964 review (Jorpes 1964) indicated that the first description was published in 1880 by Adolph Schmidt-Mulheim who carried out an investigation on the nutritional value of peptones. In the 1880–1900, a number of French scientists including Fano, Grosjean, Contejean, Cley, Pachon, Hedon, Delezenne, Apiro, and Ellinger continued with Schidt-Mulheim's work and concluded that peptones induced the formation of an anticoagulant, but they did not manage to identify or purify the anticoagulant. In 1911, Doyon, Morel, and Policard of Lyon made a serious attempt to isolate and identify the presumed antithrombin of the liver. Doyon subsequently purified "heparin" using a process that was similar to the present-day commercial process for extraction, purification of heparin. Their work was published in a series of papers in 1911–1912. However, these findings were not noted by McLean and Howell who then independently discovered heparin without the knowledge of Doyles's publications.

2 Development of Clinical Heparin Products

Barrowcliffe has provided a comprehensive review on the early development of commercial clinical heparin products (Barrowcliffe 2012). Briefly, the early products from the 1930s to the 1960s were predominantly extracted from bovine lung. Because of availability and ease of handling, the source of heparin was shifted to porcine mucosa. Concurrent with the outbreak of variant Creutzfeldt-Jakob disease (vCJD) related to the consumption of meat from infected animals, clinical heparin products from bovine sources have been discontinued in Europe and the United States since the 1990s. However, bovine heparin products are continued to be used in the Middle-East, Asia, and South America. The structure of heparin is highly heterogeneous, and products not only from different species but also from different organs and tissues of the same species have different structures, physicochemical characteristics, and specific activities (Tovar et al. 2016; St Ange et al. 2016; Bertini et al. 2017b). The availability of the international and pharmacopoeial standards for anticoagulant activity/potency and standardization of assay methods (Gray et al. 2009; PharmEur_07/2024:0333; USP_Heparin_Sodium) aid the equivalency of labelling of products in International Units (IU) from different sources and therefore provide similar antithrombotic efficacy on a unit basis (Jeske et al. 2018). However, due to the differences in specific activity, the amount of heparin by mass to obtain the same potency will be different and therefore products from different sources may not be interchangeable. Adulteration and contamination of heparin have been reported over the years (Casu et al. 1987; Coyne et al. 1998), but the most serious event was in 2007 when porcine heparin was adulterated with oversulfated chondroitin sulfate (Liu et al. 2009; Kishimoto et al. 2008). This led to global morbidity in patients. Pharmacopoeias and regulatory authorities promptly revised analytical methods to ensure the quality and safety of heparin products (Szajek et al. 2016). Since more than 50% of raw and crude porcine mucosa heparin originates from China, regulatory authorities such as the US FDA are considering diversification of the supply of heparin from different species (Keire et al. 2015; Al-Hakim 2021). The issues concerning heparin from different sources are seriously considered by the pharmacopoeias and regulatory authorities. Monographs for bovine heparin have already been published by the Brazilian Pharmacopoeia (Vilanova et al. 2019), and these monographs show different specifications from those that apply to porcine heparin.

3 Mechanism of Action

The anticoagulant and antithrombotic function of heparin has been reviewed in detail in several publications (Gray et al. 2012; Beurskens et al. 2020; Qiu et al. 2021; Hogwood et al. 2023; Sultana and Kamihira 2024). It acts mainly by potentiating the activity of antithrombin, a plasma coagulation inhibitor. Antithrombin inhibits activated coagulation factors with thrombin and factor Xa (FXa) being its major targets. As indicated in the Hogwood et al. review (Hogwood et al. 2023), heparin

Table 1 Anticoagulant activities of heparin from different sources and two different low molecular weight heparins produced by different methods

	Potency IU/mg	(95% CL)				
Assays	Porcine heparin	Bovine heparin	Bovine lung	Ovine heparin	LMWH Enoxaparin	LMWH Tinzaparin
aXa	203 187–219	135 132–138	127 123–132	179 172–186	105 103–107	104 102–106
aIIa	196 176–218	125 116–134	126 121–130	174 165–183	30 29–31	59 57–61
aXa/ aIIa	1.04 0.86–1.24	1.08 0.99–1.19	1.01 0.95–1.09	1.03 0.94–1.013	3.50 3.32–3.69	1.76 1.67–1.86
EP	199 193–204	160 157–163	138 132–147	182 177–188	32 30–33	105 97–114
APT	199 189–209	136 126–150	115 113–117	178 173–182	50 48–52	74 66–85
HCII	206 197–216	186 175–198	206 192–222	195 180–212	37 33–40	159 145–174
Mw	16,900	15,400	16,600	16,800	4,350	6,650

aXa antithrombin-dependent anti-factor Xa assay, *aIIa* antithrombin-dependent anti-factor IIa assay, *EP* European Pharmacopoeia clot method using sheep plasma, *APTT* activated partial thromboplastin time method using human plasma, *HCII* heparin cofactor dependent anti-factor IIa assay, *Mw* weight average molecular weight

will also attenuate the coagulant effect of thrombin via its binding to heparin cofactor II. It is also widely accepted that the interaction of heparin with other plasmatic and endothelial anchored proteins leads to the release of anticoagulant factors such as tissue factor pathway inhibitor (TFPI) which also contributes to its overall antithrombotic action. Although heparin was discovered in the early 1900 and its commercialization as a clinical product was in the 1930s, it was not till the 1970s that several structural elements were elucidated, and its mode of action was expounded (Lindahl et al. 1979; Choay et al. 1980). While the principal action of heparin is via the potentiation of the inhibitory activities of antithrombin, heparin from different sources have structural differences which give rise to different specific activities (Table 1). It was in 1976 that fractionated heparin was reported by Johnson et al. (1976) and shown to have in vitro and in vivo anticoagulant effects. This led to the development of several low molecular weight heparins that are now successful antithrombotics (Table 2).

Detailed reviews of the clinical uses of heparin and low molecular weight heparin (Qiu et al. 2021; Sultana and Kamihira 2024) indicate the antithrombotic action of heparin and low molecular weight heparin stems from a combination of their anticoagulant activities and their interaction with other plasmatic and endothelial factors that may provide anti-complement and anti-inflammatory actions. The antithrombotic action of heparin is in part through the inhibition of thrombin, which is a powerful platelet stimulator and through mechanisms that are unrelated to

Table 2 Low molecular weight heparins available in Europe

Low molecular weight heparin	Prepared by:	Typical molecular weight
Dalteparin	Nitrous acid depolymerization of heparin	6,000 Da
Enoxaparin	Alkaline depolymerization of the benzyl ester derivative of heparin	4,500 Da
Nadroparin	Nitrous acid depolymerization of heparin	4,650 Da
Parnaparin	Radical-catalyzed depolymerization, with hydrogen peroxide and with a cupric salt, of heparin	5,000 Da
Tinzaparin	Enzymatic depolymerization of heparin	6,500 Da

anticoagulant activity. A similar glycosaminoglycan (GAG), heparan sulfate, which is considered a less sulfated non-anticoagulant version of heparin is also an efficacious antithrombotic (Nader et al. 2004). It is likely that heparin and similar GAGs have antithrombotic activity through disruption of the interactions between the hemostatic and inflammatory systems (Stark and Massberg 2021), where they attenuate harmful proteins which link these pathways (Mulloy et al. 2016).

4 Structure of Heparin

Heparin, as a biological medicine, is probably one of the most structurally complex therapeutics in use. The structural complexity of heparin has been covered in detail elsewhere (Casu and Lindahl 2001; Mulloy 2012) and herein will be covered in brief with focus on the relationship with anticoagulant/antithrombotic activity.

Heparin is within the glycosaminoglycans (GAGs) group of polysaccharides which in mammals are linear and characterized by a repeating hexose backbone. Within this family it should be noted that heparan sulfate, a ubiquitous cell surface GAG, and heparin have structural similarities with the latter being more heavily sulfated (Gallagher 2012). The clinical product has an average molecular weight of between 14 and 18 kDa (Mulloy et al. 2000) with its polydispersity confirmed in the 1970s (Johnson and Mulloy 1976). Broadly, different heparin sources tend to show differences in their molecular weight (Fig. 1). This antithrombin-interacting sequence is the pentasaccharide, with specific carboxylate and sulfate groups interacting with positive amino acids in the structure of antithrombin, altering its conformational state which enhances its inhibitor action (Petitou and van Boeckel 2004). A review by Petitou (Petitou et al. 2003) provides an interesting sequence of events that led to the discovery of the pentasaccharide. The heavily sulfated saccharide chains giving rise to highly negative charges which facilitate interactions with other positively charged proteins unrelated to coagulation and enhance the non-anticoagulant effect of heparin (Lindahl and Hook 1978; Mulloy and Linhardt 2001; Meneghetti et al. 2015).

As discussed, heparin is heterogenous and the pentasaccharide sequence is not "uniformly" present across all the saccharide chains within a heparin preparation. In

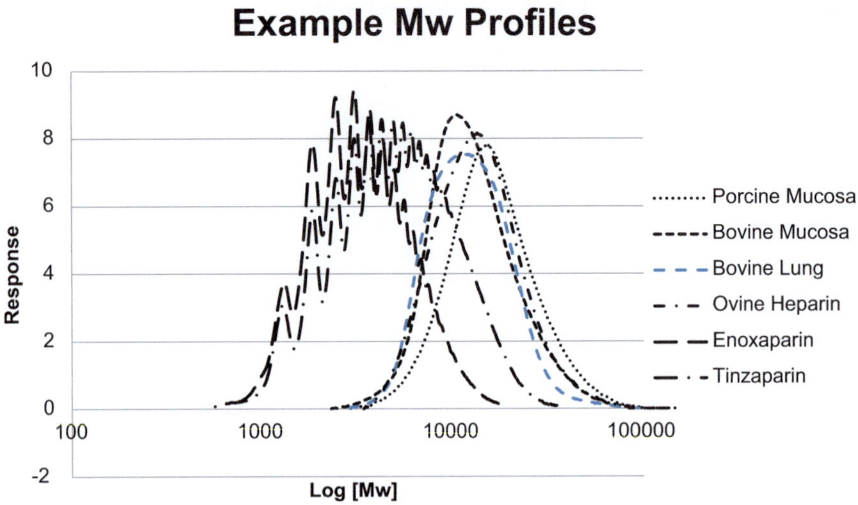

Fig. 1 Molecular weight profiles of unfractionated heparin from different species. Molecular weight distribution of 2 low molecular weight heparins: enoxaparin and tinzaparin are also shown as a comparison. Chromatograms have been generated using the broad standard method (Mulloy and Hogwoord 2022)

the 1970s, it was shown that only about a third of the molecules in heparin products contained this pentasaccharide sequence and therefore have high affinity to antithrombin (Lam et al. 1976; Andersson et al. 1976). The current heparin products manufactured from porcine mucosa can consist up to approximately 50% high-affinity material. For religious and availability reasons, in South America and some Asian countries, heparin from bovine mucosa is the preferred source of heparin. These clinical bovine mucosa heparins currently contain about 30% high affinity for antithrombin material (Hogwood et al. 2017). The fractionation of heparin, in addition to reducing the molecular weight (to between 4 and 6 kDa), lowers the specific activity of the material. This activity reduction highlights the template requirement for thrombin inhibition, where an additional 13 saccharides on the non-reducing end of the pentasaccharide are needed (Hoylaerts et al. 1984). Clinical low molecular weight heparins are prepared by different depolymerization methods (see Table 1) which each gives them a unique molecular weight and activity profile. By comparison with unfractionated heparin, low molecular weight heparins show higher inhibitory activity against FXa (anti-Xa) than against thrombin (anti-IIa). Therefore, the ratios of anti-Xa to anti-IIa activity are always greater than 1 and European pharmacopoeia specifies low molecular weight heparins must have an anti-Xa to anti-IIa ratio of greater than 1.5 (PharmEur_07/2023:0828).

It should be noted that the heterogenous properties of heparin and cell surface heparan sulfate, enable both GAGs to interact with a wide range of proteins (Wang et al. 2022; Mulloy et al. 2016; Hogwood et al. 2023). These interactions highlight a probable beneficial role beyond anticoagulation in vivo due to known anti-complement and anti-inflammatory interactions for which there is much interest in the development of heparin for non-anticoagulant indications (Mulloy 2019; Cassinelli and Naggi 2016; Casu et al. 2008; Wang et al. 2022) and contribute to the antithrombotic properties of heparin.

5 Reversal of Heparin

An advantage of heparin over LMWH is that its anticoagulant activity can be fully neutralized. Protamine, a mixture of cationic peptides extracted from fish, is commonly used clinically for reversal of heparin in cases of heparin overdose or to reduce anticoagulation after cardiac surgery (Pai and Crowther 2012). The interaction between heparin and protamine is charge-based, the cationic peptide with the anionic polysaccharide, and the neutral macromolecular salt formed has no anticoagulant activity. The capacity of protamine to neutralize heparin anticoagulant activity depends on the specific activity and molecular weight of the heparin sample (Hogwood et al. 2017). While it is generally indicated that 1 mg of protamine will neutralize 100 IU of heparin, the actual interaction is mass/mass-related. Greater amounts of protamine are required to neutralize bovine heparin than porcine heparin and this is due to a lower specific activity found with bovine heparins. Furthermore, protamine is more effective in binding to longer heparin polysaccharide chains than the shorter heparin oligosaccharides. Therefore, while it neutralizes the anti-IIa activity of LMWHs (Kouta et al. 2021), it does not completely neutralize the anti-Xa activity (Schroeder et al. 2011). Alongside limited neutralization of LMWHs, there are several potential adverse side effects of protamine (Sokolowska et al. 2016) and the possible formation of large immunogenic complexes that are similar to heparin/platelet factor 4 complexes and this may lead to heparin-induced thrombocytopenia (Bakchoul et al. 2016; Sommers et al. 2017).

Due to the recent shortages in supply of protamine, alternative agents to neutralize heparin are being considered to reduce reliance on protamine (Maneno and Ness 2021). Platelet factor 4 is an option but it has not yet received regulatory approval. An approach using recombinant human FVIIa is being considered despite the increased risk in procoagulant activity which may lead to thrombosis (Pai and Crowther 2012). New heparin-neutralizing agents are in development at various pre-clinical and clinical stages (Sokolowska et al. 2016). The enzymatic digestion of protamine sulfate to form low molecular weight protamine (LMWP) produces an agent that has been found to neutralize both UFH and LMWH, and to exhibit less antigenic potential than unfractionated protamine (He et al. 2014). The cationic peptide, poly-L-lysine, can bind to and neutralize heparin, with a MW 15,000 g/mole poly-L-lysine fraction (comparable to typical heparin in MW) identified as a possible substitute for protamine (Muralidharan-Chari et al. 2017). Another readily available cationic macromolecule is the polysaccharide chitin, which when converted to quaternized chitosan has similar neutralizing effects to protamine (Drozd et al. 2019). Some synthetic options are possible, with block co-polymers consisting of one neutral and one cationic block optimized for heparin binding in vitro (Valimaki et al. 2016) and another block copolymer termed HBC (Heparin Binding Co-polymer) which neutralizes LMWH (Kalaska et al. 2020). Lastly, more specific heparin targeting agents, not solely reliant on a charge-based interaction, are the use of a recombinant inactive antithrombin (Bianchini et al. 2018) and andaxanet, a recombinant inactivated FXa that can bind to heparin activated anti-thrombin (Maneno and Ness 2021). The former binds to the high affinity pentasaccharide in heparin, with the latter which is already approved as an antagonist to the FXa inhibitors, apixaban and rivaroxaban.

6 Clinical Use of Heparin

The primary clinical indication for heparins, both UFH and LMWH, is for the prophylaxis and treatment of venous thromboembolism (VTE). Herein, a brief overview of different VTE interventions requiring the use of heparin will be described, with more detailed reviews of specific applications being available elsewhere (Mulloy et al. 2016; Lim et al. 2018; Witt et al. 2018; Anderson et al. 2019; Ortel et al. 2020; Lyman et al. 2021). Additional non-VTE uses of heparin will also be briefly covered. It is broadly viewed that UFH, regardless of source, is a "single" type of preparation whereas LMWH as described above differs in its characteristics. As such LMWH cannot be viewed as interchangeable, with assessment and comparison of clinical trials showing a complex picture (Agnelli et al. 2015). Within this brief review, LMWH will be considered broadly as a group.

6.1 Treatment of VTE

The risk factors associated with VTE can be defined as "effects" that can disrupt the normal hemostatic balance of blood, such as age, obesity, cancer, and genetic factors such as known thrombophilia, immobility, surgery, and hormonal treatments such as HRT and oral contraception (Reitsma et al. 2012). These risks, or combinations of, predispose a patient to thrombosis. Initially, UFH was used for VTE (Barritt and Jordan 1960) but following the development of LMWHs which do not require regular monitoring (Bratt et al. 1985; Holm et al. 1986; Prandoni et al. 1992; Hull et al. 1992; Thery et al. 1992), LMWH became the preferred treatment (Cohen 2012; Kearon et al. 2012). However, in some cases such as high risk of bleeding, heparin is considered more suitable (Garcia et al. 2012; Cohen et al. 2014) because of its shorter half-life and when needed the rapid reversal of activity by protamine (Pai and Crowther 2012). It should be noted that for patients with renal impairment, heparin is the preferred treatment as LMWH clearance tends to be reduced which increases bleeding risk (Cohen et al. 2014) although with dose adjustment LMWH can be used (Leung and MacRae 2019).

Treatment approaches differ between UFH and LWMH, with UFH requiring a loading intravenous bolus followed by continuous infusion, whereas LWMH is given via subcutaneous injection. For UFH, regular monitoring typically via

APTT is required (Marlar et al. 2017), although anti-Xa assays are increasing in use (Baluwala et al. 2017). LMWH may only occasionally require monitoring by the anti-Xa assay (Garcia et al. 2012; Babin et al. 2017). A further advantage of LMWH is the fixed dose treatment regime (Quinlan et al. 2004) which is highly preferable for outpatients with conditions such as pregnancy-induced thrombosis and thrombosis associated with cancer. The length of treatment following a VTE is variable, dependent on associated factors and subject to interpretation. For example in pregnancy, treatment would occur throughout to term and beyond (Brenner et al. 2021), and in cancer patients for 6 months before reassessment of risk/benefit (Lyman et al. 2021). Individualized regimes may be required to balance the risk of recurrent VTE against the risk of side effects, the most notable of which is bleeding (Ageno et al. 2015). The choice to continue with therapy after a VTE event will depend on the patient's bleeding risk and the likelihood of VTE recurrence, whichever might be higher (Kearon et al. 2012; Kearon and Akl 2014).

6.2 VTE Prophylaxis

Heparin and LMWH are used for prophylaxis in hospitalized patients who present one or more risk factors for VTE, with immobility a significant factor. While both types of heparin will reduce the incidence of a potential deep vein thrombosis or pulmonary embolism, LMWHs tend to have a lower bleeding risk and some superiority (Alikhan et al. 2014). Generally, both heparin and LMWH are effective in medical patients with consensus that LMWH has a better safety profile (Cohen et al. 2010). However, it should be noted that underlying pathology, such a renal impairment (Cook et al. 2008), the static nature of patients reducing cardiopulmonary function, and ongoing treatments greatly increase the risk of VTE (McLeod and Geerts 2011).

Major orthopedic surgery, such as to hips or legs, by its nature presents a high risk for the development of VTE which can persist after surgery with presentation typically after discharge from the hospital (Leclerc et al. 1998; White et al. 2003). Refinement to surgical, anesthesiological, and perioperative care have reduced basal VTE risk (Falck-Ytter et al. 2012; Francis 2013; Chan et al. 2014), prophylactic treatment ensures VTE risk remains low (Chan et al. 2014), with routine prophylaxis recommended for most orthopedic patients (Falck-Ytter et al. 2012) alongside mechanical prophylaxis. Due to greater efficacy, safety, and the use of dosing schedules, LMWH is preferable to heparin (Hirsh et al. 2001). Treatment with LMWH for prevention of VTE has been shown to be effective both for hip and knee surgery and in trauma cases (Hovanessian 1999; Hirsh et al. 2001; Francis 2013), but as with treatment of VTE heparin may be preferable in cases of renal impairment. The recommended time to start prophylaxis varies with procedure, with initiation typically between 6 and 12 h after surgical closer to balance the risk of blood loss with the need for prophylaxis. As an example, delayed use of LMWH to 24 h from standard 12 h did not lower the incidence of VTE but did reduce total blood loss associated with the surgical intervention (Liu et al. 2014). It should also be noted that if pre-operative treatment for VTE is required, then prior to surgery a heparin free period is needed (Falck-Ytter et al. 2012).

In more 'minor" surgical procedures, such as upper limb, gastrointestinal, and day cases, a patient's individual risk profile is assessed to balance possible thrombosis to bleeding before considering prophylaxis. The degree of immobility is a major factor, with LMWH being first choice alongside mechanical means (Ettema et al. 2008; Testroote et al. 2008), although whether heparin is routinely needed is not fully agreed (Falck-Ytter et al. 2012). However, a meta-analysis of trials where patients have short-term reduction in mobility has shown a significant reduction in VTE, with non-significant increased risk of major bleeding with LMWH prophylaxis (Chapelle et al. 2014).

6.3 Pregnancy

Pregnancy shifts hemostasis to a hypercoagulable state and presents a unique risk factor for VTE (Berresheim et al. 2014; Guimicheva et al. 2015). There is an estimated four- to five-fold increase in risk for VTE while pregnant, which rises further during puerperium and can be further influenced by underlying material risk factors (Lussana et al. 2012; Marshall 2014). These risk factors can be pregnancy-related such as pre-eclampsia, multiple pregnancy, or hyperemesis gravidarum or unrelated such as thrombophilia. In the developed world pregnancy-associated VTE accounts for about 10% of maternal deaths (Marshall 2014). The change to a more hypercoagulable state is due to shifts in the levels of coagulation factors, with a decrease in protein S, an inhibitor, and increases in Factor VII, Factor VIII, and fibrinogen (Stirling et al. 1984; Chunilal et al. 2002; Hoke et al. 2004). In pre-eclampsia, there are also reductions in antithrombin and protein C (de Boer et al. 1989). Due to these changes in coagulation factors, and possibly further changes in plasma proteins that can bind to heparin, the response to heparin therapy can complicate treatment options (Chunilal et al. 2002).

In the treatment or prophylaxis of pregnancy-associated VTE, both heparin and LMWH are known not to cross the placenta (Forestier et al. 1987). They are considered safe for use, in contrast to other anticoagulant agents such as vitamin K antagonist, which have known teratogenicity, or for non-Vitamin K antagonist oral anticoagulants which has limited safety information (Marshall 2014). The use of LMWH is preferable and has been shown to be safe and effective (Greer and Nelson-Piercy 2005; Kher et al. 2007; Bates et al. 2012; Konstantinides 2014). Low molecular weight heparins also have an advantage over heparin as LMWH carries lower risk of osteoporosis and thrombocytopenia (Bates et al. 2012; Lussana et al. 2012) which may be important for a preferable outcome due to the protracted nature of treatment/prophylaxis needed throughout pregnancy. Although routine monitoring does not tend to be needed, adjustments in dosage may be required due to higher clearance and increase in blood volume associated with pregnancy (Kher et al. 2007).

6.4 Cancer

In relation to VTE in cancer, LMWH is preferred for prophylaxis and treatment (Carrier et al. 2014; Elyamany et al. 2014). The risk of VTE varies, depending on the site of the primary tumor, the therapeutic approach, and underlying patient characteristics, and requires an individual approach for treatment (Khorana 2010; Khorana and McCrae 2014). Cancer malignancy presents as a hypercoagulable state (Cohen et al. 2014) with a risk of VTE increased seven-fold over those without (Noble 2012; Franchini and Mannucci 2015) and occurrence between 1% and 30% (Lee et al. 2003). Chemotherapeutic treatment can further increase risk (Falanga and Zacharski 2005; Di Nisio et al. 2014) requiring prophylaxis in both inpatient (Kamphuisen and Beyer-Westendorf 2014) and outpatient settings (Khorana 2012). Observationally, this link between cancer and thrombosis is sufficiently high that testing for cancer may be warranted in patients with an unprovoked VTE to diagnose a malignancy (Robertson et al. 2015).

Cancer patients under anticoagulation have an increased risk of contracting complications, with an expected increased bleeding risk but also recurrent thrombosis due to treatment failure when compared to other patient groups (Kyrle 2014; Kamphuisen and Beyer-Westendorf 2014; Prandoni et al. 2015). Compared with vitamin K antagonist, LMWHs are more effective for thromboprophylaxis (Di Nisio et al. 2014) and at reducing recurrent thrombosis (Lee et al. 2003), providing a better survival outcome following symptomatic VTE (Zhang et al. 2015). However, as a prophylaxis for VTE in ambulatory patients undergoing chemotherapy survival was unaffected but symptomatic VTE was significantly reduced with no increased risk in bleeding events (Ben-Aharon et al. 2014). A further factor in the use of heparin in cancer patients are effects unrelated to prevention of thrombosis which complicate analysis of VTE prophylaxis on survival outcomes (Lee 2010; Noble 2012; Franchini and Mannucci 2015).

6.5 Bypass and Dialysis

Cardiopulmonary bypass was developed in the 1960s, and heparin has a major role in this procedure as it maintains blood fluidity during the operation (Hessel 2014). Apart from being an effective anticoagulant, a further advantage, as mentioned earlier, is that heparin can be readily neutralized by protamine sulfate following bypass completion (Bull et al. 1975). However, it should be noted that the development of cardiopulmonary bypass lacked the rigors of modern-day clinical trials and was in part the cause to drive effective reviews of clinical interventions (Stoney 2009; Ferraris 2002). Further refinements to extracorporeal membrane oxygenation (ECMO) machines are the incorporation of heparin coatings into the bypass circuits (Sievert et al. 2009; Hanedan et al. 2020) which have been shown to reduce complement and inflammatory responses of blood (Mathieu et al. 2024).

Hemodialysis was first developed in the 1920s with the first "artificial kidney" used successfully in the 1940s (Gottschalk and Fellner 1997). Heparin became the primary anticoagulant following the initially used hirudin (Cameron 2000). The main advantage, as with the bypass circuit mentioned above, is that heparin acts as an anticoagulant and antithrombotic and can be rapidly neutralized following dialysis completion (Gozdzikiewicz et al. 2009; Cronin and Reilly 2010). However, with the frequency of use in dialysis there are known risks of bleeding (Brunelli et al. 2019) and with repeated exposure the possible complication of HIT (Suranyi and Chow 2010). While alternative anticoagulants such as danaparoid and fondparinux could be considered when there is an occurrence of HIT, the effectiveness of heparinoids, LMWH and direct oral anticoagulants (DOACs) is not evident and such treatments are not readily neutralized post dialysis (Claudel et al. 2021).

7 Adverse Reactions to Heparin

The adverse reactions that can occur through the clinical use of heparin have been covered in detail (Alban 2012; Mulloy et al. 2016; Hogwood et al. 2023) and herein a brief description will be provided. The main adverse reaction is heparin-induced thrombocytopenia (HIT), whereby platelet activation gives rise to loss of platelets, leading to a prothrombotic state. There are two types of HIT, mild which is caused by direct interaction of heparin with platelets (Chong and Castaldi 1986) and severe which is an immune-related response following several days of heparin exposure (Martel et al. 2005). The severe form of HIT requires cessation of treatment and use of an alternative anticoagulant, such as fondaparinux or a DOAC, to maintain anticoagulation. The immune-mediated response is due to the interaction of heparin with CXCL4, in which it forms large complexes (Rauova et al. 2005; Bertini et al. 2017a) that are highly immunogenic. The binding of antibodies to heparin-CXCL4 triggers platelet activation via the FC receptor (Kelton et al. 1988), but these antibodies have also been shown to activate endothelial cells (Cines et al. 1987), immune cells (Pouplard et al. 2001; Xiao et al. 2008), and the complement system (Khandelwal et al. 2018). Other types of adverse reaction are: skin lesions (Schindewolf et al. 2009), osteoporosis (Le Templier and Rodger 2008), and alopecia (Barnes et al. 2000; Sarris et al. 2003; Wang and Po 2006).

Lastly, as with all anticoagulants, there is a risk of bleeding (Schulman et al. 2008) which in the strictest sense is not an adverse reaction. The incidence of bleeding while on heparin therapy cannot be readily defined as there can be many factors which can contribute given the array of uses that heparin anticoagulation is used for. A review of bleeding risk showed an incidence level of between 1.5% and 4.7% for UFH and LMWH across use as VTE prophylaxis/treatment and for acute coronary syndrome (Crowther and Cook 2008). These levels are much higher than those observed within clinical trials, where for example a trial for acute venous thrombosis had a cumulative incidence of major bleeding at 0.25% (Van Rein 2017). Due to the tightly controlled nature of clinical trials, patients with risk factors are often excluded. Factors that can influence the risk of bleeding include increased age, renal insufficiency, body weight, gender, anemia, and cancer (Kinnaird et al. 2003; Macie et al. 2004; Manoukian et al. 2007; Schulman et al. 2008; Ruiz-Gimenez et al.

2008; Trujillo-Santos et al. 2008). As described above, with superior pharmacokinetics, LMWHs have a broadly lower incidence of bleeding relative to heparin (Palmer et al. 1997; Mismetti et al. 2001; Riess et al. 2010). While the general risk of bleeding is low, the occurrence of bleeding is a strong predictor of mortality (Budaj et al. 2009; Eikelboom et al. 2009; Kalathottukaren et al. 2018).

8 Monitoring of Heparin

The anticoagulant action of heparin is primarily through potentiation of the inhibitory action of antithrombin on FXa and thrombin. However, traditionally, monitoring of heparin employs indirect methods that are based on the prolongation of clotting time such as the APTT assay. Recently, decrease in chromogenic signal via the anti-Xa assay has been introduced and is used in some clinical laboratories as a replacement for the APTT. Low molecular weight heparins used for prevention of thrombosis are not usually monitored and if needed, this is carried out by using anti-FXa assays. There are some limitations to both types of monitoring, as described in detail elsewhere (Marlar et al. 2017; Connell and Sylvester 2022; Thalappil et al. 2024; Baker et al. 2024) but can be explained as challenges with standard curves, assay sensitivity, ratios to control plasma, and reagent/kit composition. The need for monitoring varies for indication with frequency and potential risk of bleeding factors requiring consideration (McRae et al. 2021). An alternative method to determine patient coagulation state is the use of thromboelastography (Zmuda et al. 2000) which has been found to be useful at point of care (Dias et al. 2019; Yin et al. 2025) and involve the use of whole blood rather than plasma alone. Direct methods based on binding to dyes such as tolidine blue can be used to directly quantify sulfated polysaccharides (Shriver and Sasisekharan 2013; Copley and Whitney 1943) but these are not specific for heparin. Recently, such a diagnostic product, Heparin Red has been developed but has been found to be more relevant for monitoring of non-anticoagulant heparins (Warttinger et al. 2016) such as tafoxiparin which is under clinical development to prevent the protraction of labor (Ekman-Ordeberg et al. 2024).

9 Conclusion

Heparin was discovered over 100 years ago and its effectiveness as an anticoagulant and antithrombotic has been proven. Heparin and LMWHs are heterogeneous biologicals, with complex structures that vary among tissues and organs and across different species. The structural requirement and mechanism of action as an anticoagulant are now well understood. The next milestone for this complex biologic will most likely be the elucidation of the mode of action and the impact on pathways such as complement and inflammation.

References

Ageno W, Samperiz A, Caballero R, Dentali F, Di Micco P, Prandoni P, Becattini C, Uresandi F, Verhamme P, Monreal M, Riete investigators (2015) Duration of anticoagulation after venous thromboembolism in real world clinical practice. Thromb Res 135:666–672

Agnelli G, Prandoni P, Di Minno G, Cimminiello C, Scaglione F, Boracchi P, Molteni M, Polo Friz H, Di Minno MN, Marano G (2015) Thromboprophylaxis with low-molecular-weight heparins: an assessment of the methodological quality of studies. Semin Thromb Hemost 41: 113–132

Alban S (2012) Adverse effects of heparin. Handb Exp Pharmacol 207:211–263. https://doi.org/10.1007/978-3-642-23056-1_10. PMID: 22566227

Al-Hakim A (2021) General considerations for diversifying heparin drug products by improving the current heparin manufacturing process and reintroducing bovine sourced heparin to the US market. Clin Appl Thromb Hemost 27:10760296211052293

Alikhan R, Bedenis R, Cohen AT (2014) Heparin for the prevention of venous thromboembolism in acutely ill medical patients (excluding stroke and myocardial infarction). Cochrane Database Syst Rev 5:CD003747

Anderson DR, Morgano GP, Bennett C, Dentali F, Francis CW, Garcia DA, Kahn SR, Rahman M, Rajasekhar A, Rogers FB, Smythe MA, Tikkinen KAO, Yates AJ, Baldeh T, Balduzzi S, Brozek JL, Ikobaltzeta IE, Johal H, Neumann I, Wiercioch W, Yepes-Nunez JJ, Schunemann HJ, Dahm P (2019) American Society of Hematology 2019 guidelines for management of venous thromboembolism: prevention of venous thromboembolism in surgical hospitalized patients. Blood Adv 3:3898–3944

Andersson LO, Barrowcliffe TW, Holmer E, Johnson EA, Sims GE (1976) Anticoagulant properties of heparin fractionated by affinity chromatography on matrix-bound antithrombin iii and by gel filtration. Thromb Res 9:575–583

Babin JL, Traylor KL, Witt DM (2017) Laboratory monitoring of low-molecular-weight heparin and fondaparinux. Semin Thromb Hemost 43:261–269

Bakchoul T, Jouni R, Warkentin TE (2016) Protamine (heparin)-induced thrombocytopenia: a review of the serological and clinical features associated with anti-protamine/heparin antibodies. J Thromb Haemost 14:1685–1695

Baker P, Platton S, Arachchillage DJ, Kitchen S, Patel J, Riat R, Gomez K, Committee BSH (2024) Measurement of heparin, direct oral anti-coagulants and other non-coumarin anti-coagulants and their effects on haemostasis assays: A British Society for Haematology guideline. Br J Haematol 205:1302–1318

Baluwala I, Favaloro EJ, Pasalic L (2017) Therapeutic monitoring of unfractionated heparin - trials and tribulations. Expert Rev Hematol 10:595–605

Barnes C, Deidun D, Hynes K, Monagle P (2000) Alopecia and dalteparin: a previously unreported association. Blood 96:1618–1619

Barritt DW, Jordan SC (1960) Anticoagulant drugs in the treatment of pulmonary embolism. A controlled trial. Lancet 1:1309–1312

Barrowcliffe TW (2012) History of heparin. Handb Exp Pharmacol 207:3–22. https://doi.org/10.1007/978-3-642-23056-1_1. PMID: 22566218

Bates SM, Greer IA, Middeldorp S, Veenstra DL, Prabulos AM, Vandvik PO (2012) VTE, thrombophilia, antithrombotic therapy, and pregnancy: antithrombotic therapy and prevention of thrombosis, 9th ed: American College of Chest Physicians Evidence-Based Clinical Practice Guidelines. Chest 141:e691S–e736S

Ben-Aharon I, Stemmer SM, Leibovici L, Shpilberg O, Sulkes A, Gafter-Gvili A (2014) Low molecular weight heparin (LMWH) for primary thrombo-prophylaxis in patients with solid malignancies - systematic review and meta-analysis. Acta Oncol 53:1230–1237

Berresheim M, Wilkie J, Nerenberg KA, Ibrahim Q, Bungard TJ (2014) A case series of LMWH use in pregnancy: should trough anti-Xa levels guide dosing? Thromb Res 134:1234–1240

Bertini S, Fareed J, Madaschi L, Risi G, Torri G, Naggi A (2017a) Characterization of PF4-heparin complexes by photon correlation spectroscopy and zeta potential. Clin Appl Thromb Hemost 23:725. https://doi.org/10.1177/1076029616685430

Bertini S, Risi G, Guerrini M, Carrick K, Szajek AY, Mulloy B (2017b) Molecular weights of bovine and porcine heparin samples: comparison of chromatographic methods and results of a collaborative survey. Molecules 22:1214

Beurskens DMH, Huckriede JP, Schrijver R, Hemker HC, Reutelingsperger CP, Nicolaes GAF (2020) The anticoagulant and nonanticoagulant properties of heparin. Thromb Haemost 120: 1371–1383

Bianchini EP, Sebestyen A, Abache T, Bourti Y, Fontayne A, Richard V, Tamion F, Plantier JL, Doguet F, Borgel D (2018) Inactivated antithombin as anticoagulant reversal in a rat model of cardiopulmonary bypass: a potent and potentially safer alternative to protamine. Br J Haematol 180:715–720

Bratt G, Tornebohm E, Granqvist S, Aberg W, Lockner D (1985) A comparison between low molecular weight heparin (KABI 2165) and standard heparin in the intravenous treatment of deep venous thrombosis. Thromb Haemost 54:813–817

Brenner B, Grandone E, Makatsariya A, Khizroeva J, Bitsadze V, Tretyakova M (2021) Approach to the evaluation and treatment of venous thromboembolism in pregnancy. Semin Reprod Med 39:186–193

Brunelli SM, Cohen DE, Marlowe G, Liu D, Njord L, Van Wyck D, Aronoff G (2019) Safety and efficacy of heparin during dialysis in the context of systemic anticoagulant and antiplatelet medications. J Nephrol 32:453–460

Budaj A, Eikelboom JW, Mehta SR, Afzal R, Chrolavicius S, Bassand JP, Fox KA, Wallentin L, Peters RJ, Granger CB, Joyner CD, Yusuf S, Oasis Investigators (2009) Improving clinical outcomes by reducing bleeding in patients with non-ST-elevation acute coronary syndromes. Eur Heart J 30:655–661

Bull BS, Korpman RA, Huse WM, Briggs BD (1975) Heparin therapy during extracorporeal circulation. I. Problems inherent in existing heparin protocols. J Thorac Cardiovasc Surg 69: 674–684

Caen JP (1984) Heparin: a 70 year history from 1914 to 1984. Nouv Rev Fr Hematol (1978) 26: 209–210

Cameron JS (2000) Practical haemodialysis began with cellophane and heparin: the crucial role of William Thalhimer (1884-1961). Nephrol Dial Transplant 15:1086–1091

Carrier M, Cameron C, Delluc A, Castellucci L, Khorana AA, Lee AY (2014) Efficacy and safety of anticoagulant therapy for the treatment of acute cancer-associated thrombosis: a systematic review and meta-analysis. Thromb Res 134:1214–1219

Cassinelli G, Naggi A (2016) Old and new applications of non-anticoagulant heparin. Int J Cardiol 212(Suppl 1):S14–S21

Casu B, Lindahl U (2001) Structure and biological interactions of heparin and heparan sulfate. Adv Carbohydr Chem Biochem 57:159–206. https://doi.org/10.1016/s0065-2318(01)57017-1. PMID: 11836942

Casu B, Naggi A, Oreste P, Torri G, Pangrazzj J, Maggi A, Abbadini M, Donati MB (1987) Bleeding associated with heparin contaminants. Lancet 1:1088

Casu B, Vlodavsky I, Sanderson RD (2008) Non-anticoagulant heparins and inhibition of cancer. Pathophysiol Haemost Thromb 36:195–203

Chan NC, Siegal D, Lauw MN, Ginsberg JS, Eikelboom JW, Guyatt GH, Hirsh J (2014) A systematic review of contemporary trials of anticoagulants in orthopaedic thromboprophylaxis: suggestions for a radical reappraisal. J Thromb Thrombolysis 40:231

Chapelle C, Rosencher N, Jacques Zufferey P, Mismetti P, Cucherat M, Laporte S, Group Meta-Embol (2014) Prevention of venous thromboembolic events with low-molecular-weight heparin in the non-major orthopaedic setting: meta-analysis of randomized controlled trials. Arthroscopy 30:987–996

Choay J, Lormeau JC, Petitou M, Sinay P, Casu B, Oreste P, Torri G, Gatti G (1980) Anti-Xa active heparin oligosaccharides. Thromb Res 18:573–578

Chong BH, Castaldi PA (1986) Platelet proaggregating effect of heparin: possible mechanism for non-immune heparin-associated thrombocytopenia. Aust NZ J Med 16:715–716

Chunilal SD, Young E, Johnston MA, Robertson C, Naguit I, Stevens P, Galashan D, Oskamp ML, Brennan B, Ginsberg JS (2002) The APTT response of pregnant plasma to unfractionated heparin. Thromb Haemost 87:92–97

Cines DB, Tomaski A, Tannenbaum S (1987) Immune endothelial-cell injury in heparin-associated thrombocytopenia. N Engl J Med 316:581–589

Claudel SE, Miles LA, Murea M (2021) Anticoagulation in hemodialysis: A narrative review. Semin Dial 34:103–115

Cohen AT (2012) Long-term benefits of preventing venous thromboembolic events. Curr Med Res Opin 28:877–889

Cohen AT, Nandini B, Wills JO, Ota S (2010) VTE prophylaxis for the medical patient: where do we stand? - a focus on cancer patients. Thromb Res 125(Suppl 2):S21–S29

Cohen AT, Dobromirski M, Gurwith MM (2014) Managing pulmonary embolism from presentation to extended treatment. Thromb Res 133:139–148

Connell NT, Sylvester KW (2022) To aPTT or not to aPTT: evaluating the optimal monitoring strategy for unfractionated heparin. Thromb Res 218:199–200

Cook D, Douketis J, Meade M, Guyatt G, Zytaruk N, Granton J, Skrobik Y, Albert M, Fowler R, Hebert P, Pagliarello G, Friedrich J, Freitag A, Karachi T, Rabbat C, Heels-Ansdell D, Geerts W, Crowther M, Group Canadian Critical Care Trials (2008) Venous thromboembolism and bleeding in critically ill patients with severe renal insufficiency receiving dalteparin thromboprophylaxis: prevalence, incidence and risk factors. Crit Care 12:R32

Copley AL, Whitney DV III (1943) The standardization and assay of heparin by the toluidine blue and azure a reactions. J Lab Clin Med 28:762–770

Coyne E, Messmore HL, Walenga JM, Fareed J, Wehrmacher WH (1998) Ethylenediaminetetraacetic acid (EDTA) in heparin. Thromb Res 90:245–246

Cronin RE, Reilly RF (2010) Unfractionated heparin for hemodialysis: still the best option. Semin Dial 23:510–515

Crowther MA, Cook DJ (2008) Preventing venous thromboembolism in critically ill patients. Semin Thromb Hemost 34:469–474

de Boer K, ten Cate JW, Sturk A, Borm JJ, Treffers PE (1989) Enhanced thrombin generation in normal and hypertensive pregnancy. Am J Obstet Gynecol 160:95–100

Di Nisio M, Porreca E, Otten HM, Rutjes AW (2014) Primary prophylaxis for venous thromboembolism in ambulatory cancer patients receiving chemotherapy. Cochrane Database Syst Rev 8: CD008500

Dias JD, Lopez-Espina CG, Panigada M, Dalton HJ, Hartmann J, Achneck HE (2019) Cartridge-based thromboelastography can be used to monitor and quantify the activity of unfractionated and low-molecular-weight heparins. TH Open 3:e295–e305

Drozd NN, Logvinova YS, Shagdarova BT, Il'ina AV, Varlamov VP (2019) Analysis of the action of quaternized chitosans with different molecular weight on anticoagulant activity of heparins in vitro. Bull Exp Biol Med 167:279–283

Eikelboom JW, Quinlan DJ, O'Donnell M (2009) Major bleeding, mortality, and efficacy of fondaparinux in venous thromboembolism prevention trials. Circulation 120:2006–2011

Ekman-Ordeberg G, Hellgren-Wangdahl M, Jeppson A, Rahkonen L, Blomberg M, Pettersson K, Bejlum C, Engberg M, Ludvigsen M, Uotila J, Tihtonen K, Hallberg G, Jonsson M (2024) Tafoxiparin, a novel drug candidate for cervical ripening and labor augmentation: results from 2 randomized, placebo-controlled studies. Am J Obstet Gynecol 230:S759–SS68

Elyamany G, Alzahrani AM, Bukhary E (2014) Cancer-associated thrombosis: an overview. Clin Med Insights Oncol 8:129–137

Ettema HB, Kollen BJ, Verheyen CC, Buller HR (2008) Prevention of venous thromboembolism in patients with immobilization of the lower extremities: a meta-analysis of randomized controlled trials. J Thromb Haemost 6:1093–1098

Falanga A, Zacharski L (2005) Deep vein thrombosis in cancer: the scale of the problem and approaches to management. Ann Oncol 16:696–701

Falck-Ytter Y, Francis CW, Johanson NA, Curley C, Dahl OE, Schulman S, Ortel TL, Pauker SG, Colwell CW Jr, Physicians American College of Chest (2012) Prevention of VTE in orthopedic surgery patients: antithrombotic therapy and prevention of thrombosis, 9th ed: American College of Chest Physicians Evidence-Based Clinical Practice Guidelines. *Chest* 141:e278S–325S

Ferraris VA (2002) Heroes and evidence. J Thorac Cardiovasc Surg 124:11–13

Forestier F, Daffos F, Rainaut M, Toulemonde F (1987) Low molecular weight heparin (CY 216) does not cross the placenta during the third trimester of pregnancy. Thromb Haemost 57:234

Franchini M, Mannucci PM (2015) Low-molecular-weight heparins and cancer: focus on antitumoral effect. Ann Med 47:116–121

Francis CW (2013) Prevention of VTE in patients having major orthopedic surgery. J Thromb Thrombolysis 35:359–367

Gallagher JT (2012) Heparan sulphate. a heparin in miniature. In: Handbook of experimental pharmacology, pp 347–360

Garcia DA, Baglin TP, Weitz JI, Samama MM, Physicians American College of Chest (2012) Parenteral anticoagulants: antithrombotic therapy and prevention of thrombosis, 9th ed: American College of Chest Physicians Evidence-Based Clinical Practice Guidelines. *Chest* 141:e24S–43S

Gottschalk CW, Fellner SK (1997) History of the science of dialysis. Am J Nephrol 17:289–298

Gozdzikiewicz J, Borawski J, Mysliwiec M (2009) Pleiotropic effects of heparin and heparinoids in peritoneal dialysis. Clin Appl Thromb Hemost 15:92–97

Gray E, Hogwood J, Rigsby P, Mulloy B, Szajek A, Ambrose M, Jameison F, Hauck W, Morris T (2009) An international collaborative study to value assign the 6th [sixth] international standard for unfractionated heparin and the US pharmacopeial heparin reference standard for assay Lot F. World Health Organisation

Gray E, Hogwood J, Mulloy B (2012) The anticoagulant and antithrombotic mechanisms of heparin. Handb Exp Pharmacol 207:43–61. https://doi.org/10.1007/978-3-642-23056-1_3. PMID: 22566220

Greer IA, Nelson-Piercy C (2005) Low-molecular-weight heparins for thromboprophylaxis and treatment of venous thromboembolism in pregnancy: a systematic review of safety and efficacy. Blood 106:401–407

Guimicheva B, Czuprynska J, Arya R (2015) The prevention of pregnancy-related venous thromboembolism. Br J Haematol 168:163–174

Hanedan MO, Yuruk MA, Arslan AK, Kilic A, Sayar U, Mataraci I (2020) Heparin-coated- vs. non-coated cardiopulmonary bypass circuits: comparing immediate results with different target activated clotting time. Braz J Cardiovasc Surg 35:913–917

He H, Ye J, Liu E, Liang Q, Liu Q, Yang VC (2014) Low molecular weight protamine (LMWP): a nontoxic protamine substitute and an effective cell-penetrating peptide. J Control Release 193: 63–73

Hemker HC (2016) A century of heparin: past, present and future. J Thromb Haemost 14:2329–2338

Hessel EA 2nd (2014) A brief history of cardiopulmonary bypass. Semin Cardiothorac Vasc Anesth 18:87–100

Hirsh J, Warkentin TE, Shaughnessy SG, Anand SS, Halperin JL, Raschke R, Granger C, Ohman EM, Dalen JE (2001) Heparin and low-molecular-weight heparin: mechanisms of action, pharmacokinetics, dosing, monitoring, efficacy, and safety. Chest 119:64S–94S

Hogwood J, Mulloy B, Gray E (2017) Precipitation and neutralization of heparin from different sources by protamine sulfate. Pharmaceuticals (Basel) 10:59

Hogwood J, Mulloy B, Lever R, Gray E, Page CP (2023) Pharmacology of heparin and related drugs: an update. Pharmacol Rev 75:328–379

Hoke M, Kyrle PA, Philipp K, Pabinger I, Kaider A, Schonauer V, Quehenberger P, Eichinger S (2004) Prospective evaluation of coagulation activation in pregnant women receiving low-molecular weight heparin. Thromb Haemost 91:935–940

Holm HA, Ly B, Handeland GF, Abildgaard U, Arnesen KE, Gottschalk P, Hoeg V, Aandahl M, Haugen K, Laerum F et al (1986) Subcutaneous heparin treatment of deep venous thrombosis: a comparison of unfractionated and low molecular weight heparin. Haemostasis 16(Suppl 2): 30–37

Hovanessian HC (1999) New-generation anticoagulants: the low molecular weight heparins. Ann Emerg Med 34:768–779

Howell WH, Holt E (1918) Two new factors in blood coagulation – heparin and pro-antithrombin. Am J Phys 47:328–341

Hoylaerts M, Owen WG, Collen D (1984) Involvement of heparin chain length in the heparin-catalyzed inhibition of thrombin by antithrombin III. J Biol Chem 259:5670–5677

Hull RD, Raskob GE, Pineo GF, Green D, Trowbridge AA, Elliott CG, Lerner RG, Hall J, Sparling T, Brettell HR et al (1992) Subcutaneous low-molecular-weight heparin compared with continuous intravenous heparin in the treatment of proximal-vein thrombosis. N Engl J Med 326:975–982

Jeske W, Kouta A, Farooqui A, Siddiqui F, Rangnekar V, Niverthi M, Laddu R, Hoppensteadt D, Iqbal O, Walenga J, Fareed J (2018) Bovine mucosal heparins are comparable to porcine mucosal heparin at USP potency adjusted levels. Front Med (Lausanne) 5:360

Johnson EA, Mulloy B (1976) The molecular-weight range of mucosal-heparin preparations. Carbohydr Res 51:119–127

Johnson EA, Kirkwood TB, Stirling Y, Perez-Requejo JL, Ingram GI, Bangham DR, Brozovic M (1976) Four heparin preparations: anti-Xa potentiating effect of heparin after subcutaneous injection. Thromb Haemost 35:586–591

Jorpes JE (1964) The early history of heparin. Ann N Y Acad Sci 115:392–398

Kalaska B, Miklosz J, Kamiński K, Swieton J, Jakimczuk A, Yusa SI, Pawlak D, Nowakowska M, Szczubiałka K, Mogielnicki A (2020) Heparin-binding copolymer as a complete antidote for low-molecular-weight heparins in rats. J Pharmacol Exp Ther 373:51–61

Kalathottukaren MT, Haynes CA, Kizhakkedathu JN (2018) Approaches to prevent bleeding associated with anticoagulants: current status and recent developments. Drug Deliv Transl Res 8:928–944

Kamphuisen PW, Beyer-Westendorf J (2014) Bleeding complications during anticoagulant treatment in patients with cancer. Thromb Res 133(Suppl 2):S49–S55

Kearon C, Akl EA (2014) Duration of anticoagulant therapy for deep vein thrombosis and pulmonary embolism. Blood 123:1794–1801

Kearon C, Akl EA, Comerota AJ, Prandoni P, Bounameaux H, Goldhaber SZ, Nelson ME, Wells PS, Gould MK, Dentali F, Crowther M, Kahn SR, Physicians American College of Chest (2012) Antithrombotic therapy for VTE disease: antithrombotic therapy and prevention of thrombosis, 9th ed: American College of Chest Physicians Evidence-Based Clinical Practice Guidelines. *Chest* 141:e419S–94S

Keire DA, Mulloy B, Chase C, Al-Hakim A, Cairatti D, Gray E, Hogwood J, Morris T, Mourao P, Soares M, Szajek A (2015) Diversifying the global heparin supply chain reintroduction of bovine heparin in the United States. Pharm Technol 39:2–8

Kelton JG, Sheridan D, Santos A, Smith J, Steeves K, Smith C, Brown C, Murphy WG (1988) Heparin-induced thrombocytopenia: laboratory studies. Blood 72:925–930

Khandelwal S, Ravi J, Rauova L, Johnson A, Lee GM, Gilner JB, Gunti S, Notkins AL, Kuchibhatla M, Frank M, Poncz M, Cines DB, Arepally GM (2018) Polyreactive IgM initiates complement activation by PF4/heparin complexes through the classical pathway. Blood 132: 2431–2440

Kher A, Bauersachs R, Nielsen JD (2007) The management of thrombosis in pregnancy: role of low-molecular-weight heparin. Thromb Haemost 97:505–513

Khorana AA (2010) Venous thromboembolism and prognosis in cancer. Thromb Res 125:490–493

Khorana AA (2012) Risk assessment for cancer-associated thrombosis: what is the best approach? Thromb Res 129(Suppl 1):S10–S15

Khorana AA, McCrae KR (2014) Risk stratification strategies for cancer-associated thrombosis: an update. Thromb Res 133(Suppl 2):S35–S38

Kinnaird TD, Stabile E, Mintz GS, Lee CW, Canos DA, Gevorkian N, Pinnow EE, Kent KM, Pichard AD, Satler LF, Weissman NJ, Lindsay J, Fuchs S (2003) Incidence, predictors, and prognostic implications of bleeding and blood transfusion following percutaneous coronary interventions. Am J Cardiol 92:930–935

Kishimoto TK, Viswanathan K, Ganguly T, Elankumaran S, Smith S, Pelzer K, Lansing JC, Sriranganathan N, Zhao G, Galcheva-Gargova Z, Al-Hakim A, Bailey GS, Fraser B, Roy S, Rogers-Cotrone T, Buhse L, Whary M, Fox J, Nasr M, Dal Pan GJ, Shriver Z, Langer RS, Venkataraman G, Austen KF, Woodcock J, Sasisekharan R (2008) Contaminated heparin associated with adverse clinical events and activation of the contact system. N Engl J Med 358:2457–2467

Konstantinides SV (2014) 2014 ESC guidelines on the diagnosis and management of acute pulmonary embolism. Eur Heart J 35:3145–3146

Kouta A, Jeske W, Cera L, Farshid A, Duff R, Hoppensteadt D, Fareed J (2021) Protamine sulfate neutralization profile of various dosages of bovine, ovine and porcine UFHs and their depolymerized derivatives in non-human primates. Clin Appl Thromb Hemost 27: 10760296211005544

Kyrle PA (2014) Predicting recurrent venous thromboembolism in cancer: is it possible? Thromb Res 133(Suppl 2):S17–S22

Lam LH, Silbert JE, Rosenberg RD (1976) The separation of active and inactive forms of heparin. Biochem Biophys Res Commun 69:570–577

Le Templier G, Rodger MA (2008) Heparin-induced osteoporosis and pregnancy. Curr Opin Pulm Med 14:403–407

Leclerc JR, Gent M, Hirsh J, Geerts WH, Ginsberg JS (1998) The incidence of symptomatic venous thromboembolism during and after prophylaxis with enoxaparin: a multi-institutional cohort study of patients who underwent hip or knee arthroplasty. Canadian Collaborative Group. Arch Intern Med 158:873–878

Lee AY (2010) The roles of anticoagulants in patients with cancer. Thromb Res 125(Suppl 2):S8–S11

Lee AY, Levine MN, Baker RI, Bowden C, Kakkar AK, Prins M, Rickles FR, Julian JA, Haley S, Kovacs MJ, Gent M, Investigators Randomized Comparison of Low-Molecular-Weight Heparin versus Oral Anticoagulant Therapy for the Prevention of Recurrent Venous Thromboembolism in Patients with Cancer (2003) Low-molecular-weight heparin versus a coumarin for the prevention of recurrent venous thromboembolism in patients with cancer. N Engl J Med 349: 146–153

Leung KC, MacRae JM (2019) Anticoagulation in CKD and ESRD. J Nephrol 32:719–731

Lim W, Le Gal G, Bates SM, Righini M, Haramati LB, Lang E, Kline JA, Chasteen S, Snyder M, Patel P, Bhatt M, Patel P, Braun C, Begum H, Wiercioch W, Schunemann HJ, Mustafa RA (2018) American Society of Hematology 2018 guidelines for management of venous thromboembolism: diagnosis of venous thromboembolism. Blood Adv 2:3226–3256

Lindahl U, Hook M (1978) Glycosaminoglycans and their binding to biological macromolecules. Annu Rev Biochem 47:385–417

Lindahl U, Backstrom G, Hook M, Thunberg L, Fransson LA, Linker A (1979) Structure of the antithrombin-binding site in heparin. Proc Natl Acad Sci USA 76:3198–3202

Liu H, Zhang Z, Linhardt RJ (2009) Lessons learned from the contamination of heparin. Nat Prod Rep 26:313–321

Liu F, Chu X, Huang J, Tian K, Hua J, Tong P (2014) Administration of enoxaparin 24 h after total knee arthroplasty: safer for bleeding and equally effective for deep venous thrombosis prevention. Arch Orthop Trauma Surg 134:679–683

Lussana F, Coppens M, Cattaneo M, Middeldorp S (2012) Pregnancy-related venous thromboembolism: risk and the effect of thromboprophylaxis. Thromb Res 129:673–680

Lyman GH, Carrier M, Ay C, Di Nisio M, Hicks LK, Khorana AA, Leavitt AD, Lee AYY, Macbeth F, Morgan RL, Noble S, Sexton EA, Stenehjem D, Wiercioch W, Kahale LA, Alonso-Coello P (2021) American Society of Hematology 2021 guidelines for management of venous thromboembolism: prevention and treatment in patients with cancer. Blood Adv 5: 927–974

Macie C, Forbes L, Foster GA, Douketis JD (2004) Dosing practices and risk factors for bleeding in patients receiving enoxaparin for the treatment of an acute coronary syndrome. Chest 125:1616–1621

Maneno JN, Ness GL (2021) Andexanet alfa, the possible alternative to protamine for reversal of unfractionated heparin. Ann Pharmacother 55:261–264

Manoukian SV, Voeltz MD, Eikelboom J (2007) Bleeding complications in acute coronary syndromes and percutaneous coronary intervention: predictors, prognostic significance, and paradigms for reducing risk. Clin Cardiol 30:II24-34

Marlar RA, Clement B, Gausman J (2017) Activated partial thromboplastin time monitoring of unfractionated heparin therapy: issues and recommendations. Semin Thromb Hemost 43:253–260

Marshall AL (2014) Diagnosis, treatment, and prevention of venous thromboembolism in pregnancy. Postgrad Med 126:25–34

Martel N, Lee J, Wells PS (2005) Risk for heparin-induced thrombocytopenia with unfractionated and low-molecular-weight heparin thromboprophylaxis: a meta-analysis. Blood 106:2710–2715

Mathieu L, Beurton A, Rougier N, Flambard M, Germain C, Pernot M, Ouattara A (2024) Heparin consumption and inflammatory response according to the coating of cardiopulmonary bypass circuits in cardiac surgery: A retrospective analysis. Perfusion 39:1531–1537

McLean J (1916) The thromboplastic action of cephalin. Am J Phys 41:250–257

McLeod AG, Geerts W (2011) Venous thromboembolism prophylaxis in critically ill patients. Crit Care Clin 27:765–80, v

McRae HL, Militello L, Refaai MA (2021) Updates in anticoagulation therapy monitoring. Biomedicine 9:262

Meneghetti MC, Hughes AJ, Rudd TR, Nader HB, Powell AK, Yates EA, Lima MA (2015) Heparan sulfate and heparin interactions with proteins. J R Soc Interface 12:0589

Mismetti P, Laporte S, Darmon JY, Buchmuller A, Decousus H (2001) Meta-analysis of low molecular weight heparin in the prevention of venous thromboembolism in general surgery. Br J Surg 88:913–930

Mulloy B (2012) Structure and physicochemical characterisation of heparin. Handb Exp Pharmacol 207:77–98. https://doi.org/10.1007/978-3-642-23056-1_5. PMID: 22566222

Mulloy B (2019) The non-anticoagulant promise of heparin and its mimetics. Curr Opin Pharmacol 46:50–54

Mulloy B, Linhardt RJ (2001) Order out of complexity--protein structures that interact with heparin. Curr Opin Struct Biol 11:623–628

Mulloy B, Gray E, Barrowcliffe TW (2000) Characterization of unfractionated heparin: comparison of materials from the last 50 years. Thromb Haemost 84:1052–1056

Mulloy B, Hogwood J, Gray E, Lever R, Page CP (2016) Pharmacology of heparin and related drugs. Pharmacol Rev 68:76–141

Muralidharan-Chari V, Kim J, Mousa SA (2017) Reversal of anticoagulant activity of heparin and low molecular weight heparins by poly-l-lysine: a comparative 'in vitro' study versus protamine sulfate. Thromb Res 155:128–130

Nader HB, Lopes CC, Rocha HA, Santos EA, Dietrich CP (2004) Heparins and heparinoids: occurrence, structure and mechanism of antithrombotic and hemorrhagic activities. Curr Pharm Des 10:951–966

Noble S (2012) Low-molecular-weight heparin and survival in lung cancer. Thromb Res 129(Suppl 1):S114–S118

Ong CS, Marcum JA, Zehr KJ, Cameron DE (2019) A century of heparin. Ann Thorac Surg 108: 955–958

Ortel TL, Neumann I, Ageno W, Beyth R, Clark NP, Cuker A, Hutten BA, Jaff MR, Manja V, Schulman S, Thurston C, Vedantham S, Verhamme P, Witt DM, Florez I D, Izcovich A, Nieuwlaat R, Ross S, Schunemann H J, Wiercioch W, Zhang Y, Zhang Y (2020) American Society of Hematology 2020 guidelines for management of venous thromboembolism: treatment of deep vein thrombosis and pulmonary embolism. Blood Adv 4:4693–4738

Pai M, Crowther MA (2012) Neutralization of heparin activity. Handb Exp Pharmacol 207:265–277. https://doi.org/10.1007/978-3-642-23056-1_11. PMID: 22566228

Palmer AJ, Schramm W, Kirchhof B, Bergemann R (1997) Low molecular weight heparin and unfractionated heparin for prevention of thrombo-embolism in general surgery: a meta-analysis of randomised clinical trials. Haemostasis 27:65–74

Paschoa AF (2016) Heparin: 100 years of pleiotropic effects. J Thromb Thrombolysis 41:636–643

Petitou M, van Boeckel CA (2004) A synthetic antithrombin III binding pentasaccharide is now a drug! What comes next? Angew Chem Int Ed Engl 43:3118–3133

Petitou M, Casu B, Lindahl U (2003) 1976-1983, a critical period in the history of heparin: the discovery of the antithrombin binding site. Biochimie 85:83–89

PharmEur_07/2023:0828. Heparins, Low Molecular Mass, European Pharmacopoeia

PharmEur_07/2024:0333. Heparin sodium, European Pharmacopoeia, 07/2024:0333

Pouplard C, Iochmann S, Renard B, Herault O, Colombat P, Amiral J, Gruel Y (2001) Induction of monocyte tissue factor expression by antibodies to heparin-platelet factor 4 complexes developed in heparin-induced thrombocytopenia. Blood 97:3300–3302

Prandoni P, Lensing AW, Buller HR, Carta M, Cogo A, Vigo M, Casara D, Ruol A, ten Cate JW (1992) Comparison of subcutaneous low-molecular-weight heparin with intravenous standard heparin in proximal deep-vein thrombosis. Lancet 339:441–445

Prandoni P, Lensing AW, Prins MH, Pesavento R, Piccioli A, Sartori MT, Tormene D, Milan M, Vedovetto V, Noventa F, Villalta S, Harenberg J (2015) The impact of residual thrombosis on the long-term outcome of patients with deep venous thrombosis treated with conventional anticoagulation. Semin Thromb Hemost 41:133–140

Qiu M, Huang S, Luo C, Wu Z, Liang B, Huang H, Ci Z, Zhang D, Han L, Lin J (2021) Pharmacological and clinical application of heparin progress: an essential drug for modern medicine. Biomed Pharmacother 139:111561

Quinlan DJ, McQuillan A, Eikelboom JW (2004) Low-molecular-weight heparin compared with intravenous unfractionated heparin for treatment of pulmonary embolism: a meta-analysis of randomized, controlled trials. Ann Intern Med 140:175–183

Rauova L, Poncz M, McKenzie SE, Reilly MP, Arepally G, Weisel JW, Nagaswami C, Cines DB, Sachais BS (2005) Ultralarge complexes of PF4 and heparin are central to the pathogenesis of heparin-induced thrombocytopenia. Blood 105:131–138

Reitsma PH, Versteeg HH, Middeldorp S (2012) Mechanistic view of risk factors for venous thromboembolism. Arterioscler Thromb Vasc Biol 32:563–568

Riess H, Haas S, Tebbe U, Gerlach HE, Abletshauser C, Sieder C, Rossol S, Pfeiffer B, Schellong SM (2010) A randomized, double-blind study of certoparin vs. unfractionated heparin to prevent venous thromboembolic events in acutely ill, non-surgical patients: CERTIFY study. J Thromb Haemost 8:1209–1215

Robertson L, Yeoh SE, Stansby G, Agarwal R (2015) Effect of testing for cancer on cancer- and venous thromboembolism (VTE)-related mortality and morbidity in patients with unprovoked VTE. Cochrane Database Syst Rev 3:CD010837

Ruiz-Gimenez N, Suarez C, Gonzalez R, Nieto JA, Todoli JA, Samperiz AL, Monreal M, Riete Investigators (2008) Predictive variables for major bleeding events in patients presenting with documented acute venous thromboembolism. Findings from the RIETE Registry. Thromb Haemost 100:26–31

Sarris E, Tsele E, Bagiatoudi G, Salpigidis K, Stavrianaki D, Kaklamanis L, Siakotos M (2003) Diffuse alopecia in a hemodialysis patient caused by a low-molecular-weight heparin, tinzaparin. Am J Kidney Dis 41:E15

Schindewolf M, Schwaner S, Wolter M, Kroll H, Recke A, Kaufmann R, Boehncke WH, Lindhoff-Last E, Ludwig RJ (2009) Incidence and causes of heparin-induced skin lesions. CMAJ 181: 477–481

Schroeder M, Hogwood J, Gray E, Mulloy B, Hackett AM, Johansen KB (2011) Protamine neutralisation of low molecular weight heparins and their oligosaccharide components. Anal Bioanal Chem 399:763–771

Schulman S, Beyth RJ, Kearon C, Levine MN (2008) Hemorrhagic complications of anticoagulant and thrombolytic treatment: American College of Chest Physicians Evidence-Based Clinical Practice Guidelines (8th edition). Chest 133:257S–298S

Shriver Z, Sasisekharan R (2013) Heparin sensing: blue-chip binding. Nat Chem 5:644–646

Sievert AN, Shackelford AG, McCall MM (2009) Trends and emerging technologies in extracorporeal life support: results of the 2006 ECLS survey. J Extra Corpor Technol 41:73–78

Sokolowska E, Kalaska B, Miklosz J, Mogielnicki A (2016) The toxicology of heparin reversal with protamine: past, present and future. Expert Opin Drug Metab Toxicol 12:897–909

Sommers CD, Ye H, Liu J, Linhardt RJ, Keire DA (2017) Heparin and homogeneous model heparin oligosaccharides form distinct complexes with protamine: light scattering and zeta potential analysis. J Pharm Biomed Anal 140:113–121

St Ange K, Onishi A, Fu L, Sun X, Lin L, Mori D, Zhang F, Dordick JS, Fareed J, Hoppensteadt D, Jeske W, Linhardt RJ (2016) Analysis of heparins derived from bovine tissues and comparison to porcine intestinal heparins. Clin Appl Thromb Hemost 22:520–527

Stark K, Massberg S (2021) Interplay between inflammation and thrombosis in cardiovascular pathology. Nat Rev Cardiol 18:666–682

Stirling Y, Woolf L, North WR, Seghatchian MJ, Meade TW (1984) Haemostasis in normal pregnancy. Thromb Haemost 52:176–182

Stoney WS (2009) Evolution of cardiopulmonary bypass. Circulation 119:2844–2853

Sultana R, Kamihira M (2024) Multifaceted heparin: diverse applications beyond anticoagulant therapy. Pharmaceuticals (Basel) 17:1362

Suranyi M, Chow JS (2010) Review: anticoagulation for haemodialysis. Nephrology (Carlton) 15: 386–392

Szajek AY, Chess E, Johansen K, Gratzl G, Gray E, Keire D, Linhardt RJ, Liu J, Morris T, Mulloy B, Nasr M, Shriver Z, Torralba P, Viskov C, Williams R, Woodcock J, Workman W, Al-Hakim A (2016) The US regulatory and pharmacopeia response to the global heparin contamination crisis. Nat Biotechnol 34:625–630

Testroote M, Stigter W, de Visser DC, Janzing H (2008) Low molecular weight heparin for prevention of venous thromboembolism in patients with lower-leg immobilization. Cochrane Database Syst Rev:CD006681

Thalappil V, Anand J, Keepanasseril A, Kar R (2024) Standardization of anti-Xa assay and its comparison with activated partial thromboplastin time for monitoring unfractionated heparin therapy. Indian J Hematol Blood Transfus 40:432–436

Thery C, Simonneau G, Meyer G, Helenon O, Bridey F, Armagnac C, d'Azemar P, Coquart JP (1992) Randomized trial of subcutaneous low-molecular-weight heparin CY 216 (Fraxiparine) compared with intravenous unfractionated heparin in the curative treatment of submassive pulmonary embolism. A dose-ranging study. Circulation 85:1380–1389

Tovar AM, Santos GR, Capille NV, Piquet AA, Glauser BF, Pereira MS, Vilanova E, Mourao PA (2016) Structural and haemostatic features of pharmaceutical heparins from different animal sources: challenges to define thresholds separating distinct drugs. Sci Rep 6:35619

Trujillo-Santos J, Nieto JA, Tiberio G, Piccioli A, Di Micco P, Prandoni P, Monreal M, Riete Registry (2008) Predicting recurrences or major bleeding in cancer patients with venous thromboembolism. Findings from the RIETE Registry. Thromb Haemost 100:435–439

USP_Heparin_Sodium. Heparin Sodium, United States Pharmacopeia, USP41-NF36

Valimaki S, Khakalo A, Ora A, Johansson LS, Rojas OJ, Kostiainen MA (2016) Effect of PEG-PDMAEMA block copolymer architecture on polyelectrolyte complex formation with heparin. Biomacromolecules 17:2891–2900

van Rein J.S., Biedermann F.J.M., van der Meer S.C., Cannegieter N., Wiersma H.W., Vermaas P. H., Reitsma M.J.H.A., Kruip W.M., Lijfering (2017) Major bleeding risks of different low-molecular-weight heparin agents: a cohort study in 12 934 patients treated for acute venous thrombosis Journal of Thrombosis and Haemostasis 15(7):1386–1391. https://doi.org/10.1111/jth.13715

Vilanova E, Vairo BC, Smcg Oliveira BF, Glauser NV, Capille GRC, Santos AMF, Tovar MS, Pereira, Mourao PAS (2019) Heparins sourced from bovine and porcine mucosa gain exclusive monographs in the Brazilian pharmacopeia. Front Med (Lausanne) 6:16

Wang YY, Po HL (2006) Enoxaparin-induced alopecia in patients with cerebral venous thrombosis. J Clin Pharm Ther 31:513–517

Wang P, Chi L, Zhang Z, Zhao H, Zhang F, Linhardt RJ (2022) Heparin: an old drug for new clinical applications. Carbohydr Polym 295:119818

Wardrop D, Keeling D (2008) The story of the discovery of heparin and warfarin. Br J Haematol 141:757–763

Warttinger U, Giese C, Harenberg J, Holmer E, Kramer R (2016) A fluorescent probe assay (Heparin Red) for direct detection of heparins in human plasma. Anal Bioanal Chem 408: 8241–8251

White RH, Zhou H, Romano PS (2003) Incidence of symptomatic venous thromboembolism after different elective or urgent surgical procedures. Thromb Haemost 90:446–455

Witt DM, Nieuwlaat R, Clark NP, Ansell J, Holbrook A, Skov J, Shehab N, Mock J, Myers T, Dentali F, Crowther MA, Agarwal A, Bhatt M, Khatib R, Riva JJ, Zhang Y, Guyatt G (2018) American Society of Hematology 2018 guidelines for management of venous thromboembolism: optimal management of anticoagulation therapy. Blood Adv 2:3257–3291

Xiao Z, Visentin GP, Dayananda KM, Neelamegham S (2008) Immune complexes formed following the binding of anti-platelet factor 4 (CXCL4) antibodies to CXCL4 stimulate human neutrophil activation and cell adhesion. Blood 112:1091–1100

Yin EB, Bracey AW, Chatterjee S (2025) Thromboelastography versus thromboelastometry for unfractionated heparin monitoring in adult patients on extracorporeal membrane oxygenation. Perfusion 40:235–242

Zhang S, Zhai Z, Yang Y, Zhu J, Gong J, Xie W, Kuang T, Wang C (2015) Long-term treatment with low-molecular-weight heparin prolonged the survival time for acute pulmonary embolism patients concurrent with malignancy: an observational analysis from a long-term follow-up study. Thromb Res 135:582–587

Zmuda K, Neofotistos D, Ts'ao CH (2000) Effects of unfractionated heparin, low-molecular-weight heparin, and heparinoid on thromboelastographic assay of blood coagulation. Am J Clin Pathol 113:725–731

Comparison of the Biologic Activity of Different Species of Heparin

Walter Jeske

Contents

Abstract

Heparin and related low molecular weight heparin derivatives remain critical drugs for the prevention and treatment of thrombotic conditions. Concerns relating to the stability and sufficiency of the porcine intestinal mucosa supplies from which most heparin is currently derived have spurred an interest in identifying other sources for heparin. Commercial quantities of heparin may be obtained from cow and sheep intestine, and heparin or heparin-like material has been identified in a number of other species. Being biologic in nature, these heparins exhibit unique structural and functional profiles. This chapter summarizes our current understanding of these heparins.

Submitted to: Antithrombotics and Anti-Fibrinolytics, Gray and Hogwood, eds.

W. Jeske (✉)
Loyola University Chicago, Cardiovascular Research Institute, Maywood, IL, USA
e-mail: wjeske@luc.edu

E. Gray, J. Hogwood (eds.), *Antithrombotic and Antiplatelet Agents*, Handbook of Experimental Pharmacology 291, https://doi.org/10.1007/164_2025_781

Keywords

Anticoagulant · Antithrombotic · Biologic · Bleeding · Heparin

1 Introduction

Heparin is a complex poly-component, animal-derived drug that is comprised of linear polysaccharides varying in both length and saccharide sequence (Esko and Selleck 2002; Baytas and Linhardt 2020). A member of the glycosaminoglycan family, heparin, is composed of repeating disaccharide units comprised of hexosamine and uronic acid residues (Baytas and Linhardt 2020) which are modified with N-acetyl, N-sulfo, and O-sulfo groups at various positions affording a large number of sequence permutations (Esko and Selleck 2002).

Heparin's clinical utility is derived from its ability to prevent blood clotting. Heparin inhibits coagulation through a variety of mechanisms including (primarily) the promotion of antithrombin (AT)-mediated inhibition of coagulation proteases including factor Xa and thrombin (Middeldorp 2008), thrombin inhibition via binding to heparin cofactor II, and increasing the circulating level of TFPI. Despite the development of a variety of more targeted, orally available anticoagulants, heparin remains an important therapeutic agent for rapid treatment of thrombotic conditions (due to its ability to be administered intravenously) and for interventional procedures such as dialysis and cardiopulmonary bypass (where the ability to rapidly neutralize anticoagulant activity is desirable) (Lee et al. 2023). Heparin also serves as the starting material for the production of LMWH.

The physicochemical properties of heparin play important roles in mediating the various biologic functions of the drug. For example, it is known that a particular pentasaccharide sequence containing a central 3-O sulfated glucosamine group is required for high-affinity binding to AT (Atha et al. 1987). Beyond contributing to AT binding, the presence of a high negative charge due to 2-O, 6-O, N-sulfation influences the ability of heparin to bind HC-II (Hurst et al. 1983), release TFPI (Valentin et al. 1994), and interact with the platelet alpha-granule protein platelet factor 4 (Chudasama et al. 2010). The distribution of oligosaccharide chain lengths influences anticoagulant activity as chains shorter than 18 saccharides are unable to inhibit thrombin (Hirsh et al. 2001) and heparin chains with molecular weights greater than about 10 kDa have minimal absorption following SC administration (Emanuele and Fareed 1987).

The most used source material for pharmaceutical heparin is porcine intestinal mucosa. Recent history has demonstrated the risks of having a single-sourced material. In 2007–8, heparin contaminated with oversulfated chondroitin sulfate (OSCS) resulted in the death of many individuals. Diseases in the herds used to source porcine mucosa can also lead to heparin shortages (Al-Hakim 2021). With heparin demand currently about 100 tons per year (Douaisi et al. 2024), it has been suggested that there may be insufficient porcine raw material to meet heparin demand (Vilanova et al. 2019). For these reasons, there is interest in diversifying the sourcing of heparin (Al-Hakim 2021).

Heparin and heparin-like glycosaminoglycans have been identified in a number of species and in a number of tissues. Pharmaceutical quantities of heparin have been obtained from bovine intestinal mucosa and lung (Al-Hakim 2021), and it has been suggested that similar quantities could be derived from ovine intestinal mucosa. Heparins, or heparin-like GAGs, have also been isolated from other mammalian species (turkey, camel) as well as a variety of marine sources (clam, mollusk, shrimp, whale, and fish skin).

Isolation of heparin requires that the native tissue first be digested to release heparin from its endogenous binding sites with subsequent isolation of the raw heparin from the digestate and purification (Baytas and Linhardt 2020). Given the variety of source tissues and the harsh reaction conditions required for its isolation (Baytas and Linhardt 2020), it is not surprising that heparins derived from different sources have different chemical characteristics which can translate into differing biologic activities.

2 Structural Comparison

The molecular weight profile of heparin preparations is often characterized using size exclusion chromatography. Porcine heparin has an average molecular weight ranging from 15,000 to 19,000 Da (The United States Pharmacopeial Convention, "Heparin Sodium"). Heparin is polydisperse having a dispersity of ~1.3, with chains ranging in size from 10 to 75 disaccharide residues (Linhardt 2003). Using this technique, heparins isolated from porcine and ovine intestinal mucosa have been shown to have comparable mean molecular weights and dispersities, while heparin from bovine mucosa tends to exhibit a higher mean molecular weight (Jeske et al. 2019). Bovine lung-derived heparin which had been used clinically in the past exhibits a lower mean molecular weight than heparin from porcine mucosa, but has a comparable degree of sulfation (St Ange et al. 2016).

The degree of sulfation for glycosaminoglycan (GAG) chains has been assessed using nuclear magnetic resonance (NMR) spectroscopy and by disaccharide analysis. Heparins from porcine and bovine sources are made up of a similar array of disaccharide building blocks, although in different proportions (Oliveira et al 2025; Santos et al. 2014; Xie et al. 2018). By both methods, porcine heparin has been shown to consist of primarily tri-sulfated disaccharide with higher levels of O, N sulfation. Ovine mucosal heparin tends to have slightly higher levels of overall sulfation than porcine heparin, related to increased levels of N- and 6-O sulfation (Fu et al. 2013). The overall degree of sulfation is lower in bovine mucosal heparins compared to either porcine or ovine heparins (Song et al. 2023) with the major structural difference between bovine and porcine heparins being an increased proportion of N-sulfated glucosamine lacking 6-O sulfation in bovine heparin (Vilanova et al. 2019).

The loss of sulfation in bovine mucosal heparin relative to heparins from ovine and porcine tissues is also seen in the level of 3-O sulfation and thus, the presence of the minimal antithrombin (AT)-binding pentasaccharide (Hirsh et al. 2001). The affinities of these three heparins for antithrombin have been assessed using surface plasmon resonance (SPR). By competitive SPR, porcine heparin was shown to bind better to AT than bovine heparin (Fu et al. 2013). By LC-MS/MS, bovine mucosal heparin has lower mass percentage of oligosaccharides capable of binding to AT compared to ovine- and porcine mucosal heparins (Wang et al. 2022). Fluorescence titration studies demonstrate differential binding to AT (Santos et al. 2014). These studies have indicated a lower affinity of bovine mucosal heparin for AT. Primary component analysis using data derived from NMR spectra and disaccharide analysis performed following digestion of heparins by heparin lyases shows well-resolved separation of commercial intestinal mucosal heparins derived from pig, sheep, and cow (Ouyang et al. 2019). Recent work has shown that bovine mucosal heparin can be fractionated into low- and high-affinity fractions whereby the high-affinity fraction is structurally similar to porcine mucosal heparin (Oliveira et al. 2024).

3 Biologic Activity

3.1 In Vitro

Heparin anticoagulant potency is typically defined in terms of antithrombin-mediated anticoagulant activities; that is, its inhibition of factor Xa and thrombin and prolongation of the aPTT. Relative to the USP potency standard, porcine mucosal heparin has anti-Xa and anti-thrombin potencies of 180–200 U/mg. Ovine heparin exhibits comparable potency (Kouta et al. 2019). The potency of bovine mucosal heparin, owing to its lower level of sulfation and reduced number of AT-binding sites is weaker, with potencies reported to range from 100 to 140 U/mg (Kouta et al. 2019). An important consideration in assessing heparin potency is the assay that is utilized to determine potency as it has been shown that bovine mucosal heparin exhibits increased activity by aPTT when sheep plasma, rather than human plasma, is used (Vilanova et al. 2019). A study comparing porcine mucosal, bovine mucosal, and bovine lung heparins demonstrated that both bovine heparins had lower activity than porcine heparin when measured by aPTT, anti-Xa, and anti-IIa assays (Tovar et al. 2016). In a heparin cofactor II-mediated anti-IIa assay, porcine and bovine mucosal heparins show comparable potency (Tovar et al. 2019).

An ideal replacement for, or complement to, porcine mucosal heparin would exhibit the same activity so that the same dosing, monitoring, and neutralization protocols could be used (Oliveira et al. 2024). The lower potency of bovine mucosal heparin makes this interchangeability difficult. A number of means of addressing this issue have been assessed including potency-based dosing, fractionation of bovine heparin, and chemical modification of bovine heparin.

Heparin can be fractionated based on molecular weight or charge density. Molecular size fractionation did not make a bovine mucosal heparin equivalent to porcine mucosal heparin as even the highest molecular weight fraction of bovine heparin had lower activity, measured by aPTT, anti-Xa, or anti-IIa assays, than porcine heparin (Tovar et al. 2019). Fractionating bovine heparin using high-resolution anion-exchange chromatography, however, resulted in high and low anticoagulant fractions (Santos et al. 2014). The high antithrombin binding heparin (HABH) fraction was shown to have disaccharide composition, anionic strength, and molecular size similar to those of PMH. The HABH fraction also exhibited potencies equal to or greater than that of PMH in AT-dependent assays.

Treatment of bovine mucosal heparin with either 3-O-sulfotransferase or a combination of 3-O and 6-O-sulfotransferases results in the generation of AT binding sites as evidenced by competitive SPR assay (Fu et al. 2017). Increased tri-sulfated disaccharide content following 3-O and 6-O sulfation results in increased anti-Xa and anti-IIa activities, but also increased binding to PF4. Increased 3-O sulfation only led to increased anticoagulant activity without increasing binding to PF4, though the resulting heparin is structurally different from porcine mucosal heparin. In another study, bovine and porcine heparins were subjected to gel permeation chromatography to produce fractions with molecular weights of approximately 15 kDa; fractions of bovine lung and porcine mucosal heparins had similar activities, while the activity of fractions of bovine mucosal heparin remained lower (Tovar et al. 2016). A study comparing porcine and ovine mucosal heparins with a bovine lung heparin demonstrated that ovine heparin had comparable anti-IIa and anti-Xa potencies as porcine heparin and that both exhibited more activity than bovine lung heparin (Oliveira et al. 2022).

Tissue factor pathway inhibitor (TFPI) is the primary endogenous regulator of the extrinsic pathway of coagulation. While TFPI is normally expressed on the endothelial surface, numerous studies have demonstrated that administration of heparin or similar polyanionic drugs leads to an increase in the plasma levels of TFPI. The effect of various heparins on circulating TFPI levels has been largely tested using animal models. Overall degree of sulfation is important (Kouta et al. 2020).

The ability to neutralize the anticoagulant activity of heparin is an important feature of the drug. This is commonly achieved by the administration of polycationic protamine sulfate (or chloride) whereby heparin and protamine form a charge-based complex that is no longer able to interact with antithrombin. The concern with protamine neutralization is that protamine is not specific for AT-binding heparin chains and that given the need to administer higher amounts of bovine mucosal heparin by weight to achieve the same activity, higher doses of protamine may be necessary to completely neutralize the bovine heparin. Higher doses of protamine are needed with bovine heparin when measured as residual anti-Xa or thrombin activity (Aquino et al. 2010; Santos et al. 2014). From a clinical standpoint, this may be concerning if a protocol for porcine heparin neutralization is used for a patient treated with bovine heparin, as a lower dose of protamine may result in a delay in achieving full neutralization or may not completely neutralize the anticoagulant effect, leading to unexpected bleeding (Vilanova et al. 2019).

3.2 Animal Models

The pharmacokinetic behavior of heparin is typically measured in terms of its pharmacodynamic actions (anti-Xa and anti-IIa activities) (Brancazio et al. 1995; Delavenne et al. 2017). Fluorescent dye and LC-MS methods now exist to measure chemical levels of heparin in plasma samples (Song et al. 2023; Warttinger et al. 2016). Despite subtle differences in the disaccharide composition of porcine, bovine, and ovine mucosal heparins, comparable circulating levels were observed in non-human primates treated with equi-gravimetric amounts of these heparins, when chemical levels were measured (Song et al. 2023). The levels of heparin measured by LC-MS or by fluorescent dye method correlated well with the levels measured by functional activity, through the slope of the regression lines for porcine, bovine and ovine heparins were different reflecting the differences in their potency.

In rat models where thrombus formation was induced by a combination of hypercoagulability and stasis of flow (venous) or induced by endothelial lesion (arterial), bovine heparins required twice the dose on a weight basis to exhibit the same antithrombotic effect (Santos et al. 2014). Relative blood loss was comparable, however on gravimetric basis (Santos et al. 2014). Using a tail transection model, at doses required to achieve complete inhibition of thrombus formation (100 IU/kg), blood loss was the same for bovine and porcine heparins. At higher doses, bleeding induced by bovine heparin was significantly greater than seen with porcine heparin administration despite ex vivo anticoagulant activity measured by aPTT being higher in porcine heparin-treated animals (Aquino et al. 2010). HABH fraction which exhibited comparable in vitro potency to porcine heparin was also shown to be a comparable in terms of antithrombotic activity in a ferric chloride model of thrombosis in mice (Tovar et al. 2019), blood loss in mouse tail model, and reversibility upon protamine administration (Tovar et al. 2019). PMH has higher antithrombotic potency than bovine heparins on a weight basis, but similar antithrombotic and bleeding on a IU basis (Tovar et al. 2016; Jeske et al. 2019).

3.3 Human Studies

Few human studies have directly compared the effects of heparins derived from different species. In one study, seventeen patients underwent hemodialysis using unfractionated heparin as the anticoagulant (Tovar et al. 2013). These patients underwent multiple dialysis sessions on both porcine and bovine mucosal heparins, with each heparin administered as bolus injection of equal anticoagulant units. Dosing was rather low, ranging from 6,000 to 12,000 IU prior to the dialysis session. Although the same dosing in terms of anticoagulant units was administered, the Cmax (measured as aPTT activity) following treatment with bovine heparin was lower (1.63 ± 0.44 IU/ml) than following porcine heparin administration (2.15 ± 0.56 IU/ml) despite there being more "chemical" heparin (measured as hexuronic acid content) following bovine heparin treatment. Despite the differences in circulating heparin concentrations, bleeding time measured at the end of dialysis sessions was not significantly different between heparin treatments.

In a small, randomized trial involving 32 patients undergoing bypass surgery, patients were randomized to receive bovine or porcine mucosal heparin (Gomes et al. 2016). Equivalent doses of the two heparins were administered in terms of unitage, leading to equivalent prolongation of the activated clotting time (ACT) and the amount of post-surgical blood loss. Protamine effectively reversed the prolongation of ACT by both heparins, but as predicted by in vitro data, a higher protamine dose was required in the bovine heparin-treated group to reverse anticoagulation. A subsequent retrospective study of Brazilian patients who underwent on-pump coronary surgery while being anticoagulated with bovine mucosal heparin ($n = 204$) or porcine mucosal heparin ($n = 65$) demonstrated comparable levels of anticoagulation and blood loss (De Lima Torres et al. 2020).

3.4 HIT

The interaction of heparins with platelet factor 4 is of interest as this is a key piece leading to the development of heparin-induced thrombocytopenia. Heparin-induced thrombocytopenia is a potentially catastrophic adverse effect associated with heparin therapy which results from the development of antibodies against a complex of heparin and platelet factor 4. In some patients, these antibodies can activate platelets leading to a prothrombotic environment despite the presence of heparin.

The interaction between heparin and platelet factor 4 has been assessed using physicochemical methods such as photon correlation spectroscopy (PCS) and zeta potential as well as functionally using platelet activation assays as an indirect measure of complex formation. By PCS/zeta potential, the impact of molecular weight and degree of sulfation on complex formation was observed, with larger complexes measured with ovine heparin and smaller complexes seen with bovine heparin, relative to porcine heparin (Bertini et al. 2017). While literature has shown that larger heparin-PF4 complexes are better at mediating anti-heparin/PF4 antibody-dependent platelet activation (Rauova et al. 2005), data to show whether these larger complexes lead to a stronger immunogenic response are lacking. Functional assays show little difference in the ability of heparins derived from porcine, bovine, and ovine tissues to cause platelet activation in vitro, in the presence of anti-heparin/PF4 antibodies (Walenga et al. 2016). Bovine and porcine heparin, and the HABH were shown to interact with PF4 similarly by ELISA using anti-PF4 antibody KKO as a probe for complex formation (Tovar et al. 2019).

While all heparins are able to be incorporated into immune complexes with anti-PF4/heparin antibodies in vitro, it is less clear whether differences exist in the ability of heparins from different sources to induce the formation of HIT antibodies and/or cause clinical heparin-induced thrombocytopenia. In a study of patients scheduled to receive intravenous porcine mucosal or bovine lung heparin for at least 5 days for the prophylaxis of thromboembolism, a similar rate of thrombocytopenia was observed (Ansell et al. 1985). In a study evaluating HIT antibody generation in patients randomized to receive porcine or bovine heparin during coronary artery bypass grafting surgery, a higher percentage of patients treated with bovine lung heparin were antibody positive on post-operative days 5 and 6, although the platelet counts in these patients did not differ (Francis et al. 2003). A second study in CABG patients randomized to either porcine mucosal or bovine lung heparin did not show significant differences in the incidences of HIT measured in terms of either ELISA or serotonin-release assay positivity (Konkle et al. 2001). Comparative studies utilizing bovine mucosal heparin have not been reported. Overall, the available studies are likely too small to adequately control for a wide range of potential confounding factors such as differing definitions of thrombocytopenia, the duration and dose of heparin, and the patient population being tested (Ansell et al. 1985).

4 Conversion to LMWHs

An important use of heparin is as a source material for the production of low molecular weight heparins (LMWHs). Commercially available LMWHs are produced from porcine heparin (Liu et al. 2017). A number of research studies have applied the same depolymerization technologies to the cleavage of bovine and ovine heparins and assessed the resultant LMWHs. It has been shown that with some modification to the reaction conditions, nitrous acid cleavage of ovine mucosal heparin or bovine lung heparin can result in LMWHs that meet EP monograph specifications (molecular weight, potency) for dalteparin (Xie et al. 2018). Structural differences seen in bovine lung heparin (higher sulfation) are carried over to the depolymerized products. In contrast, a study has shown that LMWHs produced from bovine and ovine intestinal mucosal heparin by beta-elimination are biosimilar to their porcine counterpart (St Ange et al. 2016). LMWHs generated by beta-elimination from bovine lung or mucosal heparins starting material show comparable mean molecular weight, anti-Xa, and anti-IIa activities to Lovenox (Liu et al. 2017). Despite notable differences in disaccharide composition, LMWHs produced from ovine mucosal heparin by a beta-elimination reaction exhibited comparable mean molecular weights and bioactivity in terms of anti-Xa and anti-IIa activity (Chen et al. 2019). Ovine LMWH produced by beta-elimination showed comparable pharmacokinetic-pharmacodynamic behavior as Lovenox when measured using anti-Xa and anti-IIa assays following SC administration to primates (Jeske et al. 2018).

5 Other "Minor" Sources of Heparin

Heparins and heparin-like materials have been isolated and characterized from a variety of other mammalian and marine species (Hovingh et al. 1986). These heparins vary widely in size, degree of sulfation, and anticoagulant activity (Table 1). These sources seem unlikely to be exploited to produce pharmaceutically relevant quantities of heparin.

Table 1 Minor sources of heparin

Marine sources		
Mollusk *A. brasiliana*	Higher AT-binding fraction compared to BMH (45% vs. 25%) Anticoagulant potency ~twofold that of BLH/BMH	Paiva et al. (1995), Pejler et al. (1987), Dietrich et al. (1985)
Mollusk *M. mercenaria*	High AT-affinity fraction has M.W. ~18 kDa ~2.5 sulfate/disaccharide Potency: >300 USP U/mg	Jordan and Marcum (1986)
Mollusk *T. phylippinarum*	Increased trisulfated disaccharide content and AT-binding region M.W. ~15 kDa Potency (aPTT and anti-Xa): >300 U/mg	Cesaretti et al. (2004)
Mollusk *T. mactroides*	Increased 3-O sulfation relative to PMH and BLH Increased anti-IIa activity relative to anti-Xa activity	Pejler et al. (1987)
Mollusk *C. Chione*	85% fast-moving heparin, decreased trisulfated disaccharide M.W. ~11 kDa Potency: 95 IU/mg (aPTT), 52 IU/mg (anti-Xa)	Luppi et al. (2005)
Mollusk *A. pleuronectus*	M.W.: 6.5–7.5 kDa Potency: 95 IU/mg (aPTT)	Saravanan and Shanmugam (2010)
Mollusk *M. meretrix*	M.W.: ~15 kDa Potency: 72 IU/mg (aPTT)	Saravanan et al. (2010)
Mollusk *A. anodata*	Degree of sulfation comparable to BMH Potency: 120 IU/mg (anti-Xa); 137 IU/mg (aPTT)	Volpi and Maccari (2005)
Shrimp *P. brasiliensis*	M.W.: 8.5 kDa Potency: 95 IU/mg USP potency	Dietrich et al. (1999)
Mammals		
Camel intestine	Degree of sulfation ~2/3^{rds} that of PMH Potency: 50–60 anti-Xa U/mg (raw heparin)	Warda et al. (2003a)
Turkey intestine	Low activity: ~17 IU/mg (anti-Xa)	Warda et al. (2003b)

6 Synthetic Heparin "Species"

In an attempt to avoid or minimize the variability observed with biologic drugs, the production of synthetic heparins has been evaluated by a number of groups. Such heparins have been produced purely synthetically (Yu et al. 2012), semi-synthetically by modification of bacterial GAGs (Douaisi et al. 2024), or via cell culture (Thacker et al. 2022). Following attempts to produce heparin with reasonable levels of anticoagulant activity using common bioproduction cell lines such as CHO and HEK293, it has been demonstrated that overexpression of genes for

3-O-sulfotransferase, 6-O-sulfotransferase, and N-deacetylase/N-sulfotransferase in a human mastocytoma cell line can yield a highly sulfated GAG closely resembling heparin in terms of the degree of sulfation and in biologic activity (Thacker et al. 2022). The ability to alter the expression of genes involved in heparin production also suggests that possibility of fine-tuning the structure to enhance desired activities and reduce those that may contribute to unwanted side-effects (such as reducing PF4 binding), potentially leading to a lowered incidence of HIT and lowered degree of variability when such heparins are used in conditions where platelet activation (and hence high circulating PF4 levels) is expected.

The idea of using bacterial-derived heparosan as a starting material for heparin production goes back to the early 1990s (Casu et al. 1994). A bioengineered heparin using *E coli* K5 heparosan as the starting material has recently been described (Douaisi et al. 2024). The heparosan is N-deacetylated, depolymerized, and N-sulfated followed by epimerization and 2-O, 3-O, and 6-O sulfation reactions. The resulting bioengineered heparin met USP heparin standards. Additionally, when this bioengineered heparin was depolymerized using chemical ß-elimination, the resultant product met USP enoxaparin specifications in terms of mean molecular weight, molecular weight distribution, 1,6-anhydro content, and anti-Xa/anti-IIa potency.

The chemical synthesis of heparin oligosaccharides has been limited to relatively small molecules and at relatively low yields (Yu et al. 2024). The basic synthetic scheme involves building the oligosaccharide backbone and then exposing that backbone to a variety of enzymes to incorporate sulfate groups and convert glucuronic acid to iduronic acid. Dodecasaccharides produced in this manner that express high levels of anti-Xa activity have been described (Xu et al. 2017). Unlike smaller saccharide chains, the anti-Xa activity of the dodecasaccharides can be neutralized by protamine. On a gravimetric basis, the dodecasaccharides were able to reduce thrombus formation in animal models more effectively than enoxaparin.

7 Conclusions

Most studies to date have characterized the similarities and differences among various species of heparin in terms of physicochemical composition (molecular weight, degree of sulfation, sulfation pattern) and AT-mediated anticoagulant potency. As ~80% of chains do not bind AT (Bal dit Sollier et al. 2020), it may be interesting to evaluate the similarities/differences among various species of heparin in terms of their non-AT-mediated anticoagulation pathways such as activation of HC-II and release of TFPI. Additionally, it is known that heparin chains have a number of other biologic actions beyond anticoagulation (Mulloy et al. 2015) including binding to growth factors, interfering with the interaction between P-selectin and PSGL-1, interfering with the formation and functioning of NETs, contributing to passivation of matrix surfaces, and exhibiting anti-inflammatory or anti-metastatic effects. Studies comparing the effects of different heparins on these various pleiotropic actions have not been reported. Based on the totality of available data, it appears that simple substitution of one species of heparin for another isn't easily achieved. It has been suggested that a strategy similar to that used for characterizing generic enoxaparins may be useful for defining comparability of unfractionated heparin preparations (Bezerra et al. 2023).

References

Al-Hakim A (2021) General considerations for diversifying heparin drug products by improving the current heparin manufacturing process and reintroducing bovine sourced heparin to the US market. Clin Appl Thromb Hemost 27:1–14

Ansell JE, Price JM, Shah S, Beckner RR (1985) Heparin-induced thrombocytopenia. What is the real frequency? Chest 88(6):878–882

Aquino RS, Pereira MS, Vairo BC, Cinelli LP, Santos GRC, Fonseca RJC, Mourao PAS (2010) Heparins from porcine and bovine intestinal mucosa: are they similar drugs? Thromb Haemost 103:1005–1015

Atha DH, Lormeau JC, Petitou M, Rosenberg RD, Choay J (1987) Contribution of 3-O- and 6 O-sulfated glucosamine residues in the heparin-induced conformational change in antithrombin III. Biochemistry 26:6454–6461

Bal dit Sollier C, Dillinger JG, Drouet L (2020) Anticoagulant activity and pleiotropic effects of heparin. JMV-J Med Vasc 45:147–157

Baytas SN, Linhardt RJ (2020) Advances in the preparation and synthesis of heparin and related products. Drug Discov Today 25(12):2095–2109

Bertini S, Fareed J, Madaschi RG, Torri G, Naggi A (2017) Characterization of PF4-Heparin complexes by photon correlation spectroscopy and zeta potential. Clin Appl Thromb Hemost 23(7):725–734

Bezerra FF, Oliviera SNMCG, Sales RA, Piquet AA, Capille NV, Vilanova A, Tovar AMF, Mourao PAS (2023) Approaches to assure similarity between pharmaceutical heparins from two different manufacturers. Pharmaceutics 15:1115

Brancazio LR, Roperti KA, Stierer R, Laifer SA (1995) Pharmacokinetics and pharmacodynamics of subcutaneous heparin during the early third trimester of pregnancy. Am J Obstet Gynecol 173(4):1240–1245

Casu B, Grazioli G, Razi N, Guerrini M, Naggi A, Totti G, Oreste P, Tursi F, Zoppetti G, Lindahl U (1994) Heparin-like compounds prepared by chemical modification of capsular polysaccharide from E coli K5. Carbohydr Res 263(2):271–284

Cesaretti M, Luppi E, Maccari F, Volpi N (2004) Isolation and characterization of a heparin with high anticoagulant activity from the clam *Tapes phylippinarum*: evidence for the presence of a high content of antithrombin III binding site. Glycobiology 14(12):1275–1284

Chen J, Yu Y, Fareed J, Hoppensteadt D, Jeske W, Kouta A, Jin C, Jin Y, You Y, Xia K, Zhang F, Chen S, Ye X, Linhardt RJ (2019) Comparison of low-molecular-weight heparins prepared from ovine heparins with enoxaparin. Clin Appl Thromb Hemost 25:1–9

Chudasama SL, Espinasse B, Hwang F, Qi R, Joglekar M, Afonina G, Wiesner MR, Welsby IJ, Ortel TL, Arepally GM (2010) Heparin modifies the immunogenicity of positively charged proteins. Blood 116(26):6046–6053

De Lima Torres FA, Torres ACB, Ribeiro A, Maia CO, Almeida FP, Roceto J, Matkovski JA, Kovalski MG, Pizato VA, Cordeiro TMG (2020) A retrospective study on unfractionated bovine heparin safety in in-pump cardiac surgery. Int J Cardiovasc Sci 33(3):235–242

Delavenne X, Ollier E, Chollet S, Sandri S, Lanoiselée J, Hodin S, Montmartin A, Fuzellier JF, Mismetti P, Gergelé L (2017) Pharmacokinetic/pharmacodynamic model for unfractionated heparin dosing during cardiopulmonary bypass. Br J Aenesth 118(5):705–712

Dietrich CP, de Paiva JF, Moraes CT, Takahashi HK, Porcionatto MA, Nader HB (1985) Isolation and characterization of a heparin with high anticoagulant activity from *Anomalocardia brasiliana*. Biochem et Biophys Acta 843:1–7

Dietrich CP, Paiva JF, Castro RAB, Chavante SF, Jeske W, Fareed J, Gorin PAJ, Mendes A, Nader HB (1999) Structural features and anticoagulant activities of a novel natural low molecular weight heparin from the shrimp *Penaeus brasiliensis*. Biochem Biophys Acta 1428:273–283

Douaisi D, Paskaleva EE, Fu L, Grover N, McManaman CL, Varghese S, Brodfuehrer PR, Gibson JM, de Joode I, Xia K, Brier MI, Simmons TJ, Datta P, Zhang F, Onishi A, Hirakane M, Mori D, Linhardt RJ, Dordick JS (2024) Synthesis of bioengineered heparin chemically and biologically similar to porcine-derived products and convertible to low MW heparin. PNAS 121(14): e2315586121

Emanuele RM, Fareed J (1987) The effect of molecular weight on the bioavailability of heparin. Thromb Res 48:591–596

Esko JD, Selleck SB (2002) Order out of chaos: assembly of ligand binding sites in heparan sulfate. Annu Rev Biochem 71:435–471

Francis JL, Palmer GJ, Moroose R, Drexler A (2003) Comparison of bovine and porcine heparin in heparin antibody formation after cardiac surgery. Ann Thorac Surg 75(1):17–22

Fu L, Li G, Yang B, Onishi A, Li L, Sun P, Zhang F, Linhardt RJ (2013) Structural characterization of pharmaceutical heparins prepared from different animal tissues. J Pharm Sci 102(5): 1447–1457

Fu L, Mori D, Hirakane M, Lin L, Grover N, Datta P, Yu Y, Zhao J, Zhang F, Yalcin M, Mousa SA, Dordick JS, Linhardt RJ (2017) Enzymatic generation of highly anticoagulant bovine intestinal heparin. J Med Chem 60:8673–8679

Gomes WJ, Leal JC, Braile DM, Guimaraes JA, Lopes RD, Lima MA, Nader HB (2016) A Brazilian perspective foe the use of bovine heparin in open heart surgery. Int J Cardiol 223: 611–612

Hirsh J, Anand SS, Halperin JL, Fuster V (2001) Mechanism of action and pharmacology of unfractionated heparin. Arterioscler Thromb Vasc Biol 21(7):1094–1096

Hovingh P, Piepkorn M, Linker A (1986) Biologic implications of the structural, antithrombin affinity and anticoagulant activity relationships among vertebrate heparins and heparan sulphates. Biochem J 237:573–581

Hurst RE, Poon MC, Griffith MJ (1983) Structure-activity relationships of heparin. Independence of heparin charge density and antithrombin-binding domains in thrombin inhibition by antithrombin and heparin cofactor II. J Clin Invest 72(3):1042–1045

Jeske W, Kouta A, Duff R, Rangnekar V, Niverthi M, Hoppensteadt D, Fareed J, Yao Y (2018) Comparative pharmacokinetic profile of 3 batches of ovine low-molecular-weight heparin and 1 batch of branded enoxaparin. Clin Appl Thromb Hemost 24(9S):150S–156S

Jeske W, Kouta A, Farooqui A, Siddiqui F, Rangnekar V, Niverthi M, Laddu R, Hoppensteadt D, Iqbal O, Walenga J, Fareed J (2019) Bovine mucosal heparins are comparable to porcine mucosal heparin at USP potency adjusted levels. Front Med 5:360. https://doi.org/10.3389/fmed.2018.00360

Jordan RE, Marcum JA (1986) Anticoagulantly active heparin from clam (*Mercenaria mercenaria*). Arch Biochem Biophys 248(2):690–695

Konkle BA, Bauer TL, Arepally G, Cines DB, Poncz M, McNulty S, Edie RN, Mannion JD (2001) Heparin-induced thrombocytopenia: bovine versus porcine heparin in cardiopulmonary bypass surgery. Ann Thorac Surg 71:1920–1924

Kouta A, Jeske W, Hoppensteadt D, Iqbal O, Yao Y, Fareed J (2019) Comparative pharmacological profiles of various bovine, ovine and porcine heparins. Clin Appl Thromb Hemost 25:1–9

Kouta A, Hoppensteadt D, Bontekoe E, Jeske W, Duff R, Cera L, Fareed J (2020) Studies on tissue factor pathway inhibitor antigen release by bovine, ovine and porcine heparins following intravenous administration to non-human primates. Clin Appl Thromb Hemost 26:1–8

Lee MH, Beck M, Shann K (2023) Protamine dose to neutralize heparin at the completion of cardiopulmonary bypass can be reduced significantly without affecting post-operative bleeding. J Extra Corpor Technol 55:105–111

Linhardt RJ (2003) Claude S. Hudson award address in carbohydrate chemistry. Heparin: structure and activity. J Med Chem 46(3):2551–2564

Liu X, St. Ange K, Fareed J, Hoppensteadt D, Jeske W, Kouta A, Chi L, Jin C, Jin Y, Yao Y, Linhardt RJ (2017) Comparison of low-molecular-weight heparins prepared from bovine heparins with enoxaparin. Clin Appl Thromb Hemost 23(6):542–553

Luppi E, Cesaretti M, Volpi N (2005) Purification and characterization of heparin from the Italian clam *Callista chione*. Biomacromolecules 6:1672–1678

Middeldorp S (2008) Heparin: from animal organ extract to designer drug. Thromb Res 122:753–762

Mulloy B, Hogwood J, Gray E, Lever R, Page CP (2015) Pharmacology of heparin and related drugs. Pharmacol Rev 68:76–141

Oliveira SNMCG, Tovar AMF, Bezerra FF, Piquet AA, Capille NV, Santos PS, Vilanova E, Mourao PAS (2022) Anticoagulant activity of heparins from different animal sources are driven by a synergistic combination of physical-chemical factors. TH Open 6:e309–e322

Oliveira SNMCG, Bezerra FF, Piquet AA, Sales RA, Valle GCT, Capille NV, Tovar AMF, Mourao PAS (2024) A unique enoxaparin derived from bovine intestinal heparin: a single purification step of the starting material assures a bovine enoxaparin like the standard from porcine origin. ACS Omega 9:23111–23120

Oliviera SNMCG, Bezerra FF, Pereira MS, Tovar AMF, Aquino RS, Mourao PAS (2025) Global use of bovine heparin: challenges and opportunities. Proteoglycan Res 3:e70025

Ouyang Y, Han X, Yu Y, Chen J, Fu L, Zhang F, Linhardt RJ, Fareed J, Hoppensteadt D, Jeske W, Kouta A, Zhang Z, Xia K (2019) Chemometric analysis of porcine, bovine and ovine heparins. J Pharam Biomed Anal 164:345–352

Paiva JF, Santos EA, Jeske W, Fareed J, Nader HB, Dietrich CP (1995) A comparative analysis on the mechanism of the anticoagulant action of mollusc and mammalian heparins. Comp Biochem Physiol 111A:495–499

Pejler G, Danielsson A, Bjork I, Lindahl U, Nader HB, Dietrich CP (1987) Structure and antithrombin-binding properties of heparin isolated from the clams *Anomalocardia brasiliana* and *Tivela mactroides*. J Biol Chem 262(24):11413–11421

Rauova L, Poncz M, McKenzie SE, Reilly MP, Arepally G, Weisel JW, Nagaswami C, Cines DB, Sachais BS (2005) Ultralarge complexes of PF4 and heparin are central to the pathogenesis of heparin-induced thrombocytopenia. Blood 105:131–138

Santos GRC, Tovar AMF, Capille NVM, Pereira MS, Pomin VH, Mourao PAS (2014) Structural and functional analyses of bovine and porcine intestinal heparins confirm they are different drugs. Drug Discov Today 19(11):1801–1807

Saravanan R, Shanmugam A (2010) Isolation and characterization of low molecular weight glycosaminoglycans from marine mollusc *Amussium pleuronectus* (Linne) using chromatography. Appl Biochem Biotechnol 160:791–799

Saravanan R, Vairamani S, Shanmugam A (2010) Glycosaminoglycans from marine clam *Meretrix meretrix* (Linne.) are an anticoagulant. Prep Biochem Biotechnol 40:305–315

Song Y, Kouta A, Cera LM, Xia K, Zhang F, Kraemer R, Fareed J, Linhardt RJ, Jeske W (2023) Absolute pharmacokinetics of heparin in primates. Carbohydr Polym 311:120779

St Ange K, Onishi A, Fu L, Sun X, Lin L, Mori D, Zhang F, Dordick JS, Fareed J, Hoppensteadt D, Jeske W, Linhardt RJ (2016) Analysis of heparins derived from bovine tissues and comparison to porcine intestinal heparins. Clin Appl Thromb Hemost 22(6):520–527

Thacker BE, Thorne KJ, Cartwright C, Park J, Glass K, Chea A, Kellman BP, Lewis NE, Wang Z, Di Nardo A, Sharfstein ST, Jeske W, Walenga J, Hogwood J, Gray E, Mulloy B, Esko JD, Glass CA (2022) Multiplex genome editing of mammalian cells for producing recombinant heparin. Metab Eng 70:155–165

Tovar AMF, Teixeira LAC, Rembold SM, Leite M, Lugon JR, Mourao PAS (2013) Bovine and porcine heparins: different drugs with similar effects on human haemodialysis. BMC Res Notes 6:230

Tovar AMF, Santos GRC, Capille NV, Piquet AA, Glauser BF, Pereira MS, Vilanova E, Mourao PAS (2016) Structural and haemostatic features of pharmaceutical heparins from different animal sources: challenges to define thresholds separating distinct drugs. Sci Rep 6:35619

Tovar AMF, Vairo BC, Oliveira SNMCG, Glauser BF, Santos GRC, Capille NV, Piquet AA, Santana PS, Micheli KVA, Pereira MS, Vilanova E, Mourao PAS (2019) Converting the distinct heparins sourced from bovine or porcine mucosa into a single anticoagulant drug. Thromb Haemost 119:618–632

Valentin S, Larnkjer A, Ostergaard P, Nielsen JI, Nordfang O (1994) Characterization of the binding between tissue factor pathway inhibitor and glycosaminoglycans. Thromb Res 75(2): 173–183

Vilanova E, Vairo BC, Oliveira SNMCG, Glauser BF, Capille NV, Santos GRC, Tovar AMF, Pereira MS, Mourao PAS (2019) Heparins sourced from bovine and porcine mucosa gain exclusive monographs in the Brazilian pharmacopeia. Front Med 6:16

Volpi N, Maccari F (2005) Glycosaminoglycans composition of the large freshwater mollusc bivalve *Anodonta anodonta*. Biomacromolecules 6:3174–3180

Walenga J, Jeske W, Bertini S, Risi G, Sung M, Farooqui A, Bacher C, Hoppensteadt D, Iqbal O, Lewis B, Bakhos M (2016) Bovine heparin demonstrates the same interaction with HIT antibodies as porcine heparin. Blood 134(Suppl 1):2351

Wang Z, Arnold K, Dhurandahare VM, Xu Y, Pagadala V, Labra E, Jeske W, Fareed J, Gearing M, Liu J (2022) Analysis of 3-O-sulfated heparan sulfate using isotopically labeled oligosaccharide calibrants. Anal Chem 94:2950–2957

Warda M, Gouda EM, Toida T, Chi L, Linhardt RJ (2003a) Isolation and characterization of raw heparin from dromedary intestine: evaluation of a new source of pharmaceutical heparin. Comp Biochem Physiol Part C 136:357–365

Warda M, Mao W, Toida T, Linhardt RJ (2003b) Turkey intestine as a commercial source of heparin? Comparative structural studies of intestinal avian and mammalian glycosaminoglycans. Comp Biochem Physiol Part B 134:189–197

Warttinger U, Giese C, Harenberg J, Holmer E, Krämer R (2016) A fluorescent probe assay (Heparin Red) for direct detection of heparins in human plasma. Anal Bioanal Chem 408(28): 8241–8251

Xie S, Guan Y, Zhu P, Yu M, Linhardt RJ, Chi L, Jin L (2018) Preparation of low molecular weight heparins from bovine and ovine heparins using nitrous acid degradation. Carbohydr Polym 197: 83–91

Xu Y, Chandarajoti K, Zhang X, Pagadala V, Dou W, Hoppensteadt DM, Sparkenbaugh EM, Cooley B, Daily S, Key NS, Severynse-Stevens D, Fareed J, Linhardt RJ, Pawlinski R, Liu J (2017) Synthetic oligosaccharides can replace animal-sourced low-molecular weight heparins. Sci Transl Med 9(406). https://doi.org/10.1126/scitranslmed.aan5954

Yu Y, Pempe EH, Liu J (2012) Chemoenzymatic synthesis of heparin oligosaccharides with both anti-factor Xa and anti-factor IIa activities. J Biol Chem 287(34):29054–29061

Yu Y, Song Y, Zhao Y, Wang N, Wei B, Linhardt RJ, Dordick JS, Zhang F, Wang H (2024) Quality control, safety assessment and preparation approaches of low molecular weight heparin. Carbohydr Polym 339:122216

Part III

Direct Anticoagulants

Direct Oral Anticoagulant Inhibitors: Mode of Action, Clinical Aspects

Eman Hassan and Will Lester

Contents

E. Hassan (✉) · W. Lester
Department of Cardiovascular Sciences, College of Medicine and Health, University of Birmingham, Birmingham, UK

Department of Haematology, Queen Elizabeth Hospital, Birmingham, UK
e-mail: eman.hassan@uhb.nhs.uk; will.lester@uhb.nhs.uk

E. Gray, J. Hogwood (eds.), *Antithrombotic and Antiplatelet Agents*, Handbook of Experimental Pharmacology 291, https://doi.org/10.1007/164_2025_786

Abstract

This chapter provides a comprehensive overview of direct oral anticoagulants (DOACs), focusing on their mechanisms of action, clinical utility, and practical considerations in anticoagulation management. DOACs have revolutionised anticoagulation by selectively targeting thrombin and activated factor X (FXa), offering improved safety, predictable pharmacokinetics, and reduced need for monitoring. The chapter covers their indications, contraindications, dosing, perioperative management, reversal, and use in special populations, including those with renal or hepatic impairment, cancer-associated thrombosis, and extreme body weights. It provides clinicians with practical guidance for the effective application of DOACs in various clinical settings.

Keywords

Anticoagulation therapy · Atrial fibrillation · Cancer-associated thrombosis · Direct oral anticoagulants · DOACs · Extreme body weight · Factor Xa inhibitors · Hepatic impairment · Perioperative management · Renal impairment · Thrombin inhibitors · Venous thromboembolism

1 Introduction

For more than six decades, Vitamin K antagonists (VKAs) were the only available oral anticoagulants, representing a breakthrough in the management of venous thromboembolism (VTE) and atrial fibrillation (AF), as well as enabling the use of mechanical heart valve replacements for patients with severe valvular disease. Despite their effectiveness, VKAs have significant limitations, including multiple food and drug interactions, unpredictable anticoagulant effects, a narrow therapeutic range requiring regular monitoring, and an increased risk of serious bleeding even in patients with well-controlled anticoagulation (Aronis and Hylek 2018). This has constrained the broader uptake of VKAs and fuelled research into more convenient and safer oral anticoagulants.

Direct oral anticoagulants (DOACs) have emerged as the first viable alternatives to VKAs, offering targeted inhibition of specific coagulation factors. They have

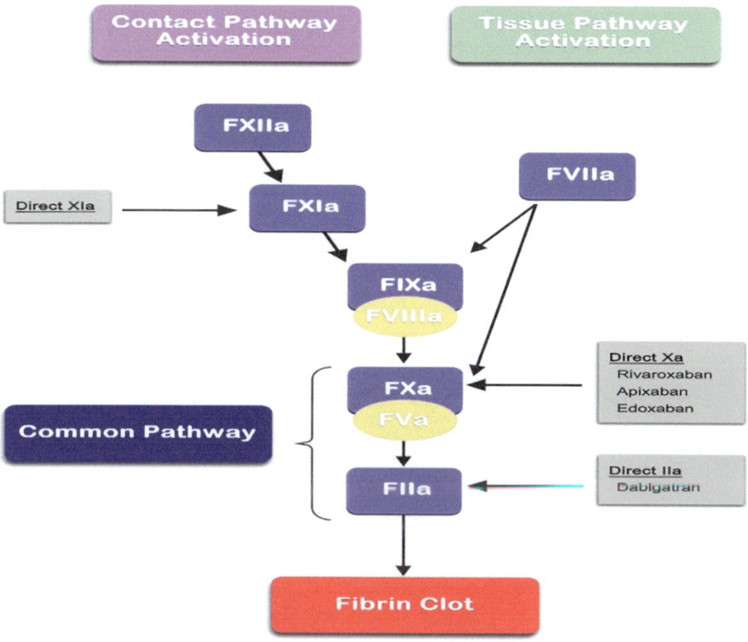

Fig. 1 Diagram showing a simplified coagulation cascade and the site of action of DOACs. F factor

demonstrated superiority or noninferiority to anticoagulation with VKAs and low-molecular-weight heparins (LMWHs), in reducing risk of thromboembolic complications with similar or reduced bleeding risk (Ruff et al. 2014; van der Hulle et al. 2014). DOACs are currently categorized into two classes: direct thrombin inhibitors and direct activated factor X (FXa) inhibitors (Fig. 1). Direct thrombin inhibitors, such as dabigatran, act by selectively binding to the active site of thrombin, preventing the conversion of fibrinogen to fibrin. Its activity leads to a downstream inhibition of fibrin and disruption in stable fibrin clot formation. Dabigatran also reduces thrombin-mediated platelet activation, which is essential for clot stabilisation (Comin and Kallmes 2012). On the other hand, FXa inhibitors, including rivaroxaban, apixaban, and edoxaban, work by directly binding to the active site of FXa. In addition to inhibiting free FXa, these agents also block FXa within the prothrombinase complex, which assembles on activated platelets and converts prothrombin to thrombin, thereby reducing thrombin generation and clot formation (Kim et al. 2018). Compared to VKAs, DOACs provide several advantages, including rapid onset and offset of action, fewer food and drug interactions, a favourable pharmacological profile and less intensive monitoring requirements, making them advantageous in both routine and periprocedural care (Rose and Bar 2018).

Over the past decade, DOACs have been widely used in clinical practice. Despite having a better safety profile than VKAs in terms of certain bleeding risks, e.g. intracranial bleeding (ICH), DOACs still carry a non-negligible risk of bleeding and can result in increased gastrointestinal, urothelial, and mucosal bleeding in comparison to VKAs and LMWH. Research has increasingly focused on coagulation factor XI (FXI), activated FXI (FXIa), and factor XII as promising targets. The next class of DOACs under development targets FXI/FXIa in the intrinsic pathway of coagulation, aiming to uncouple thrombosis from haemostasis and potentially reduce bleeding risks. Clinical observations over the past 70 years in patients with FXI deficiency suggest that inhibiting this protein may provide effective anticoagulation with a lower risk of severe bleeding; therefore, these anticoagulants will be potentially safer than current DOACs (Fredenburgh and Weitz 2023).

2 Indications and Contraindications for DOAC Use

Indications
Prevention of stroke and systemic embolism in AF (non-valvular)
Treatment and prevention of recurrent DVT and PE
Prevention of VTE in patients undergoing orthopaedic surgery
Secondary prevention of atherothrombotic events in patients with coronary artery disease or symptomatic peripheral artery disease (low-dose rivaroxaban with aspirin)
Contraindications
Active major bleeding
Mechanical heart valves
Severe renal impairment (creatinine clearance <15 mL/min for most DOACs, <30 mL/min for dabigatran)
Advanced hepatic disease associated with coagulopathy and bleeding risk
Pregnancy and breastfeeding (due to limited safety data)
Hypersensitivity
DOACs are not recommended in antiphospholipid syndrome (particularly triple positivity cases)
Cautions
Use with strong inhibitors or inducers of p-glycoprotein (p-gp) or CYP3A4 enzymes
Increased bleeding risk in elderly patients (>75 years), low body weight, or concurrent antiplatelet therapy

3 DOAC Initiation

Initiating a DOAC requires a comprehensive evaluation to ensure safety and efficacy. Before starting a DOAC, it is essential to assess the risks and benefits of anticoagulation and carefully consider the suitability of DOACs vs VKA and LMWH. This includes evaluating the patient's overall clinical status, co-morbidities, risk of bleeding, and reviewing all concurrent medications to identify potential drug interactions. Baseline investigations must include a full blood count

(FBC), renal and liver function tests, and a formal calculation of Cockcroft-Gault creatinine clearance (CrCl), as reliance on eGFR alone is insufficient. Contraindications to DOAC use must be thoroughly evaluated.

4 DOAC Dosing

Unlike VKAs, DOACs offer a simplified approach to anticoagulation therapy with fixed dosing regimens tailored to specific clinical indications and CrCl. Table 1 provides dosing recommendations for DOACs.

Table 1 Dosing recommendations for DOACs according to indication and CrCl

Indication	DOAC	Normal renal function (CrCl ≥50 mL/min)	Moderate impairment (CrCl 30–49 mL/min)	Severe impairment (CrCl <30 mL/min)
Stroke prevention in AF	Dabigatran	150 mg TWICE daily	110 mg TWICE daily	Avoid
	Rivaroxaban	20 mg ONCE daily	15 mg ONCE daily	15 mg ONCE daily if CrCl 15–29; contraindicated <15
	Apixaban	5 mg TWICE daily	2.5 mg TWICE daily if ≥2 risk factors[a]	2.5 mg TWICE daily if CrCl 15–29; Avoid in CrCl <15[b]
	Edoxaban	60 mg ONCE daily	30 mg ONCE daily	30 mg ONCE daily if CrCl 15–29; contraindicated if CrCl<15
VTE treatment	Dabigatran	150 mg TWICE daily after 5 days parenteral anticoagulation	110 mg TWICE daily after 5 days parenteral anticoagulation	Avoid
	Rivaroxaban	15 mg TWICE daily for 21 days, then 20 mg ONCE daily	15 mg TWICE daily for 21 days, then 15 mg ONCE daily	15 mg ONCE daily if CrCl 15–29; contraindicated <15
	Apixaban	10 mg TWICE daily for 7 days, then 5 mg TWICE daily	10 mg TWICE daily for 7 days, then 5 mg TWICE daily	No clear guidance in CrCl 15–29; contraindicated if CrCl <15
	Edoxaban	60 mg ONCE daily after 5 days parenteral anticoagulation	30 mg ONCE daily after 5 days parenteral anticoagulation	30 mg ONCE daily if CrCl 15–29; contraindicated <15

AF atrial fibrillation, *CrCl* indicates Cockcroft-Gault creatinine clearance, *DOAC* direct oral anticoagulant, *VTE* venous thromboembolism

[a]Age ≥ 80 years, Cr ≥133 μmol/L, and body weight ≤ 60 kg

[b]Lower dose of apixaban is under investigations for AF patients with CrCl<15

4.1 Renal Impairment

Patients with renal dysfunction face distinct challenges when using DOACs due to their dependence on renal clearance for elimination, which varies among agents. Dabigatran is the most renally eliminated, accountable for 80% of its clearance, followed by edoxaban, rivaroxaban, and apixaban 50%, 35%, and 27%, respectively. Impaired renal function increases the risk of drug accumulation, potentially elevating bleeding risks. Randomised controlled trials (RCTs) assessing DOACs in VTE or AF generally excluded patients with severe renal impairment (CrCl <30 mL/min), leaving a gap in evidence in this population. Regulatory agencies have approved certain DOACs for patients with CrCl as low as 15 mL/min based on pharmacokinetic (PK) studies, but the lack of robust clinical trial evidence emphasises the need for further research, particularly for those with end-stage renal disease undergoing dialysis.

Emerging evidence suggests that apixaban may have a lower, or at least comparable, risk of major bleeding compared to warfarin in patients with AF and advanced chronic kidney disease (CKD); therefore, some AF guidelines suggest apixaban as potential option for patients with end-stage renal disease and those who are on dialysis (January et al. 2019). Conversely, the use of rivaroxaban in severe CKD or dialysis patients remains a topic of debate. Clinical studies have provided mixed results regarding its bleeding risk compared to warfarin (Kumar et al. 2019). In the absence of robust studies with hard clinical end points, the routine use of DOACs in those with CrCl <15 mL/min as well as in patients on dialysis is better avoided (Kumar et al. 2019).

Contrary to other DOACs, edoxaban displays a decrease in efficacy compared with warfarin in patients with CrCl 95 mL/min or above, which led to regulatory bodies warning about the use of this agent in individuals with normal-high CrCl. However, a post hoc analysis of the trial of edoxaban versus warfarin in patients with AF showed that edoxaban remained safe and effective in patients with high CrCl (Bohula et al. 2016).

4.2 Dose Reduction

For extended VTE prevention, there is evidence that reduced doses of apixaban and rivaroxaban are as effective as full anticoagulation for prevention of recurrent VTE while reducing the risk of bleeding (Vasanthamohan et al. 2018). Apixaban dose can be reduced to a lower dose of 2.5 mg twice daily and rivaroxaban to 10 mg once daily after 6 months of treatment; however, higher doses may be recommended for patients at high risk of recurrence. In contrast, doses of dabigatran and edoxaban continue for VTE prevention.

In patients with AF, the efficacy of apixaban dose reduction was established in clinical studies which demonstrated that patients meeting at least two of the following criteria

- Age ≥ 80 years
- Body weight ≤ 60 kg
- Serum creatinine ≥133 μmol/L

benefitted from a reduced dose of 2.5 mg twice daily, which maintained efficacy in stroke prevention with lower risk of bleeding (Alexander et al. 2016; Zeitouni et al. 2020). This dose adjustment has been incorporated into clinical practice guidelines and approved by major regulatory agencies.

5 DOAC Monitoring

After DOAC initiation, patients' follow-up should occur every 1–3 months and then every 6–12 months, with more frequent follow-ups as needed based on patient-specific factors. Each follow-up should include a review of the patient's health status, adherence to treatment, and any bleeding or thromboembolic events. Additionally, adverse effects and medication interactions should be carefully assessed.

Routine coagulation and level monitoring of DOACs are not required when used according to license, but measuring drug concentration can add value in some circumstances, including renal impairment, use of interacting drugs, extremes of body weight, severe acute haemorrhage, assessment of compliance, suspected overdose, uncertainty about the last dose before a high-bleeding-risk procedure, gastrointestinal conditions affecting absorption, and non-standard dosing (Baker et al. 2024).

6 Switching Between Anticoagulants

Switching between DOACs and other anticoagulants is sometimes required due to different factors such as patient preference, evolving co-morbid conditions, or complications like breakthrough thrombosis, bleeding, or the need for procedures. The ultimate goal of switching between anticoagulants is to limit the interruption of therapeutic anticoagulation to minimise the risk of thrombosis. Table 2 provides detailed guidance on switching between anticoagulants to minimise risks of under- or over-anticoagulation (Raval et al. 2017).

7 Challenges in the Use of DOACs

Despite extensive evaluation of DOACs in RCTs, significant uncertainties and challenges in their clinical use remain.

Table 2 Guidance for anticoagulation switching

From	To	Guidance
VKA	DOAC	Stop VKA and check INR to start DOAC INR ≤ 2.0 for dabigatran and Apixaban INR ≤ 3.0 for rivaroxaban (AF) INR ≤ 2.5 for rivaroxaban (VTE) and edoxaban
LMWH or UFH	DOAC	UFH: Start DOAC 0 to 2 h after stopping UFH LMWH: Stop LMWH and start DOAC at the same time that the next dose of LMWH would have been given
Dabigatran	VKA	CrCl >50 mL/min: Start VKA and stop Dabigatran 3 days later CrCl 31–50 mL/min: Start VKA and stop Dabigatran 2 days later CrCl 15–30 mL/min: Start VKA and stop Dabigatran 1 day later
Rivaroxaban or apixaban	VKA	If bridging is required: Start VKA and stop DOAC 3 days later If bridging is not required: Stop DOAC and start LMWH and VKA at the time DOAC would have been due, then stop LMWH when INR is within the therapeutic range
Edoxaban	VKA	Start VKA and stop DOAC 3 days later If continuous anticoagulation is required: reduce edoxaban by 50% and start warfarin concomitantly and stop Edoxaban when INR ≥2
DOAC	DOAC	Stop current DOAC regimen and begin the new DOAC agent at the time the next dose of DOAC is due
DOAC	LMWH or UFH	Stop DOAC and start parenteral anticoagulant at the same time that the next dose of DOAC would have been given

Source: Summary of Product Characteristics EMC (2024a, b) and Chen et al. (2020)
CrCl indicates Cockcroft-Gault creatinine clearance, *DOAC* direct oral anticoagulant, *INR* International Normalised Ratio, *LMWH* low-molecular-weight heparin, *UFH* unfractionated heparin; and *VKA* vitamin K antagonist

8 DOACs in Liver Disease

DOAC elimination involves varying degrees of non-renal pathways – apixaban (75%), rivaroxaban (65%), edoxaban (50%), and dabigatran (20%) – which can be significantly affected by hepatic impairment (Steffel et al. 2021). Liver disease can lead to reduced synthesis of coagulation factors, altered plasma protein binding, and impaired metabolism, all of which may influence the anticoagulant effect. Furthermore, in conditions like hepatorenal syndrome, compromised renal function can exacerbate these effects, leading to unpredictable drug levels and increased bleeding risks.

The use of DOACs in individuals with liver impairment is primarily determined by the Child-Pugh classification system, which evaluates the extent of liver dysfunction. All DOACs are contraindicated in severe hepatic impairment (Child-Pugh C). For individuals with mild-to-moderate liver dysfunction (Child-Pugh A or B), DOACs without dose adjustments are appropriate. The International Society on Thrombosis and Haemostasis recommends DOACs as the preferred treatment for

AF due to superior safety and efficacy and suggests their use as an option for VTE treatment (Carlin et al. 2024). Current PK studies and clinical trial data are insufficient to definitively support or oppose the use of specific DOACs in liver cirrhosis. Since liver cirrhosis is a dynamic condition with the potential for changes in hepatic function over time, it is recommended to obtain blood tests to evaluate hepatic function and coagulation parameters before initiating and periodically throughout DOAC therapy.

9 DOACs in Cancer-Associated Thrombosis

Cancer is a significant risk factor for VTE, accounting for approximately 20% of all VTE cases. The introduction of DOACs has broadened treatment options for cancer-associated thrombosis (CAT). As LMWH was the standard treatment for CAT, several RCTs have since emerged comparing the efficacy and safety of DOACs in this setting. Evidence comparing DOACs to LMWH shows that rivaroxaban is superior to LMWH in reducing VTE recurrence but is associated with higher rates of both major and clinically relevant non-major bleeding (Young et al. 2018). Similarly, edoxaban and apixaban were found to be non-inferior to LMWH in preventing VTE recurrence (McBane 2nd et al. 2020; Agnelli et al. 2020; Raskob et al. 2018). While edoxaban demonstrated increased bleeding risks in patients with gastrointestinal cancers, apixaban maintained comparable rates of major bleeding to LMWH.

The use of DOACs for the prevention of VTE in patients with cancer has also been investigated in clinical trials. Evidence supports the use of these agents in cancer patients receiving ambulatory chemotherapy with intermediate-high VTE risk and low bleeding risk (Khorana et al. 2019; Riva and Ageno 2021).

Special considerations are necessary for patients with luminal gastrointestinal or genitourinary malignancies, as these populations exhibit higher rates of bleeding when treated with DOACs. Furthermore, drug–drug interactions between DOACs and cancer therapies should be considered. DOACs depend on the p-gp system for uptake and the CYP3A4 system for metabolism, necessitating caution when co-administered with cancer treatments that act as strong inducers or inhibitors of p-gp or CYP3A4 pathways. In patients with active cancer and VTE, secondary thrombo-prophylaxis is recommended and can be effectively maintained with DOACs until cancer remission is achieved.

10 DOACs in Extremes of Weight

10.1 Obesity

Obesity (BMI $\geq$30 kg/m^2) is a significant risk factor for VTE and non-valvular AF, with risks escalating further in morbid obesity (BMI $\geq$40 kg/m^2 or weight $>$ 120 kg) (Ageno et al. 2008; Wanahita et al. 2008).

10.1.1 VTE Treatment

Despite that obese patients being under-represented in DOAC VTE clinical trials, rivaroxaban and apixaban at standard doses have demonstrated a favourable PK and pharmacodynamic (PD) profile, with efficacy and safety outcomes comparable to standard therapies (Kubitza et al. 2007; Harkness et al. 2022). Limited evidence exists for dabigatran, and a lack of clinical data on edoxaban discourages its use in this group.

Current data do not provide clear thresholds or correlations between drug levels and clinical outcomes in this population; therefore, monitoring peak or trough drug-specific DOAC levels in obese patients is not currently recommended (Martin et al. 2021).

10.1.2 Secondary Prophylaxis

The available data are insufficient to establish evidence-based recommendations regarding DOAC dose reduction after the initial 6 months of full-dose treatment for extended VTE management; however, currently available data suggest that dose reduction may be an option.

10.1.3 Stroke Prevention in Non-valvular AF

The existing efficacy and safety data for rivaroxaban and apixaban at standard doses comparable to those used in nonobese patients support their routine use over warfarin (Talerico et al. 2024). While edoxaban may be an option, additional research is required to confirm its safety profile in this population. Currently, no data are available to support the use of dabigatran in morbidly obese patients.

10.2 Underweight

In underweight patients (≤60 kg), apixaban at standard doses for non-underweight patients and reduced-dose edoxaban have demonstrated consistent efficacy and safety compared with warfarin. In contrast, dabigatran has been associated with an increased risk of bleeding in this population (Talerico et al. 2024). While evidence for rivaroxaban in underweight patients is limited, its established efficacy and safety in the paediatric population suggest that weight-based dosing, as applied in paediatric settings, may be a viable approach for underweight adults.

11 Unusual Site of Thrombosis

Unusual-site VTE include thrombosis in the abdominal veins (such as renal, splanchnic, and ovarian veins), cerebral veins, and dural venous sinuses, as well as upper extremity venous thrombosis. Evidence for the use of DOACs in managing unusual-site VTE is still limited, mostly drawn from a small number of RCTs and observational studies (Riva and Ageno 2021; Riat and Gomez 2022). The rarity and severity of these conditions make conducting large trials challenging. However, current data indicate that DOACs may provide comparable effectiveness and potentially enhanced safety profiles compared to VKAs in selected patients.

12 DOACs in Antiphospholipid Syndrome

Thrombotic antiphospholipid syndrome (APS) poses unique challenges in anticoagulation management due to its association with both venous and arterial, as well as microvascular, thrombotic events. The role of DOACs in APS has been a topic of investigation. Rivaroxaban and apixaban have been evaluated in patients with thrombotic APS through open-label RCTs (Cohen et al. 2016; Pengo et al. 2018; Ordi-Ros et al. 2019; Woller et al. 2022). In a follow-up of the trial of rivaroxaban in APS, patients with triple-positive APS who continued rivaroxaban experienced higher rates of thromboembolic events compared to those who switched to or remained on warfarin. The increased thromboembolic risk led to the trial's early termination (Pengo et al. 2021). A comprehensive systematic review and meta-analysis of these studies revealed that DOACs are associated with a significantly increased risk of arterial thrombosis, particularly strokes, compared to warfarin (Khairani et al. 2023). While DOACs did not show a significant difference in the risk of venous thrombotic events or major bleeding when compared to warfarin, the findings raised concerns about their safety in APS patients. As a result, current guidance worldwide advises against using DOACs for secondary thrombosis prevention in APS, particularly in those with triple positivity or arterial thrombosis history (Tektonidou et al. 2019; Cohen et al. 2020; Zuily et al. 2020). For patients with single- or double-positive APS, the data remain less conclusive.

13 DOACs in Heparin-Induced Thrombocytopenia

DOACs have emerged as a potential option for managing patients with heparin-induced thrombocytopenia (HIT) over the past decade, supported by evidence from observational studies, cohort analyses, and case reports (Warkentin et al. 2017; Albuloushi et al. 2022). Both oral Xa inhibitors (rivaroxaban, apixaban, edoxaban) and the thrombin inhibitor dabigatran have been used in cases of HIT, both with and without associated thrombosis. A key aspect of their use is that treatment often begins with a parenteral anticoagulant, with a transition to a DOAC once the acute phase is managed.

14 DOACs in Thrombophilia

The use of DOACs in patients with severe thrombophilia remains an area of limited evidence and ongoing investigation. The evidence which is based only on cohort and single-centre studies suggests that full-dose DOACs have similar efficacy and safety to VKAs in the secondary prevention of VTE, with a low hazard ratio for recurrent

VTE. However, challenges arise in patients with specific severe thrombophilia conditions, such as protein S deficiency with levels below 20% and homozygous antithrombin deficiency, where higher rates of recurrence and treatment failure have been observed (Kovac et al. 2024). The lack of RCTs and data on genetic and functional severity further complicates personalised anticoagulation in this population. Until more robust evidence emerges, clinical judgement remains paramount, with full-dose DOACs being favoured over reduced doses due to the absence of supporting data for low dose DOACs in severe thrombophilia cases.

15 DOACs in the Setting of Bariatric Surgery and Colectomy

Bariatric surgery alters the absorption of DOACs by disrupting or bypassing the absorptive surface of the proximal small intestine, altering drug metabolism by CYP3A4 and p-gp enzymes, changing intestinal transit times. It also affects drug solubility by increasing gastric pH due to reduced stomach size and by decreasing the effective intestinal surface area. Additionally, the reduced oral caloric intake immediately after surgery may further impact the bioavailability of DOACs. Absorption sites of DOACs and its alteration are summarised in Table 3. There is a lack of high-quality evidence to guide the optimal use of DOACs after bariatric surgery, and data are limited to PK/PD studies with small patient cohorts or case reports (Martin et al. 2021; Leong et al. 2022). Despite the uncertainty surrounding their efficacy and safety, DOACs remain an attractive alternative to VKAs in this context. Current guidance suggests that in the early or acute post-operative period, prescribers should consider the potential impact of altered gastrointestinal anatomy, malabsorption, and reduced oral intake. A cautious approach involves initiating treatment with a parenteral anticoagulant, such as LMWH or fondaparinux, followed by a transition to a DOAC during the stable post-acute phase.

Table 3 Site of DOACs absorption and potential impact of surgical procedures on absorption

		Surgical procedure and potential effect on absorption			
DOAC	Site of absorption	Adjustable gastric banding	Sleeve gastrectomy	Roux-en-Y gastric bypass	Colectomy
Apixaban	Primarily upper GI tract; limited colon absorption	Unlikely affected	Unlikely affected	Possibly reduced	Possibly reduced
Dabigatran	Lower stomach and proximal small intestine	Possibly reduced	Possibly reduced	Possibly reduced	Unlikely affected
Edoxaban	Proximal small intestine[a]	Possibly reduced	Possibly reduced	Possibly reduced	Unlikely affected
Rivaroxaban	Primarily stomach, some small intestine	Possibly reduced	Possibly reduced	Possibly reduced	Unlikely affected

Source: Martin et al. (2021)
[a]Dependant on acidic environment

16 DOACs in Elderly and Frail Patients

The prevalence of AF and the associated use of DOACs are rapidly increasing among older adults. While robust evidence supports the use of DOACs in vital older patients with nonvalvular AF, data remain limited for frail patient populations as this group was often under-represented or excluded in RCTs due to their high bleeding risk and potential overexposure to DOACs (Spruit et al. 2024). This led to a gap in evidence-based guidance for managing anticoagulation in these vulnerable patients.

Across various subgroups in key clinical trials, the relative effects of DOACs compared to warfarin on major outcomes have generally been consistent. Some factors, including age, renal function, body mass index, other medical conditions, concurrent medications, prior exposure to warfarin, and variations in therapeutic range control, have influenced outcomes in specific contexts with certain DOACs. These variations have not led to substantial changes in treatment guidelines (American Geriatrics Society 2023). Apixaban is generally preferred in elderly patients over rivaroxaban due to its better safety profile, lower bleeding risk, and similar effectiveness in stroke prevention (Martinez et al. 2018). For frail patients already on VKA, transitioning to long-term DOAC use may offer comparable reductions in haemorrhagic stroke, overall stroke, and mortality, as observed in larger trials. However, frail elderly individuals who are stable on VKAs may face a heightened risk of gastrointestinal bleeding when switching to DOACs (Joosten et al. 2024). Treatment decisions should therefore be personalised, involving discussions about balancing the convenience and reduced risks of intracranial bleeding, stroke, and the improved potential for increased gastrointestinal bleeding. Regardless of the choice between VKAs and DOACs, the overarching priority for frail elderly patients with AF and high stroke risk is maintaining consistent oral anticoagulation.

17 DOACs in Children

Based on the safety and efficacy of rivaroxaban and dabigatran in the clinical trials, they are currently licensed for the treatment and prevention of VTE in children (Male et al. 2020; Halton et al. 2021). The approval of DOACs has revolutionised paediatric anticoagulation. DOACs are more practical and attractive option for the paediatric population due to their oral administration, child-friendly formulations, and reduced monitoring requirements.

In addition to VTE treatment, DOACs have been evaluated for VTE prevention in children with congenital and acquired heart disease. This broadens their potential applications and adds to the growing number of paediatric patients treated with DOACs (Pina et al. 2019; Payne et al. 2019). However, DOACs paediatric trials excluded preterm and low-birth-weight infants and those having had less than a defined period of oral feeding, while patients with liver or renal impairment, neonates, and those with cancer were under-represented. Paediatric formulations, such as powders or granules for suspension, were used in clinical trials, with weight-based dosing from tablets or capsules used for older children. For younger children, bodyweight-adjusted dosing relies on liquid formulations, which are not yet widely accessible. While DOACs do not require therapeutic monitoring, challenges such as restricted access to testing and reversal agents continue to limit their use in specific scenarios.

18 Perioperative Management

The perioperative management of DOACs requires a tailored approach that balances the risk of bleeding with thromboembolic protection. The timing of interruption is primarily dictated by the bleeding risk of the procedure, the patient's renal function, and drug-specific half-lives. DOACs have half-lives ranging from 9 to 14 h. Withholding DOACs for two full days – corresponding to approximately 60–68 h or four to five half-lives – provides adequate clearance for high-risk procedures and major surgeries (Douketis et al. 2016), while withholding DOACs for one full day, corresponding to a 30-to-36-h interruption interval (approximately three DOAC half-lives), typically leaves a minimal residual anticoagulant effect. This residual effect is considered clinically acceptable for procedures with a lower risk of bleeding. Due to the rapid onset and offset of DOACs, periprocedural bridging is generally not required; however, careful attention should be given to the appropriate timing for withholding and resuming DOAC therapy around procedures to minimise bleeding and thrombotic risks. The recommended duration of DOAC interruption before and resumption after procedures, based on the type of DOAC and the bleeding risk of the procedure, is detailed in Table 4. In high-risk patients, such as those with coronary stents, specialist advice should be sought when planning invasive procedures to ensure optimal management of antithrombotic therapy.

18.1 Perioperative Measurement of DOAC Levels

Studies demonstrate stable and low residual anticoagulant levels (<50 ng/mL in 98.8% of cases) when adhering to recommended timing intervals, making routine pre-procedure DOAC level measurements unnecessary (Douketis et al. 2019).

19 DOAC Reversal

Bleeding remains the most common complication of DOACs, though the risk of serious bleeding, particularly ICH, is lower than with VKAs. Most bleeding events can be managed by temporarily withholding the anticoagulant and providing supportive care to maintain haemodynamic stability and enhance renal clearance. However, in cases of trauma, life-threatening or severe bleeding, urgent surgeries that cannot be delayed, or high bleeding risk procedures, rapid anticoagulation reversal is essential to prevent exsanguination and reduce mortality.

Table 4 DOAC peri-procedural management recommendations

Bleeding risk	DOAC	Recommended interval of interruption prior to the procedure	DOAC resumption after the procedure
Low-to-moderate bleeding risk procedures	Direct Xa inhibitors (rivaroxaban, apixaban, edoxaban) Dabigatran (CrCl $\geq$50 mL/min)	1 day	DOACs can be restarted the day after the procedure[a]
	Dabigatran (CrCl $<$50 mL/min)	2 days	
Certain low-risk procedures (e.g. minor dental, endoscopic, minor surgical interventions)	All	Continuing DOACs or omitting the morning dose has been shown to be safe with appropriate local haemostatic measures	
High bleeding risk procedures	Direct Xa inhibitors (rivaroxaban, apixaban, edoxaban) Dabigatran (CrCl $\geq$50 mL/min)	2 days	2–3 days to ensure adequate haemostasis
	Dabigatran (CrCl $<$50 mL/min)	3–4 days	

Source: Douketis and Spyropoulos (2024)

DOAC direct oral anticoagulant, *CrCl* creatinine clearance

[a] If the procedure allows immediate and complete haemostasis, such as a soft tissue biopsy without significant vascular injury, DOACs can be restarted 6–8 h later, ideally aligning with the next scheduled dose (Heidbuchel et al. 2015)

The choice of reversal strategy depends on multiple factors, including the specific DOAC involved, timing of the last dose, bleeding severity, and patient-specific considerations such as age, weight, renal and hepatic function, frailty, indication for anticoagulation, and prior thrombotic or bleeding events. The decision to reverse anticoagulation should weigh the benefits of stabilising haemostasis against the potential risk of post-reversal thrombosis. Ongoing research continues to refine reversal strategies, with studies evaluating both existing and emerging reversal agents to improve safety and efficacy.

19.1 Specific Reversal Agents

19.1.1 Idarucizumab

Dabigatran has low protein binding (about 35%), making it amenable to clearance through dialysis or haemofiltration. However, this method has been largely replaced following the approval of idarucizumab, a humanised monoclonal antibody Fab fragment that rapidly and specifically binds to dabigatran, neutralising its effects within minutes. Its anticoagulant reversal begins in less than 5 min, with a half-life of approximately 45 min in patients with normal kidney function. Within 4 h, less than 4% of its peak plasma concentration remains (Levy et al. 2018). Idarucizumab is the only approved reversal agent for dabigatran before urgent procedures in non-bleeding patients.

The 30-day risk of thromboembolism following idarucizumab administration has been reported at 4.8%, which is comparable to the incidence observed in patients receiving 4-factor prothrombin complex concentrates. The majority of these thrombotic events occurred in patients who had not resumed their baseline anticoagulation (Pollack Jr. et al. 2017).

19.1.2 Andexanet Alfa

Andexanet alfa (andexanet) is a recombinant, inactive FXa variant specifically designed to reverse the effects of FXa inhibitors. As a modified recombinant FXa decoy molecule, it temporarily binds and sequesters FXa inhibitors, preventing them from interacting with endogenous FXa, thereby rapidly diminishing their anticoagulant effects. In patients receiving FXa inhibitors, andexanet rapidly reduces anti-FXa activity and free drug levels while restoring thrombin generation (Apostel et al. 2021; Siegal et al. 2015).

Andexanet received approval in the United States in 2018 and in Europe in 2019 through an expedited review process (Heo 2018; Patel and Steen 2016). It is specifically indicated for adults treated with apixaban or rivaroxaban, who require urgent anticoagulation reversal due to life-threatening or uncontrolled bleeding. Its use in surgical patients remains off-label.

Andexanet is administered as an initial bolus followed by a continuous infusion, with the dosage determined by factors such as the time since the last dose, the type of FXa inhibitor used, and its dosage. Findings from randomised trials indicate that andexanet is effective in achieving excellent or good haemostatic efficacy at 12 h by lowering anti-FXa activity. However, andexanet use is associated with an elevated risk of thrombotic complications (Siegal et al. 2015; Connolly et al. 2019). The risk of thrombosis associated with andexanet is linked to its interaction with tissue factor pathway inhibitor (TFPI) (Siegal et al. 2015). Under normal physiological conditions, TFPI functions as an endogenous anticoagulant by binding to and inhibiting FXa, which in turn suppresses the FVIIa–tissue factor complex. However, andexanet sequesters TFPI, impairing its natural anticoagulant activity and potentially promoting a prothrombotic state. At a 30-day follow-up, thrombotic events were reported in 10% of patients, with most occurring before anticoagulation was restarted (Connolly et al. 2019; Milling Jr. et al. 2023). Therefore, regulatory agencies have issued warnings about potential risks, including thromboembolic events, ischemic complications, cardiac arrest, and sudden death, emphasising the importance restarting anticoagulation as soon as it is clinically appropriate.

19.2 Nonspecific Reversal Agents

19.2.1 Prothrombin Complex Concentrates (PCCs)

PCCs are plasma-derived products containing coagulation factors II (prothrombin), IX, X, and VII in varying concentrations. PCCs include 3- or 4-factor PCC [3F-PCC or 4F-PCC] and activated PCC (aPCC). Among PCCs, 4F-PCCs are the most commonly used for DOAC reversal. These concentrates provide all four vitamin K–dependent coagulation factors, along with small amounts of protein C and S. 4F-PCCs are believed to counteract the anticoagulant effects of DOACs by enhancing thrombin generation through the replenishment of coagulation proteins (Connolly et al. 2024).

Evaluating the efficacy and safety of PCCs for DOAC reversal in patients with major bleeding or those requiring urgent invasive procedures remains challenging due to the lack of RCTs (Heubner et al. 2023). 4F-PCCs have generally been effective in achieving haemostasis in patients with major bleeding and has been associated with reduced mortality compared to no reversal treatment in cases of traumatic ICH (Milling and Pollack 2020; Dybdahl et al. 2019). Other studies considered their effect on mortality and disability in patients with ICH to be minimal (Lazo-Langner et al. 2013).

The risk of thromboembolic complications with PCCs in this setting appears to be low. Pooled data and meta-analysis have confirmed an overall efficacy of 80%, with a maximum thromboembolism rate of 4% based on available data (Piran et al. 2019; Milioglou et al. 2021). In addition to the thrombotic risk, 4F-PCCs have been shown to restore thrombin generation only when FXa inhibitor levels are low (Gómez-Outes et al. 2021). Therefore, 4F-PCC may be considered a haemostatic option when specific reversal agents like andexanet or idarucizumab are unavailable or their use is not authorised for a particular indication.

4F-PCC can be administered for DOAC reversal as either a fixed dose (2000 IU) or a weight-based dose (25–50 IU/kg), with studies showing no significant differences in efficacy, thromboembolic risk, or mortality between the two strategies, though the fixed dose generally results in a lower total drug exposure (Chiasakul et al. 2023).

aPCC contains varying amounts of activated clotting factors, with the majority of activation occurring with FVII. It is primarily used to manage bleeding in patients with haemophilia A or B who have developed inhibitors and has been shown to enhance thrombin generation (Shaw et al. 2023). A retrospective study found that aPCC had a 56% success rate in achieving haemostasis for DOAC-associated major bleeding and 84% in surgical patients, with a 6% risk of thromboembolism (Shaw et al. 2020).

19.2.2 Recombinant FVIIa

Recombinant FVIIa (rFVIIa) enhances thrombin generation by binding to tissue factor at sites of injury. It is approved for use in haemophilia A or B patients with inhibitors; however, there is no evidence supporting its efficacy in managing DOAC-associated bleeding, and its safety in this context remains uncertain.

Fresh frozen plasma is not a reversal agent for DOACs and should only be used to manage dilutional coagulopathy in cases of massive haemorrhage. *Tranexamic acid* has no formal role in DOAC reversal but may serve as a supportive adjunct in patients with major bleeding or requiring urgent surgery.

19.3 Reversal of New Direct FXIa Inhibitors

In patients requiring urgent surgery, intravenous tranexamic acid may help reduce bleeding risk. For serious bleeding, tranexamic acid and low-dose rFVIIa are suggested, based on experience in managing FXI deficiency. If rFVIIa is unavailable or ineffective, aPCC may be considered as an alternative. However, there is no evidence to support the use of PCC or FFP for reversing oral FXIa inhibitors (Chan and Weitz 2023).

19.4 Reversal Strategies Under Investigation

Several novel reversal strategies for DOACs are under investigation. *Ciraparantag*, initially developed for heparin reversal, was later found to bind DOACs and has shown efficacy in reversing whole blood clotting time in early studies (Ansell et al. 2017). *VMX-C001*, a FXa variant resistant to FXa inhibitors, is being evaluated for its ability to restore coagulation with lower risk of thrombosis (Verhoef et al. 2017). *Extracorporeal hemadsorption*, using a sorbent-based filtration system, has demonstrated high efficacy in removing FXa inhibitors, particularly in cardiac surgery settings (Tripathi et al. 2022).

References

Ageno W, Becattini C, Brighton T, Selby R, Kamphuisen PW (2008) Cardiovascular risk factors and venous thromboembolism: a meta-analysis. Circulation 117(1):93–102. https://doi.org/10.1161/circulationaha.107.709204

Agnelli G, Becattini C, Meyer G et al (2020) Apixaban for the treatment of venous thromboembolism associated with cancer. N Engl J Med 382(17):1599–1607. https://doi.org/10.1056/NEJMoa1915103

Albuloushi A, Rhoten M, Kelly J, Sylvester KW, Grandoni J, Connors JM (2022) Evaluation of the use of direct oral anticoagulants for the management of heparin-induced thrombocytopenia. J Thromb Thrombolysis 54(4):597–604. https://doi.org/10.1007/s11239-022-02705-6

Alexander JH, Andersson U, Lopes RD et al (2016) Apixaban 5 mg twice daily and clinical outcomes in patients with atrial fibrillation and advanced age, low body weight, or high creatinine: a secondary analysis of a randomized clinical trial. JAMA Cardiol 1(6):673–681. https://doi.org/10.1001/jamacardio.2016.1829

American Geriatrics Society (2023) American Geriatrics Society 2023 updated AGS Beers Criteria® for potentially inappropriate medication use in older adults. J Am Geriatr Soc 71(7):2052–2081. https://doi.org/10.1111/jgs.18372

Ansell JE, Bakhru SH, Laulicht BE et al (2017) Single-dose ciraparantag safely and completely reverses anticoagulant effects of edoxaban. Thromb Haemost 117(2):238–245. https://doi.org/10.1160/th16-03-0224

Apostel H, Winckers K, Bidar E, Schreiber JU (2021) Successful antithrombin administration in andexanet alfa-associated heparin resistance. J Cardiothorac Vasc Anesth 35(3):904–907. https://doi.org/10.1053/j.jvca.2020.10.042

Aronis KN, Hylek EM (2018) Evidence gaps in the era of non-vitamin K Oral anticoagulants. J Am Heart Assoc 7(3):e007338. https://doi.org/10.1161/jaha.117.007338

Baker P, Platton S, Arachchillage DJ, Kitchen S, Patel J, Riat R, Gomez K, Committee tB (2024) Measurement of heparin, direct oral anti-coagulants and other non-coumarin anti-coagulants and their effects on haemostasis assays: a British Society for Haematology Guideline. Br J Haematol 205(4):1302–1318. https://doi.org/10.1111/bjh.19729

Bohula EA, Giugliano RP, Ruff CT, Kuder JF, Murphy SA, Antman EM, Braunwald E (2016) Impact of renal function on outcomes with edoxaban in the ENGAGE AF-TIMI 48 trial. Circulation 134(1):24–36. https://doi.org/10.1161/circulationaha.116.022361

Carlin S, Cuker A, Gatt A et al (2024) Anticoagulation for stroke prevention in atrial fibrillation and treatment of venous thromboembolism and portal vein thrombosis in cirrhosis: guidance from the SSC of the ISTH. J Thromb Haemost 22(9):2653–2669. https://doi.org/10.1016/j.jtha.2024.05.023

Chan NC, Weitz JI (2023) New therapeutic targets for the prevention and treatment of venous thromboembolism with a focus on factor XI inhibitors. Arterioscler Thromb Vasc Biol 43(10):1755–1763. https://doi.org/10.1161/atvbaha.123.318781

Chen A, Stecker E, Warden BA (2020) Direct Oral anticoagulant use: a practical guide to common clinical challenges. J Am Heart Assoc 9(13):e017559. https://doi.org/10.1161/jaha.120.017559

Chiasakul T, Crowther M, Cuker A (2023) Four-factor prothrombin complex concentrate for the treatment of oral factor Xa inhibitor-associated bleeding: a meta-analysis of fixed versus variable dosing. Res Pract Thromb Haemost 7(2):100107. https://doi.org/10.1016/j.rpth.2023.100107

Cohen H, Hunt BJ, Efthymiou M et al (2016) Rivaroxaban versus warfarin to treat patients with thrombotic antiphospholipid syndrome, with or without systemic lupus erythematosus (RAPS): a randomised, controlled, open-label, phase 2/3, non-inferiority trial. Lancet Haematol 3(9):e426–e436. https://doi.org/10.1016/s2352-3026(16)30079-5

Cohen H, Cuadrado MJ, Erkan D et al (2020) 16th international congress on Antiphospholipid antibodies task force report on Antiphospholipid syndrome treatment trends. Lupus 29(12):1571–1593. https://doi.org/10.1177/0961203320950461

Comin J, Kallmes DF (2012) Dabigatran (Pradaxa). AJNR Am J Neuroradiol 33(3):426–428. https://doi.org/10.3174/ajnr.A3000

Connolly SJ, Crowther M, Eikelboom JW et al (2019) Full study report of Andexanet Alfa for bleeding associated with factor Xa inhibitors. N Engl J Med 380(14):1326–1335. https://doi.org/10.1056/NEJMoa1814051

Connolly SJ, Sharma M, Cohen AT et al (2024) Andexanet for factor Xa inhibitor-associated acute intracerebral hemorrhage. N Engl J Med 390(19):1745–1755. https://doi.org/10.1056/NEJMoa2313040

Douketis JD, Spyropoulos AC (2024) Perioperative management of patients taking direct oral anticoagulants: a review. JAMA 332(10):825–834. https://doi.org/10.1001/jama.2024.12708

Douketis J, Schulman S, Syed S (2016) Reply to Dr Lessire et al. Reg Anesth Pain Med 41(6):788. https://doi.org/10.1097/aap.0000000000000478

Douketis JD, Spyropoulos AC, Duncan J et al (2019) Perioperative management of patients with atrial fibrillation receiving a direct oral anticoagulant. JAMA Intern Med 179(11):1469–1478. https://doi.org/10.1001/jamainternmed.2019.2431

Dybdahl D, Walliser G, Chance Spalding M, Pershing M, Kincaid M (2019) Four-factor prothrombin complex concentrate for the reversal of factor Xa inhibitors for traumatic intracranial hemorrhage. Am J Emerg Med 37(10):1907–1911. https://doi.org/10.1016/j.ajem.2019.01.008

EMC (2024a) Xarelto 20mg film-coated tablets. https://www.medicines.org.uk/emc/product/2793/smpc#gref. Accessed Dec 2024

EMC (2024b) Lixiana 60mg film-coated tablets. https://www.medicines.org.uk/emc/product/6905/smpc#gref. Accessed Dec 2024

Fredenburgh JC, Weitz JI (2023) News at XI: moving beyond factor Xa inhibitors. J Thromb Haemost 21(7):1692–1702. https://doi.org/10.1016/j.jtha.2023.04.021

Gómez-Outes A, Alcubilla P, Calvo-Rojas G, Terleira-Fernández AI, Suárez-Gea ML, Lecumberri R, Vargas-Castrillón E (2021) Meta-analysis of reversal agents for severe bleeding associated with direct Oral anticoagulants. J Am Coll Cardiol 77(24):2987–3001. https://doi.org/10.1016/j.jacc.2021.04.061

Halton J, Brandão LR, Luciani M et al (2021) Dabigatran etexilate for the treatment of acute venous thromboembolism in children (DIVERSITY): a randomised, controlled, open-label, phase 2b/3, non-inferiority trial. Lancet Haematol 8(1):e22–e33. https://doi.org/10.1016/s2352-3026(20)30368-9

Harkness W, Pipitone O, Joss J, Schiedler M, Shagavah S, Moore R, Hsing J (2022) Observed Apixaban anti-Xa levels in obese patients. Ann Pharmacother. https://doi.org/10.1177/10600280221077158

Heidbuchel H, Verhamme P, Alings M et al (2015) Updated European Heart Rhythm Association Practical Guide on the use of non-vitamin K antagonist anticoagulants in patients with non-valvular atrial fibrillation. Europace 17(10):1467–1507. https://doi.org/10.1093/europace/euv309

Heo YA (2018) Andexanet Alfa: first global approval. Drugs 78(10):1049–1055. https://doi.org/10.1007/s40265-018-0940-4

Heubner L, Vicent O, Beyer-Westendorf J, Spieth PM (2023) Bleeding management in patients with direct oral anticoagulants. Minerva Anestesiol 89(7-8):707–715. https://doi.org/10.23736/s0375-9393.23.17230-0

January CT, Wann LS, Calkins H et al (2019) 2019 AHA/ACC/HRS focused update of the 2014 AHA/ACC/HRS guideline for the Management of Patients with Atrial Fibrillation: a report of the American College of Cardiology/American Heart Association Task Force on Clinical Practice Guidelines and the Heart Rhythm Society. J Am Coll Cardiol 74(1):104–132. https://doi.org/10.1016/j.jacc.2019.01.011

Joosten LPT, van Doorn S, van de Ven PM et al (2024) Safety of switching from a vitamin K antagonist to a non-vitamin K antagonist Oral anticoagulant in frail older patients with atrial fibrillation: results of the FRAIL-AF randomized controlled trial. Circulation 149(4):279–289. https://doi.org/10.1161/circulationaha.123.066485

Khairani CD, Bejjani A, Piazza G et al (2023) Direct Oral anticoagulants vs vitamin K antagonists in patients with Antiphospholipid syndromes: meta-analysis of randomized trials. J Am Coll Cardiol 81(1):16–30. https://doi.org/10.1016/j.jacc.2022.10.008

Khorana AA, Soff GA, Kakkar AK et al (2019) Rivaroxaban for Thromboprophylaxis in high-risk ambulatory patients with cancer. N Engl J Med 380(8):720–728. https://doi.org/10.1056/NEJMoa1814630

Kim PY, Yeh CH, Dale BJ, Leslie BA, Stafford AR, Fredenburgh JC, Hirsh J, Weitz JI (2018) Mechanistic basis for the differential effects of rivaroxaban and Apixaban on global tests of coagulation. TH Open 2(2):e190–e201. https://doi.org/10.1055/s-0038-1649507

Kovac M, Ignjatovic V, Orlando C, Bereczky Z, Hunt BJ (2024) The use of direct oral anticoagulants in the secondary prevention of venous thromboembolism in patients with severe thrombophilia: communication from the ISTH SSC Subcommittee on Physiological Anticoagulants and Thrombophilia. J Thromb Haemost 22(11):3322–3329. https://doi.org/10.1016/j.jtha.2024.08.006

Kubitza D, Becka M, Zuehlsdorf M, Mueck W (2007) Body weight has limited influence on the safety, tolerability, pharmacokinetics, or pharmacodynamics of rivaroxaban (BAY 59-7939) in healthy subjects. J Clin Pharmacol 47(2):218–226. https://doi.org/10.1177/0091270006296058

Kumar S, Lim E, Covic A, Verhamme P, Gale CP, Camm AJ, Goldsmith D (2019) Anticoagulation in concomitant chronic kidney disease and atrial fibrillation: JACC review topic of the week. J Am Coll Cardiol 74(17):2204–2215. https://doi.org/10.1016/j.jacc.2019.08.1031

Lazo-Langner A, Lang ES, Douketis J (2013) Clinical review: clinical management of new oral anticoagulants: a structured review with emphasis on the reversal of bleeding complications. Crit Care 17(3):230. https://doi.org/10.1186/cc12592

Leong R, Chu DK, Crowther MA, Mithoowani S (2022) Direct oral anticoagulants after bariatric surgery-what is the evidence? J Thromb Haemost 20(9):1988–2000. https://doi.org/10.1111/jth.15823

Levy JH, Douketis J, Weitz JI (2018) Reversal agents for non-vitamin K antagonist oral anticoagulants. Nat Rev Cardiol 15(5):273–281. https://doi.org/10.1038/nrcardio.2017.223

Male C, Lensing AWA, Palumbo JS et al (2020) Rivaroxaban compared with standard anticoagulants for the treatment of acute venous thromboembolism in children: a randomised, controlled, phase 3 trial. Lancet Haematol 7(1):e18–e27. https://doi.org/10.1016/s2352-3026(19)30219-4

Martin KA, Beyer-Westendorf J, Davidson BL, Huisman MV, Sandset PM, Moll S (2021) Use of direct oral anticoagulants in patients with obesity for treatment and prevention of venous thromboembolism: updated communication from the ISTH SSC subcommittee on control of anticoagulation. J Thromb Haemost 19(8):1874–1882. https://doi.org/10.1111/jth.15358

Martinez BK, Sood NA, Bunz TJ, Coleman CI (2018) Effectiveness and safety of Apixaban, dabigatran, and rivaroxaban versus warfarin in frail patients with Nonvalvular atrial fibrillation. J Am Heart Assoc 7(8). https://doi.org/10.1161/jaha.118.008643

McBane RD 2nd, Wysokinski WE, Le-Rademacher JG et al (2020) Apixaban and dalteparin in active malignancy-associated venous thromboembolism: the ADAM VTE trial. J Thromb Haemost 18(2):411–421. https://doi.org/10.1111/jth.14662

Milioglou I, Farmakis I, Neudeker M, Hussain Z, Guha A, Giannakoulas G, Kotoula V, Papaioannou M (2021) Prothrombin complex concentrate in major bleeding associated with DOACs; an updated systematic review and meta-analysis. J Thromb Thrombolysis 52(4):1137–1150. https://doi.org/10.1007/s11239-021-02480-w

Milling TJ Jr, Middeldorp S, Xu L et al (2023) Final study report of Andexanet Alfa for major bleeding with factor Xa inhibitors. Circulation 147(13):1026–1038. https://doi.org/10.1161/circulationaha.121.057844

Milling TJ, Pollack CV (2020) A review of guidelines on anticoagulation reversal across different clinical scenarios - is there a general consensus? Am J Emerg Med 38(9):1890–1903. https://doi.org/10.1016/j.ajem.2020.05.086

Ordi-Ros J, Sáez-Comet L, Pérez-Conesa M et al (2019) Rivaroxaban versus vitamin K antagonist in Antiphospholipid syndrome: a randomized noninferiority trial. Ann Intern Med 171(10):685–694. https://doi.org/10.7326/m19-0291

Patel S, Steen D (2016) Widening the path and window of opportunity for FDA approval of non-vitamin K oral anticoagulant specific antidotes and reversal agents. J Thromb Thrombolysis 41(2):285–292. https://doi.org/10.1007/s11239-015-1272-9

Payne RM, Burns KM, Glatz AC et al (2019) A multi-national trial of a direct oral anticoagulant in children with cardiac disease: design and rationale of the safety of ApiXaban on pediatric heart disease on the preventioN of embolism (SAXOPHONE) study. Am Heart J 217:52–63. https://doi.org/10.1016/j.ahj.2019.08.002

Pengo V, Denas G, Zoppellaro G et al (2018) Rivaroxaban vs warfarin in high-risk patients with antiphospholipid syndrome. Blood 132(13):1365–1371. https://doi.org/10.1182/blood-2018-04-848333

Pengo V, Hoxha A, Andreoli L et al (2021) Trial of rivaroxaban in AntiPhospholipid syndrome (TRAPS): two-year outcomes after the study closure. J Thromb Haemost 19(2):531–535. https://doi.org/10.1111/jth.15158

Pina LM, Dong X, Zhang L et al (2019) Rivaroxaban, a direct factor Xa inhibitor, versus acetylsalicylic acid as thromboprophylaxis in children post-Fontan procedure: rationale and design of a prospective, randomized trial (the UNIVERSE study). Am Heart J 213:97–104. https://doi.org/10.1016/j.ahj.2019.04.009

Piran S, Khatib R, Schulman S, Majeed A, Holbrook A, Witt DM, Wiercioch W, Schünemann HJ, Nieuwlaat R (2019) Management of direct factor Xa inhibitor-related major bleeding with prothrombin complex concentrate: a meta-analysis. Blood Adv 3(2):158–167. https://doi.org/10.1182/bloodadvances.2018024133

Pollack CV Jr, Reilly PA, van Ryn J et al (2017) Idarucizumab for dabigatran reversal – full cohort analysis. N Engl J Med 377(5):431–441. https://doi.org/10.1056/NEJMoa1707278

Raskob GE, van Es N, Verhamme P et al (2018) Edoxaban for the treatment of cancer-associated venous thromboembolism. N Engl J Med 378(7):615–624. https://doi.org/10.1056/NEJMoa1711948

Raval AN, Cigarroa JE, Chung MK et al (2017) Management of Patients on non-vitamin K antagonist Oral anticoagulants in the acute care and Periprocedural setting: a scientific statement from the American Heart Association. Circulation 135(10):e604–e633. https://doi.org/10.1161/cir.0000000000000477

Riat R, Gomez K (2022) Addendum to guidelines on the investigation and management of venous thrombosis at unusual sites (Br. J. Haematol. 2012;159:28–38): use of direct Oral anticoagulants. Br J Haematol 198(1):46–49. https://doi.org/10.1111/bjh.18189

Riva N, Ageno W (2021) Direct oral anticoagulants for unusual-site venous thromboembolism. Res Pract Thromb Haemost 5(2):265–277. https://doi.org/10.1002/rth2.12480

Rose DK, Bar B (2018) Direct Oral anticoagulant agents: pharmacologic profile, indications, coagulation monitoring, and reversal agents. J Stroke Cerebrovasc Dis 27(8):2049–2058. https://doi.org/10.1016/j.jstrokecerebrovasdis.2018.04.004

Ruff CT, Giugliano RP, Braunwald E et al (2014) Comparison of the efficacy and safety of new oral anticoagulants with warfarin in patients with atrial fibrillation: a meta-analysis of randomised trials. Lancet 383(9921):955–962. https://doi.org/10.1016/s0140-6736(13)62343-0

Shaw JR, Carrier M, Dowlatshahi D, Chakraborty S, Tokessy M, Buyukdere H, Castellucci LA (2020) Activated prothrombin complex concentrates for direct oral anticoagulant-associated bleeding or urgent surgery: hemostatic and thrombotic outcomes. Thromb Res 195:21–28. https://doi.org/10.1016/j.thromres.2020.06.044

Shaw JR, Castellucci LA, Siegal D, Carrier M (2023) DOAC-associated bleeding, hemostatic strategies, and thrombin generation assays – a review of the literature. J Thromb Haemost 21(3):433–452. https://doi.org/10.1016/j.jtha.2022.11.029

Siegal DM, Curnutte JT, Connolly SJ et al (2015) Andexanet Alfa for the reversal of factor Xa inhibitor activity. N Engl J Med 373(25):2413–2424. https://doi.org/10.1056/NEJMoa1510991

Spruit JR, de Vries TAC, Hemels MEW, Pisters R, de Groot JR, Jansen R (2024) Direct Oral anticoagulants in older and frail patients with atrial fibrillation: a decade of experience. Drugs Aging 41(9):725–740. https://doi.org/10.1007/s40266-024-01138-5

Steffel J, Collins R, Antz M et al (2021) 2021 European heart rhythm association practical guide on the use of non-vitamin K antagonist Oral anticoagulants in patients with atrial fibrillation. Europace 23(10):1612–1676. https://doi.org/10.1093/europace/euab065

Talerico R, Pola R, Klok FA, Huisman MV (2024) Direct-acting Oral anticoagulants in patients at extremes of body weight: a review of pharmacological considerations and clinical implications. TH Open 8(1):e31–e41. https://doi.org/10.1055/s-0043-1776989

Tektonidou MG, Andreoli L, Limper M et al (2019) EULAR recommendations for the management of antiphospholipid syndrome in adults. Ann Rheum Dis 78(10):1296–1304. https://doi.org/10.1136/annrheumdis-2019-215213

Tripathi R, Morales J, Lee V et al (2022) Antithrombotic drug removal from whole blood using Haemoadsorption with a porous polymer bead sorbent. Eur Heart J Cardiovasc Pharmacother 8(8):847–856. https://doi.org/10.1093/ehjcvp/pvac036

van der Hulle T, Kooiman J, den Exter PL, Dekkers OM, Klok FA, Huisman MV (2014) Effectiveness and safety of novel oral anticoagulants as compared with vitamin K antagonists

in the treatment of acute symptomatic venous thromboembolism: a systematic review and meta-analysis. J Thromb Haemost 12(3):320–328. https://doi.org/10.1111/jth.12485
Vasanthamohan L, Boonyawat K, Chai-Adisaksopha C, Crowther M (2018) Reduced-dose direct oral anticoagulants in the extended treatment of venous thromboembolism: a systematic review and meta-analysis. J Thromb Haemost 16(7):1288–1295. https://doi.org/10.1111/jth.14156
Verhoef D, Visscher KM, Vosmeer CR, Cheung KL, Reitsma PH, Geerke DP, Bos MA (2017) Engineered factor Xa variants retain procoagulant activity independent of direct factor Xa inhibitors. Nat Commun 8(1):528. https://doi.org/10.1038/s41467-017-00647-9
Wanahita N, Messerli FH, Bangalore S, Gami AS, Somers VK, Steinberg JS (2008) Atrial fibrillation and obesity--results of a meta-analysis. Am Heart J 155(2):310–315. https://doi.org/10.1016/j.ahj.2007.10.004
Warkentin TE, Pai M, Linkins LA (2017) Direct oral anticoagulants for treatment of HIT: update of Hamilton experience and literature review. Blood 130(9):1104–1113. https://doi.org/10.1182/blood-2017-04-778993
Woller SC, Stevens SM, Kaplan D et al (2022) Apixaban compared with warfarin to prevent thrombosis in thrombotic antiphospholipid syndrome: a randomized trial. Blood Adv 6(6):1661–1670. https://doi.org/10.1182/bloodadvances.2021005808
Young AM, Marshall A, Thirlwall J et al (2018) Comparison of an Oral factor Xa inhibitor with low molecular weight heparin in patients with cancer with venous thromboembolism: results of a randomized trial (SELECT-D). J Clin Oncol 36(20):2017–2023. https://doi.org/10.1200/jco.2018.78.8034
Zeitouni M, Giczewska A, Lopes RD et al (2020) Clinical and pharmacological effects of Apixaban dose adjustment in the ARISTOTLE trial. J Am Coll Cardiol 75(10):1145–1155. https://doi.org/10.1016/j.jacc.2019.12.060
Zuily S, Cohen H, Isenberg D et al (2020) Use of direct oral anticoagulants in patients with thrombotic antiphospholipid syndrome: Guidance from the Scientific and Standardization Committee of the International Society on thrombosis and Haemostasis. J Thromb Haemost 18(9):2126–2137. https://doi.org/10.1111/jth.14935

Laboratory Testing of Direct Oral Anticoagulants

Christopher Reilly-Stitt

Contents

Abstract

Direct oral anticoagulants (DOACs), also referred to as non-vitamin K oral anticoagulants (NOACs), have revolutionised anticoagulant therapy since their introduction in the late 2000s. These agents – dabigatran (a direct thrombin inhibitor) and the factor Xa inhibitors apixaban, edoxaban, and rivaroxaban – offer more predictable pharmacokinetics, fewer food and drug interactions, and do not typically require routine laboratory monitoring, unlike traditional anticoagulants such as warfarin and heparin. Despite these advantages, laboratory assessment of DOAC activity remains clinically important in specific circumstances, including bleeding, thrombosis during therapy, emergency surgery, renal or hepatic impairment, and suspected non-compliance.

C. Reilly-Stitt (✉)
UK NEQAS (Blood Coagulation), Sheffield, UK
e-mail: christopher.reilly-stitt@nhs.net

E. Gray, J. Hogwood (eds.), *Antithrombotic and Antiplatelet Agents*, Handbook of Experimental Pharmacology 291, https://doi.org/10.1007/164_2025_783

This chapter reviews the pharmacology, clinical applications, and laboratory evaluation of DOACs, outlining available assays and their principles. The gold standard for quantification is liquid chromatography-tandem mass spectrometry (LC-MS/MS), though chromogenic anti-Xa and dilute thrombin time (DTT) or ecarin-based assays are more commonly used in clinical laboratories. The impact of DOACs on routine coagulation tests such as PT, APTT, and TT is variable and reagent dependent, underscoring the need for drug-specific calibrators and assay validation.

Quality assurance through both internal quality control (IQC) and external quality assessment (EQA) is essential to maintain assay accuracy and reproducibility, in accordance with ISO 15189:2022 standards. Furthermore, DOACs can interfere with other haemostasis assays – including factor assays, antithrombin, and lupus anticoagulant testing – leading to potential diagnostic errors. Recent studies demonstrate that activated charcoal-based reagents, such as DOAC Remove™ and DOAC Stop™, can effectively neutralise DOAC interference in such assays.

In conclusion, while DOACs have largely supplanted warfarin in the management of non-valvular atrial fibrillation and venous thromboembolism due to their safety and convenience, laboratory testing retains a critical role in ensuring safe and effective patient management under specific clinical scenarios.

Keywords

Anticoagulant therapy · Anti-Xa assay · Atrial fibrillation · Dilute thrombin time (DTT) · Direct oral anticoagulants (DOACs) · Direct thrombin inhibitor · Ecarin clotting time (ECT) · External Quality Assessment (EQA) · Factor Xa inhibitors · Internal Quality Control (IQC) · LC-MS/MS · Venous thromboembolism (VTE)

1 What Are DOACs?

Vitamin K antagonists (VKAs), notably warfarin, have been the mainstay for anticoagulation in stroke prevention in AF and treatment/prevention of VTE. Direct oral anticoagulants (DOACs)—also called non-vitamin K oral anticoagulants (NOACs)—include direct thrombin inhibitors (dabigatran) and factor Xa inhibitors (rivaroxaban, apixaban and edoxaban). They have more predictable pharmacokinetics, fewer interactions and do not require the need for routine monitoring in most clinical settings.

Direct oral anticoagulants (DOACs) are a relatively new class of anticoagulants licensed for clinical use since 2008 for Rivaroxaban and Dabigatran (UK), 2011 for Apixaban (European Union) and 2015 for Edoxaban (European Union), compared to warfarin (1954) and heparin (1930s). Unlike warfarin or heparin they act on free and bound serine proteases. This ability to inactivate bound serine proteases means that the anticoagulant nature of DOACs is more accomplished than warfarin or heparin. DOACs have changed anticoagulant therapy, particularly for non-valvular atrial

Table 1 Summary table of DOACs in clinical use

Anticoagulant Trade name	Inhibits	Half-life (h)	Size g/mol	Method of clearance
Dabigatran Pradaxa	IIa	12–17	471.52	Renal 80% Hepatobiliary 20%
Apixaban Eliquis	Xa	8–15	459.90	Renal 25% Hepatobiliary 75%
Edoxaban Lixiana/Savaysa	Xa	10–14	548.06	Renal 50% Hepatobiliary 50%
Rivaroxaban Xarelto	Xa	5–9	435.88	Renal 33% Hepatic 67%

fibrillation (AF) and venous thromboembolism (VTE). Clinical trials including RE-LY (Connolly et al. 2009); ROCKET-AF (Patel et al. 2011); ARISTOTLE (Granger et al. 2011) and ENGAGE-AF-TIMI 48 (Giugliano et al. 2013) have demonstrated non-inferiority or superiority over warfarin for stroke prevention in AF. DOACs have favourable bleeding profiles in many respects, as in the case of intracranial haemorrhages in comparison to warfarin. However, risks still exist for DOACs in gastrointestinal bleeding; dose adjustment; renal and hepatic impairment and in certain patient groups.

The DOACs we will be reviewing are dabigatran; apixaban; edoxaban and rivaroxaban. Table 1 shows a summary of each of their characteristics.

The main advantages that DOACs have compared to warfarin and heparin are: they do not require regular monitoring; have more immediate drug onset and offset effects; have fewer drug and food interactions (Chen et al. 2020) and they have multiple clearance mechanisms. However, DOACs do have different pharmacokinetics when compared to warfarin. For all DOACs, there are differences in absorption and half-life; renal clearance is different for dabigatran (higher dependence on renal excretion) and edoxaban needs dose adjustments for renal function and certain drug interactions.

Drug–drug interactions that can effect DOAC concentration include: P-glycoprotein (P-gp) inhibitors can increase Dabigatran, Apixaban, Edoxaban and Rivaroxaban concentrations; P-gp inducers decrease Dabigatran, Apixaban, Edoxaban and Rivaroxaban concentrations; strong CYP3A4 inhibitors can increase concentrations of Apixaban and Rivaroxaban and strong CYP3A4 inducers can significantly decrease concentrations of Apixaban and Rivaroxaban (Chen et al. 2020).

DOACs are prescribed to: prevent strokes associated with atrial fibrillation; treat existing thrombotic events such as deep vein thrombosis (DVT) or pulmonary embolism(PE) or reduce the risk of venous thromboembolism (VTE) following orthopaedic surgery. The current guidelines from the European Society of Cardiology recommend DOACs as first-line over warfarin in non-valvular AF, except in those patients with mechanical heart valves or moderate/severe mitral stenosis (www.escardio.org/staticfile/Escardio/Guidelines/Products/Essential%20Messages/2024%20EM/Essential%20Messages_2024%20CCS.pdf).

2 Clinical Uses

DOACs are indicated for exhaustive list of clinical scenarios and conditions. Compiled in Table 2 are some of the approved clinical uses and key contraindications or cautions for dabigatran, apixaban, edoxaban and rivaroxaban.

3 Therapeutic Ranges

There are no therapeutic ranges available for DOACs; however, Table 3 shows the dosing strategies for stroke prevention in non-valvular atrial fibrillation and treatment (Tx) for PE or VTE and included are the medians and ranges of results obtained (Gosselin et al. 2018).

4 Assays Available to Measure Levels, Including Calibration and Methodology

Methods to measure DOACs include: liquid chromatography tandem mass spectrometry (LC-MS/MS); dilute thrombin time; ecarin methods (clot based and chromogenic) and chromogenic anti-Xa assays.

Table 2 Summary of approved clinical use and contraindications of DOACs

Drug	Approved clinical uses	Key contraindications/cautions
Dabigatran	Stroke prevention in non-valvular AF DVT/PE treatment & prevention Post-hip replacement thromboprophylaxis	Mechanical prosthetic heart valves (↑ risk of thrombosis/bleeding – RE-ALIGN trial) Severe renal impairment (CrCl < 30 mL/min) Significant active bleeding
Rivaroxaban	Stroke prevention in non-valvular AF DVT/PE treatment & secondary prevention Post-hip/knee replacement prophylaxis CAD/PAD (low dose + aspirin)	Mechanical valves Severe renal impairment (CrCl < 15 mL/min) Severe hepatic disease with coagulopathy
Apixaban	Stroke prevention in non-valvular AF DVT/PE treatment & secondary prevention Post-hip/knee replacement prophylaxis	Mechanical valves Severe hepatic impairment Caution in severe renal impairment (CrCl < 15 mL/min)
Edoxaban	Stroke prevention in non-valvular AF (not if CrCl > 95 mL/min due to ↓ efficacy) DVT/PE treatment after 5–10 days of parenteral anticoagulant	CrCl > 95 mL/min (less effective in AF) Mechanical valves Severe hepatic disease Severe renal impairment (CrCl < 15 mL/min)

Table 3 Dosing strategies for stroke prevention in non-valvular atrial fibrillation (NVAF) and treatment for pulmonary embolism (PE) or venous thromboembolism (VTE)

	Dabigatran		Rivaroxaban		Apixaban		Edoxaban	
Indication	Stroke prevention in NVAF	Tx PE/VTE	Stroke prevention in NVAF	Tx PE/VTE	Stroke prevention in NVAF	Tx PE/VTE	Stroke prevention in NVAF	Tx PE/VTE
Dose	150 mg bid	150 mg bid	20 mg qd	20 mg qd	5 mg bid	5 mg bid	60 mg qd	60 mg qd
Peak median Conc range ng/ml	175 (117–275)	175 (117–275)	249 (184–343)	270 (180–419)	171 (91–321)	132 (59–302)	170 (125–245)	234 (149–317)
Trough median Conc range ng/ml	91 (61–143)	60 (39–95)	44 (12–137)	26 (6–87)	103 (41–230)	63 (22–177)	36 (19–62)	19 (10–39)

The gold-standard method is LC-MS/MS demonstrating good accuracy and precision over a broad concentration range; however, this test is offered in a small number of laboratories (Schmitz et al. 2014). More rapid methods more suited to clinical laboratories where testing is required in an urgent clinical setting including the dilute thrombin time (DTT), ecarin methods and chromogenic anti-Xa assays are suitable means to measure DOACs. These rapid methods employ commercial calibrators and controls specific for the DOAC being measured as there are no international standards for any of the DOACS. In the USA, the FDA has not approved kits or calibrators for DOAC measurement.

5 Drug Specific Assays

In the NEQAS BC DOAC programme season 2025–2026, of which there are approximately 200 registered participants, there are no centres using the LC-MS/MS for dabigatran, apixaban, edoxaban or rivaroxaban measurement. Dabigatran plasma concentration can be assessed on automated platforms, using a variety of assays including a dilute thrombin time; an ecarin clotting time or ecarin chromogenic assay as long as each assay employs a specific dabigatran standard curve. In order to measure direct anti-Xa either apixaban, edoxaban or rivaroxaban the modified chromogenic anti-Xa assays, once again on automated platforms, can be employed provided drug-specific calibrators are used to derive the standard curve.

DOACs have a predictable anticoagulant effect and therefore they do not require routine monitoring. However, measuring DOAC levels may be required clinically, if a patient receiving DOAC therapy presents with: bleeding symptoms; a thrombotic event; requires emergency surgery or if there are concerns of drug compliance. Table 4 outlines how each DOAC affects routine haemostasis assays and which quantitation assay should be employed to measure drug concentration. Each laboratory should undertake testing of their routine haemostasis assays to check the

Table 4 Influence of DOACs on routine coagulation assays

Anticoagulant	PT	APTT	TT	Quantitation assay
Dabigatran	–/↑	↑↑	If normal excludes clinically relevant concentration	Dilute TT (DTI assay), ECT, chromogenic IIa assay
Apixaban	–/↑	–/↑/↑↑	Insensitive	Anti Xa assay using Apixaban Calibrator
Edoxaban	–/↑	↑	Insensitive	Anti Xa assay using Edoxaban Calibrator
Rivaroxaban	↑	↑↑	Insensitive	Anti Xa assay using rivaroxaban calibrator

Key: – = Most likely no effect on assay; ↑ = Possible effect on assay (i.e., at supratherapeutic levels or could also be reagent specific); ↑↑ = Likely effect at therapeutic levels.
APTT activated partial thromboplastin time, *DTI* direct thrombin inhibitor, *ECT* ecarin clotting time, *PT* prothrombin time, *TT* thrombin time (Baker et al. 2024).

sensitivity of their reagents to the different DOACs prescribed in primary or secondary care. Recommendations from the BSH guideline (Baker et al. 2024) includes: if measuring dabigatran, use dTT, ECT, ECA or a IIa calibrated for dabigatran; when measuring rivaroxaban, apixaban or edoxaban, anti-Xa assays with separate traceable calibrators and controls should be used for each drug; PT- and APTT-based assays should not be used to measure apixaban, edoxaban or rivaroxaban levels and further recommend against, routine monitoring of apixaban, edoxaban, rivaroxaban and dabigatran.

6 Assay Principles

Liquid chromatography mass spectrometry (LC-MS/MS) can be broken down to four phases. Firstly, the sample (blood) undergoes a clean-up process, to isolate the DOAC to be measured and remove interfering substances. The second stage involves injecting the sample into a liquid chromatograph, where the DOACs are separated based on their chemical properties.

Following which is the DOAC molecules then enter a mass spectrometer, which identifies and quantifies them by their unique mass-to-charge ratio and fragmentation patterns. The final output provides a direct measurement of the DOAC concentration in the original sample.

7 DOAC Xa Assay

A patient with an unknown level of DOAC is assayed by adding a chromogenic substrate and an excess of Xa. Depending on the level of the Anti-Xa drug (either apixaban, edoxaban or rivaroxaban) this binds to the Xa in the assay mixture. Any excess Xa then cleaves the chromogenic substrate to produce the colour change, indirectly proportional to the level of the Anti-Xa drug. Therefore, if there is a high concentration of DOAC, less FXa is available to cleave the substrate, resulting in less colour being produced and detected by the analyser and if there is a low concentration of DOAC, more FXa is present to cleave the chromogenic substrate, leading to more colour being produced.

8 Direct Thrombin Inhibitor (DTI) Assay

The DTI assay is a modified thrombin time assay performed on citrate plasma. The patient's plasma, with an unknown level of dabigatran, is first diluted in normal plasma to reduce any analytical variables or interferences. A fixed concentration of bovine or human thrombin is then added which will convert fibrinogen to fibrin to form a clot, detected by the automated analyser. The time for the clot to form is compared against a dabigatran reference curve and is directly proportional to the dabigatran concentration.

9 Ecarin Chromogenic or Clotting Assay for Dabigatran

The Ecarin assays use the snake venom toxin ecarin, from the *Echis carinatus* snake to convert prothrombin to meizothrombin. These assays are calibrated with known concentrations of dabigatran. Dabigatran present in the patient's plasma will bind to the meizothrombin, and the residual meizothrombin will cleave the chromogenic substrate to produce the colour change that is indirectly proportional to the level of dabigatran. In the case of the clot-based Ecarin assay the only difference is that the residual meizothrombin converts fibrinogen to fibrin to achieve a clotting time. The clotting time that is prolonged indicates an increased level of dabigatran and therefore a shorter clotting time indicates a lower level of dabigatran.

10 Quality Control

Ensuring that quality control is in place for DOAC measurement is the responsibility of the laboratory performing the assay. The quality control should be two pronged, with both internal quality control (IQC) and external quality assessment (EQA) being performed, in line with accreditation standards ISO 15189 2022 (ISO 15189 2022 Edition 4). IQC that performs well indicates whether the assay is performing the same as it was when last tested, so therefore measuring precision. The IQC samples provided for DOAC assays are at levels within the linear range of the assay. They are manufactured in most instances by the IVD company supplying the DOAC assay. It would be beneficial to have IQC at therapeutic levels, however since we do monitor patients on DOACs it is difficult to provide therapeutic ranges for the different dosing strategies required by the various clinical scenarios patient receive DOACs for. IQC should be performed when a new lot of the assay kit has been calibrated as a minimum. Then it is up to the clinical or laboratory scientific team to define the frequency of IQC. The frequency of IQC is determined by: the assay validation performed before the DOAC assay is introduced to the laboratory testing repertoire; adherence to an accreditation standard or good laboratory practice. The IQC material normally comes with a data sheet to indicate the expected range of IQC values that verify the assay is performing with an acceptable range. The IQC needs to be monitored for any drift away from the expected range and target values. Plus they should also perform to manufacturers' specifications: for target mean; standard deviation (SD) and coefficient of variation (CV). It is the initial assay validation that should provide data to confirm the assay is fit for purpose. EQA is primarily concerned with is my result the same as others using the same assay. EQA samples are independent of the IVD companies supplying the kit. The material distributed for EQA should: behave the same as patient samples; test the linear range of the assay and require interpretation of numerical data as in the case of DOAC measurement. There are a number of EQA schemes available to laboratories to sign up to cover the DOAC assays they offer.

11 Testing Effected by the Presence of DOACs

We have already described the effect that therapeutic and supratherapeutic levels of DOACs have on routine haemostasis assays. However, other assays employed in the investigation of bleeding and thrombotic episodes can be affected by the presence of DOACs.

Table 5 is a summary of the other assays that can be affected by DOAC levels.

The laboratory scientific staff must be informed as to which DOAC the patient is receiving and when the last dose was given prior to the blood sample being taken. Without accurate clinical information with regard to DOAC therapy assays may underestimate as in the case of one-stage factor assays by PT or APTT methods for any of the DOACs. In the case of patients receiving either: rivaroxaban; apixaban or edoxaban and requiring an antithrombin assay, it is worth noting that the antithrombin assay using Xa will likely overestimate the level.

Recently, the use of activated charcoal has been shown to neutralise clinically significant levels of dabigatran, apixaban, edoxaban and rivaroxaban up to 500 ng/ml (DOAC Remove IFU - RUO; DOAC Stop 630da0e2134c38768faa0451_LH1.12 - DOAC-Stop_Web eIFU.pdf). This can allow for more reliable measurement of haemostasis parameters, when stopping DOAC therapy is not clinically indicated. National External Quality Assessment Scheme for Blood Coagulation (NEQAS BC) ran an exercise in January 2025, that had Rivaroxaban plasma donation in the Lupus programme for DRVVT testing. In the presence of rivaroxaban, (concentration

Table 5 Summary of the potential influence of DOACs on coagulation assays

Anticoagulant	Dabigatran	Apixaban	Rivaroxaban	Edoxaban
Assay				
PT based Factor assays	↓	↓↓	↓↓	↓↓
APTT based Factor assay	↓↓	↓	↓	↓
Chromogenic Factor assay	–/↓	↓	↓	↓
Protein C Chromogenic assay	–	–	–	–
Free Protein S Antigen assay	–	–	–	–
Anti–Thrombin (IIa)	↑	–	–	–
Anti-Thrombin (Xa)	–	↑↑	↑↑	↑↑
Dilute Russell Viper Venom Time (DRVVT) (Clot based)	↑↑	↑↑	↑↑	↑↑

Key: – = Most likely no effect on assay; ↑ or ↓ = Possible effect on assay (i.e. at supratherapeutic levels or could also be reagent specific); ↑↑ or ↓↓ = Likely effect at therapeutic levels; ↑↑↑ or ↓↓↓ = Substantial effect (Schmitz et al. 2014)

215 ng/ml) DRVVT testing is expected to be prolonged and it was in 98.7% of returns (235/238) sample 25:01. DRVVT testing is used for the detection of anti-phospholipid antibodies. A significant prolongation of the DRVVT could be due to antiphospholipid antibodies. A total of 72% of participants reported false positive for the sample with rivaroxaban (the plasma did not have anti-phospholipid antibodies present). As part of the same exercise a volume of the plasma was treated with DOAC Remove™ (5-DIAGNOSTICS, Switzerland) 25:02 and the same volume of plasma was treated with DOAC Stop™ (HEMATEX, Australia) 25:03 and when tested by DRVVT the samples were within the normal range for 98.8% and 99.2% respectively for results returned, no evidence of anti-phospholipid antibodies.

A review of anticoagulants prescribed in the UK in 2019 has DOACS outstripping warfarin in terms of prescriptions issued, having a combined total for: dabigatran; apixaban; edoxaban and rivaroxaban of 61.8% against 38.1% for warfarin, this is compared to 16.3% for DOACs against 83.6% for warfarin in 2015 (Afzal et al. 2021).

References

Afzal S, Zaidi STR, Merchant HA et al (2021) Prescribing trends of oral anticoagulants in England over the last decade: a focus on new and old drugs and adverse events reporting. J Thromb Thrombolysis 52:646–653. https://doi.org/10.1007/s11239-021-02416-4

Baker P, Platton S, Arachchillage DJ, Kitchen S, Patel J, Riat R et al (2024) Measurement of heparin, direct oral anti-coagulants and other non-coumarin anti-coagulants and their effects on haemostasis assays: a British Society for Haematology guideline. Br J Haematol 205(4): 1302–1318. https://doi.org/10.1111/bjh.19729

Chen A, Stecker E, Warden BA (2020) Direct Oral anticoagulant use: a practical guide to common clinical challenges. J Am Heart Assoc 9(13):e017559. https://doi.org/10.1161/JAHA.120.017559. Epub 2020 Jun 15. PMID: 32538234; PMCID: PMC7670541

Connolly SJ, Ezekowitz MD, Yusuf S, Eikelboom J, Oldgren J, Parekh A, Pogue J, Reilly PA, Themeles E, Varrone J, Wang S, Alings M, Xavier D, Zhu J, Diaz R, Lewis BS, Darius H, Diener HC, Joyner CD, Wallentin L, RE-LY Steering Committee and Investigators (2009) Dabigatran versus warfarin in patients with atrial fibrillation. N Engl J Med 361(12):1139–1151. https://doi.org/10.1056/NEJMoa0905561. Epub 2009 Aug 30. Erratum in: N Engl J Med. 2010 Nov 4;363(19):1877

DOAC Remove IFU - RUO

DOAC Stop 630da0e2134c38768faa0451_LH1.12 - DOAC-Stop_Web eIFU.pdf

Giugliano RP, Ruff CT, Braunwald E, Murphy SA, Wiviott SD, Halperin JL, Waldo AL, Ezekowitz MD, Weitz JI, Špinar J, Ruzyllo W, Ruda M, Koretsune Y, Betcher J, Shi M, Grip LT, Patel SP, Patel I, Hanyok JJ, Mercuri M, Antman EM, ENGAGE AF-TIMI 48 Investigators (2013) Edoxaban versus warfarin in patients with atrial fibrillation. N Engl J Med 369(22): 2093–2104. https://doi.org/10.1056/NEJMoa1310907. Epub 2013 Nov 19

Gosselin RC, Adcock DM, Bates SM, Douxfils J, Favaloro EJ, Gouin-Thibault I, Guillermo C, Kawai Y, Lindhoff-Last E, Kitchen S (2018) International Council for Standardization in Haematology (ICSH) recommendations for laboratory measurement of direct oral anticoagulants. Thromb Haemost 118(3):437–450. https://doi.org/10.1055/s-0038-1627480. Epub 2018 Feb 12

Granger CB, Alexander JH, McMurray JJ, Lopes RD, Hylek EM, Hanna M, Al-Khalidi HR, Ansell J, Atar D, Avezum A, Bahit MC, Diaz R, Easton JD, Ezekowitz JA, Flaker G, Garcia D, Geraldes M, Gersh BJ, Golitsyn S, Goto S, Hermosillo AG, Hohnloser SH,

Horowitz J, Mohan P, Jansky P, Lewis BS, Lopez-Sendon JL, Pais P, Parkhomenko A, Verheugt FW, Zhu J, Wallentin L, ARISTOTLE Committees and Investigators (2011) Apixaban versus warfarin in patients with atrial fibrillation. N Engl J Med 365(11):981–992. https://doi.org/10.1056/NEJMoa1107039. Epub 2011 Aug 27

ISO 15189 2022 Edition 4

Patel MR, Mahaffey KW, Garg J, Pan G, Singer DE, Hacke W, Breithardt G, Halperin JL, Hankey GJ, Piccini JP, Becker RC, Nessel CC, Paolini JF, Berkowitz SD, Fox KA, Califf RM, ROCKET AF Investigators (2011) Rivaroxaban versus warfarin in nonvalvular atrial fibrillation. N Engl J Med 365(10):883–891. https://doi.org/10.1056/NEJMoa1009638. Epub 2011 Aug 10

Schmitz EM, Boonen K, van den Heuvel DJ, van Dongen JL, Schellings MW, Emmen JM, van der Graaf F, Brunsveld L, van de Kerkhof D (2014) Determination of dabigatran, rivaroxaban and apixaban by ultra-performance liquid chromatography – tandem mass spectrometry (UPLC-MS/MS) and coagulation assays for therapy monitoring of novel direct oral anticoagulants. J Thromb Haemost 12(10):1636–1646. https://doi.org/10.1111/jth.12702

www.escardio.org/staticfile/Escardio/Guidelines/Products/Essential%20Messages/2024%20EM/Essential%20Messages_2024%20CCS.pdf

Part IV

Platelets

Platelet Membrane Receptors and Signalling Pathways

Alice Y. Pollitt, Craig E. Hughes, and Chris I. Jones

Contents

A. Y. Pollitt · C. E. Hughes · C. I. Jones (✉)
School of Biological Sciences, University of Reading, Reading, UK
e-mail: c.i.jones@reading.ac.uk

E. Gray, J. Hogwood (eds.), *Antithrombotic and Antiplatelet Agents*, Handbook of Experimental Pharmacology 291, https://doi.org/10.1007/164_2025_787

Abstract

Platelets are central mediators of haemostasis, responding rapidly to vascular injury through tightly regulated activation and inhibitory mechanisms. This response is mediated by a range of agonists, membrane receptors, and associated signalling pathways, enabling platelets to respond rapidly and specifically to stimuli. This chapter outlines the processes of platelet activation following vascular damage, highlighting the roles of collagen, von Willebrand factor, and secondary agonists such as ADP, thromboxane A_2, and thrombin, alongside endothelial-derived inhibitory signals that restrain excessive activation. It focuses on tyrosine kinase–linked receptors, detailing immunoreceptor tyrosine-based activatory (ITAM and hemITAM) and inhibitory (ITIM/ITSM) pathways, with emphasis on key kinases including Src family kinases, Syk, and Tec family members, and receptors such as GPVI, FcγRIIA, CLEC-2, PECAM-1, and G6b-B. Adhesion receptors, particularly integrins αIIbβ3 and α2β1 and the GPIb- IX-V complex, are examined with respect to inside-out and outside-in signalling and mechanotransduction. Finally, the G-protein-coupled receptors that amplify or inhibit platelet responses are discussed, including PARs, purinergic receptors, thromboxane, and prostaglandin receptors, along with emerging concepts in the regulation of platelets by GPCRs and in therapeutic targeting. The activatory and inhibitory pathways outlined here work together to maintain a balance between haemostasis and thrombosis. This enables a rapid and coordinated platelet response to vascular damage while preventing inappropriate and excessive activation. This maintains vascular integrity while preventing excessive bleeding and pathological thrombosis.

1 Introduction

Platelets respond rapidly to vascular damage, enabling the formation of stable thrombi that prevent excessive bleeding. This response is coordinated through an array of membrane receptors and associated signalling pathways that enable platelets to react rapidly and specifically to the stimuli they encounter.

1.1 Platelet Activation

Upon vascular damage, platelets adhere to the sub-endothelial matrix via the binding of von Willebrand factor (VWF) to exposed collagen, mediated by the receptor complex GPIb-V-IX (Alevriadou et al. 1993; Ruggeri 2003; Wu et al. 2000). The stable binding and activation of this first layer of adherent platelets are promoted by the binding of GPVI and integrin $\alpha_2\beta_1$ to exposed collagens (Siljander et al. 2004), promoting intracellular signalling cascades that lead to calcium mobilisation from both internal stores and the extracellular space into the cytoplasm, platelet shape change, degranulation and a change in the affinity of integrin $\alpha_{IIb}\beta_3$ for vWF and fibrinogen (Varga-Szabo et al. 2009; Hartwig 2006; Coppinger et al. 2004; Italiano Jr. et al. 2008; Ma et al. 2007). This promotes the recruitment of additional platelets to the site of damage via integrin $\alpha_{IIb}\beta_3$ (Nesbitt et al. 2009), the binding of fibrinogen to which both supports aggregation (Pytela et al. 1986; Bennett 2001) and further stimulates platelets by the activation of integrins (Shattil and Newman 2004; Law et al. 1999; Clark et al. 1994). Platelets recruited to the growing thrombus are further stimulated by activation by agonists that are either released upon platelet degranulation (e.g. ADP) (Gachet et al. 1997), generated and secreted by activated platelets (e.g. thromboxane A_2) (Siess et al. 1983a, b) or synthesised on the platelet surface or at the site of thrombus formation (e.g. thrombin) (Bevers et al. 1982; Coughlin 2000).

1.2 Platelet Inhibition

Whilst platelet activation must occur rapidly at the site of vascular damage, inappropriate or excessive activation must also be prevented. This is primarily achieved through nitric oxide (NO) and prostacyclin (PGI_2), which are released not only by endothelial cells but also through receptors such as PECAM-1 (Jones et al. 2012, 2014a).

This chapter will discuss platelet membrane receptors and their signalling pathways, focusing on (1) tyrosine kinase-linked receptors: ITAM and ITIM pathways, (2) adhesion receptors and (3) G-protein coupled receptors (GPCRs).

2 Tyrosine Kinase-Linked Receptors: ITAM and ITIM Pathways

2.1 Tyrosine Kinases

The overwhelming majority of protein phosphorylation that occurs in cells is on serine and threonine residues, but although less common, tyrosine phosphorylation is a key mechanism of platelet activation. When phosphorylated by a tyrosine kinase, phospho-tyrosine is able to bind, with high affinity, to Src homology 2 (SH2) domains, or the less common phospho-tyrosine binding (PTB) domains. This high-affinity interaction underpins the activation and assembly of signalling pathways and signalosomes to ultimately activate effector proteins.

The two classes of these kinases are receptor tyrosine kinases (RTK) and non-receptor tyrosine kinases (nRTK). The former are membrane-bound receptor molecules and the latter are cytoplasmic proteins with the ability to move and localise with receptors, adaptor molecules and effector proteins; this is important in the regulation and kinetics of platelet activation.

RTKs are a large group, being sub-categorised into 20 different classes, although platelets only express a small number, with relatively minor roles in platelet function. Three of these are c-Kit (CD117; stem cell factor receptor), platelet-derived growth factor receptor α (PDGFR) and the insulin receptor β (CD220; INSR). Although their expression has been previously reported, their expression levels are very low, with only the insulin receptor being detectable in proteomic analyses of human or mouse platelets (Zeiler et al. 2014; Burkhart et al. 2012).

In addition to these three RTKs, platelets also express three members of the Eph kinase family of RTKs, namely EphA4, EphB1 and EphB2, although these are not detected in proteomic analyses of human or mouse platelets (Zeiler et al. 2014; Burkhart et al. 2012; Vaiyapuri et al. 2015; Prevost et al. 2002; Berrou et al. 2018). The mechanisms by which these RTKs regulate platelet function are not fully understood, but they have been implicated in promoting platelet activation by integrins, GPCRs and GPVI, and contribute to thrombus growth and stability (Vaiyapuri et al. 2015; Berrou et al. 2018; Prevost et al. 2002, 2004, 2005). Their ligands are ephrins, which are themselves transmembrane proteins capable of signalling. Platelets express EphrinB1, which suggests a role for Eph/Ephrins in platelet-platelet crosstalk, although contact-independent function has also been described (Prevost et al. 2002).

Non-receptor tyrosine kinases are more numerous and abundant than the RTKs. For example, Burkhart reported Src expression at 10,000 copies per platelet compared to the insulin receptor which was only detectable after an enrichment process (Burkhart et al. 2012). The best studied tyrosine kinase signalling pathways in platelets are the immunoreceptor tyrosine-based activatory motif (ITAM), and integrin signalling pathways, which centre on three key families of nRTKs, namely the Src family, Tec family kinases and Syk kinase.

The ITAM pathway is opposed by the immunoreceptor tyrosine-based inhibitory motif (ITIM) pathway which involves both tyrosine kinases and tyrosine phosphatases. These will be the focus of this section, although it should be noted that other examples of nRTKs are present in platelets, for example the thrombopoietin receptor, c-Mpl, which signals through Janus kinase 2 (JAK2). Although this does contribute to platelet activation, it is thought to be most relevant in haematopoietic stem cells where the JAK2-STAT signalling pathway regulates gene expression and megakaryopoiesis.

2.1.1 Src Family Kinases (SFK)

Platelets express several Src family kinases. In humans, Src (20,000 copies), Fyn (6,800 copies), Lyn (10,000 copies), Yes (6,300 copies) and Fgr (2,600 copies) are expressed, and in mouse, Src (25,000 copies), Fyn (4,100 copies), Lyn (1,700 copies), and Fgr (450 copies) are expressed (Zeiler et al. 2014; Burkhart et al. 2012). The evidence suggests that Src plays a major role in signalling downstream of integrin αIIbβ3, whereas Lyn and to a lesser extent Fyn play the major role downstream of the collagen receptor GPVI (Severin et al. 2012; Ezumi et al. 1998; Quek et al. 2000). Roles for Fgr and Yes appear to be minor in comparison (Severin et al. 2012; Quek et al. 2000). Lyn is unique, with both activatory and inhibitory function, as shown using knock-out mice which demonstrate delayed, but enhanced activation downstream of both receptors (Quek et al. 2000; Maxwell et al. 2004).

Most SFKs (notably Fyn and Lyn, but not Src) have palmitoylation and myristoylation sites at their N-terminal disordered domain, which, when palmitoylated/myristoylated, anchors these kinases to the plasma membrane and may contribute to their interaction with membrane receptors (Koegl et al. 1994; Honda et al. 2000). Further receptor interaction is brought about by other protein-protein interactions; Fyn and Lyn are able to associate with GPVI via their SH3 domains and a poly-proline sequence in the cytoplasmic tail of GPVI, and Src associates with the cytoplasmic tail of the integrin β3 subunit via an atypical interaction between its SH3 domain and a RGT sequence at the C-terminus (Arias-Salgado et al. 2003). Fyn and Lyn associate with β3 via a classical SH3-poly-proline interaction, but this is not localised to the C-terminus in the same way as Src (Arias-Salgado et al. 2003). These receptor interactions are crucial for SFK activation following ligand binding and receptor clustering (Bori-Sanz et al. 2003; Suzuki-Inoue et al. 2002; Schmaier et al. 2009).

SFKs have two key tyrosine residues which contribute to their level of activity. The 'inhibitory' tyrosine in the C-terminal disordered domain, when phosphorylated, is bound to by an intramolecular bond with its SH2 domain. Under resting conditions, the inhibitory tyrosine is phosphorylated by the kinases C-terminal Src kinase (Csk) or Csk homologous kinase (Chk), holding the kinase in an inactive, closed conformation. Following ligand binding and receptor clustering, Csk/Chk dissociate, and the inhibitory tyrosine is dephosphorylated by protein tyrosine phosphatase 1b (PTP1b) and CD148. Clustering induces further activation by trans-autophosphorylation from neighbouring SFKs on the 'activatory' tyrosine in the active site of the kinase domain resulting in fully active SFK. This process is reviewed in detail by Senis et al (2014).

2.1.2 Syk

Spleen tyrosine kinase (Syk) is highly expressed in both mouse (23,000 copies) and human platelets (4,900 copies) (Zeiler et al. 2014; Burkhart et al. 2012). Syk plays a critical role in both ITAM and hemITAM signalling, being required for signalling by GPVI, the Fc receptor γ IIA (FcγRIIA, CD32A) and CLEC-2. It also plays an important role in outside-in signalling by αIIbβ3, although its role here is less well defined than for the (hem)ITAM-containing receptors, with some researchers arguing for a direct role in integrin signalling (Clark et al. 1994; Hughes et al. 2015; Gao et al. 1997; Woodside et al. 2002), and others proposing that its role downstream of the integrin is indirect, and rather a contribution of FcγRIIA to αIIbβ3 signalling (Boylan et al. 2008; Zhi et al. 2013).

Syk contains a pair of SH2 domains (tandem-SH2) which are appropriately spaced for high affinity binding to the dual phosphotyrosine in an ITAM motif (Grucza et al. 1999). Following ligand binding and SFK activation, SFKs phosphorylate the ITAM tyrosines allowing Syk to bind. This binding is thought to be sufficient to induce Syk activation through conformational changes to the kinase domain (Tsang et al. 2008). However, in addition to this, Syk is able to be activated by phosphorylation by SFKs and by autophosphorylation on a number of regulatory tyrosines, including two key residues in the active site (Futterer et al. 1998; Brdicka et al. 2005; Arias-Palomo et al. 2007; Deindl et al. 2007). Interestingly, the mechanism differs in integrin signalling; while the β3 cytoplasmic tail contains a pair of tyrosine residues, these are not in an ITAM, and while Syk has been shown to interact with these, their phosphorylation causes Syk to disassociate (Woodside et al. 2001, 2002).

2.1.3 Tec Family Kinases

Platelets express two Tec family kinases, the eponymous Tec and Bruton's tyrosine kinase (Btk). In humans, Btk is the most highly expressed, with 11,100 copies compared to Tec at 1,300 copies (Burkhart et al. 2012). Similarly, in mice, Btk is again the more highly expressed family member with 12,100 copies compared to 500 copies of Tec (Zeiler et al. 2014). In both species, Tec is significantly lower in number and thought to play a much less significant role than Btk.

The mechanisms of Btk activation are unclear. Btk contains a PH domain allowing it to associate with the plasma membrane, as well as SH2 and SH3 domains allowing association with other signalling molecules. It contains a tyrosine residue in its active site, which when phosphorylated is associated with increased activity (Dinh et al. 2007; Lin et al. 2009). Evidence suggests that this is phosphorylated by an autophosphorylation step, although SFKs are also able to phosphorylate this tyrosine, suggesting an initial activation by SFKs and positive feedback by trans-autophosphorylation. Btk also contains a tyrosine in the SH3 domain, which is autophosphorylated, although, as shown in another Tec family member, this appears to have only a modest effect on activity (Joseph et al. 2007, 2009).

Interestingly, despite its widely accepted role as a tyrosine kinase in ITAM signalling, there is evidence that it functions instead as an adaptor molecule, as studies with a kinase-dead mutant showed that signalling was not significantly affected (Nicolson et al. 2018; Tomlinson et al. 2001; Saito et al. 2003). While this was seen for GPVI, it was not the case for the hemITAM-containing CLEC-2, for which kinase activity of Btk was required for signalling (Nicolson et al. 2021).

2.1.4 (hem)ITAM Pathways

An immunoreceptor tyrosine-based activatory motif (ITAM) is an amino acid sequence containing dual tyrosine residues which, when phosphorylated by SFKs, provide a docking site for the tandem-SH2 domains of Syk. They have a $YxxL/Ix_{6-12}YxxL/I$ consensus sequence with the two YxxL/I sequences being separated by

6–12 amino acids, depending on the receptor. ITAMs are present in a number of immune cell receptors and in platelets; GPVI associates with the ITAM-containing Fc receptor γ chain (FcRγ), and in primates, platelets also express Fc receptor γ IIA (FcγRIIA, (CD32) A – is absent from the mouse genome).

Ligand binding and subsequent clustering of ITAM-containing receptors lead to activation of SFKs, in part by exclusion of inhibitory phosphatases, preventing dephosphorylation of the activatory tyrosine. SFKs then phosphorylate the ITAM tyrosines, allowing Syk recruitment and activation (Poole et al. 1997). These two kinases then contribute to the phosphorylation of several adaptor molecules, including the integral membrane adaptor protein, linker for activation of T cells (LAT). Containing nine tyrosines, LAT acts as a scaffold around which a signalosome forms, which, in addition to other adaptor molecules (such as Gads, Grb2, SLP-76, ADAP and SKAP-HOM), also includes other tyrosine kinases (such as Btk and Tec), the lipid kinase phosphatidylinositol-3 kinase (PI3K, p85/p110) and the Vav family of guanine exchange factors (Pearce et al. 2002, 2004; Gross et al. 1999a; Atkinson et al. 2003; Quek et al. 1998; Hughes et al. 2008; Gibbins et al. 1998; Pasquet et al. 1999; Dutting et al. 2014; Jarvis et al. 2012). The end effector of this pathway is the activation of phospholipase C γ2 (PLCγ2) which, when activated, causes increased intracellular calcium via breakdown of phosphatidylinositol-(3,4,5)-trisphosphate (PIP_3) (Gross et al. 1999b). The rise in intracellular calcium results in platelet activation via secretion and integrin activation.

The signalling pathway of the hemITAM containing receptor CLEC-2 is largely identical downstream of Syk, with the exception of a lesser of a role for SLP-76, and the differential function of Btk noted above (Nicolson et al. 2018, 2021; Fuller et al. 2007). The significant difference is that the hemITAM sequence, which is essentially half of an ITAM sequence, is split over two molecules and, therefore, the tandem-SH2 domains of Syk cross-link a CLEC-2 dimer (Hughes et al. 2010a; Watson et al. 2009). The activation of Syk is also slightly different with a more prominent role for autophosphorylation, and evidence that Syk itself, not an SFK, is responsible for phosphorylating the hemITAM tyrosine (Hughes et al. 2013; Spalton et al. 2009). It has also been suggested that Btk may also play a role in the phosphorylation of Syk and the hemITAM (Manne et al. 2015). The hemITAM sequence also differs with the presence of a tri-acidic amino acid sequence immediately before the tyrosine (consensus (D/E)(D/E)(D/E)xYxxL) which is important for Syk binding (Hughes et al. 2013).

2.1.5 ITIM Pathways

An immunoreceptor tyrosine-based inhibitory motif (ITIM) and the related immunoreceptor tyrosine-based switch motif (ITSM) are amino acid sequences with many parallels with the (hem)ITAM sequence. They contain a single tyrosine residue in a YxxL motif which when phosphorylated allows the binding of SH2 domains (ITIM consensus (L/I/V/S)xYxx(L/V), ITSM consensus TxYxxV/I). Although these are single tyrosine-containing motifs, they are usually found in a pair, albeit separated by a less well-defined number of amino acids ranging from 15 to 30 residues (Daeron 1995; D'Ambrosio et al. 1995). Following ligand binding and SFK activation, Fyn and Lyn are able to phosphorylate these ITIM/ITSM tyrosine residues and allow binding of either the tyrosine phosphatases SH2 domain containing phosphatase-1 (SHP-1) and SHP-2, or the inositol phosphatases SH2 domain containing inositol phosphatase-1 (SHIP-1) and SHIP-2. SHP-1/2 have tandem-SH2 domains like Syk and can therefore bind to both tyrosines, whereas SHIP-1/2 have only a single SH2 domain (Billadeau and Leibson 2002).

As ITIMs recruit and allow activation of tyrosine and inositol phosphatases which largely function to deactivate the ITAM signalling pathway, their major role is considered to be inhibitory, acting in opposition to the activatory ITAM-containing receptors or, alternatively, in maintaining resting levels of activation in the absence of ITAM signalling. The ITSM however has been proposed to also have an activatory role in other cells via the adaptor protein SH2 domain protein 1A (SH2D1A) and CD150, although there is no evidence for these proteins in platelets (Sidorenko and Clark 2003). Other potentially activatory roles for ITIM/ITSM-containing receptors have been proposed in platelets, positively regulating integrin outside-in signalling, although the mechanisms are currently unknown (Mazharian et al. 2013; Alshahrani et al. 2016; Wee and Jackson 2005; Yip et al. 2016).

2.2 (hem)ITAM- and ITIM-Containing Receptors

2.2.1 GPVI and FcRγ Chain

Glycoprotein (GP) VI is a collagen receptor and member of the immunoglobulin (Ig) superfamily of receptors, containing two extracellular Ig domains, a transmembrane domain and a short cytoplasmic domain (Clemetson et al. 1999). The cytoplasmic tail contains binding sites for SFKs and calmodulin, and the transmembrane domain contains a crucial arginine residue which forms a salt bridge with the Fc receptor γ (FcRγ) chain (Bori-Sanz et al. 2003; Suzuki-Inoue et al. 2002; Clemetson et al. 1999; Berlanga et al. 2007; Locke et al. 2003; Andrews et al. 2002).

The FcRγ chain, expressed as a homodimer, contains the ITAM sequence and is required for surface expression of GPVI; FcRγ-deficient mice do not express GPVI at the platelet surface (Nieswandt et al. 2000). GPVI expression levels have been reported to range from 4,000 to 9,600 using both flow cytometric approaches with a range of antibodies, and by proteomics (Zeiler et al. 2014; Burkhart et al. 2012; Furihata et al. 2001; Best et al. 2003; Senis et al. 2009; Samaha et al. 2004; Dunster et al. 2020).

Under resting conditions, GPVI is present in both monomeric and dimeric forms (Horii et al. 2006; Clark et al. 2021; Jung et al. 2012). Collagen binding initiates higher order clustering of monomers and dimers which allows sustained signalling by preventing GPVI from activation-induced shedding (Pallini et al. 2021; Poulter et al. 2017). The degree of clustering appears to correlate with the degree of platelet activation under flow conditions with larger clusters being required for thrombus formation and phosphatidyl-serine exposure (Jooss et al. 2023).

GPVI binding to collagen is via the specific epitope of GPO (glycine-proline-hydroxyproline) (Knight et al. 1999). The spacing of these GPO sequences allows clustering of GPVI when binding to collagen fibres. A synthetic collagen-related peptide (CRP) which contains 10 consecutive GPO repeats is a particularly potent, GPVI-specific platelet agonist (Asselin et al. 1997; Morton et al. 1995). In addition to these, a number of other, non-collagen-based ligands have been described for GPVI. Perhaps the most interesting clinically is fibrin. Fibrin, and in mice both fibrin and fibrinogen, has been shown to activate platelets via GPVI, and not $\alpha IIb\beta 3$ alone (Mangin et al. 2018; Alshehri et al. 2015a; Mammadova-Bach et al. 2015). It is proposed that this GPVI-fibrin interaction is important for thrombus growth and stability, but not for the initiation of a thrombus, which is via GPVI-collagen, making it a prime candidate for anti-platelet therapies as it could reduce thrombus size, without increasing bleeding risk (Alshehri et al. 2015a; Mangin et al. 2023). Other GPVI endogenous ligands include laminin, galectin-9, reelin, histones, and adiponectin, although biological roles for these are less well defined, and exogenous ligands include convulxin (snake venom toxin), JAQ1 (antibody) and diesel particles (Clemetson et al. 1999; Zhi et al. 2022; Inoue et al. 2006; Alshehri et al. 2015b; Krueger et al. 2020; Riba et al. 2008).

2.2.2 FcγRIIA

FcγRIIA (CD32A) is a member of the Ig superfamily, containing two extracellular Ig domains, a transmembrane domain and a cytoplasmic tail which contains its ITAM sequence. FcγRIIA is a low-affinity receptor for immunoglobulin G (IgG) and as such contributes to platelet activation in a number of immune conditions. For example, COVID-19 related thrombosis, heparin-induced thrombotic thrombocytopenia (HITT), vaccine-induced thrombotic thrombocytopenia (VITT) all involve platelet activation via FcγRIIA (Greinacher et al. 2021; Favaloro et al. 2022; Meier et al. 2024; Smith et al. 2021; Bye et al. 2021; McKenzie and Reilly 2004; Reilly et al. 2001).

Interestingly, FcγRIIA is only found in the genome of humans and other primates and is expressed at a relatively low level compared to GPVI, with 1,000 copies per platelet (Burkhart et al. 2012). It is absent from the mouse genome, although a humanised mouse model has been developed (McKenzie and Reilly 2004; Reilly et al. 2001).

In addition to a role as an IgG receptor, it has also been proposed that FcγRIIA contributes to $\alpha IIb\beta 3$ signalling, providing an ITAM for outside-in signalling by the integrin, although in this model, it is not clear how the two receptors link nor what the ligand for FcγRIIA might be (Boylan et al. 2008; Zhi et al. 2013). Others have argued that $\alpha IIb\beta 3$ signalling is ITAM independent (Hughes et al. 2015).

2.2.3 CLEC-2

C-type lectin 2 (CLEC-2) is a C-type lectin/C-type lectin-like domain (CTL/CTLD) superfamily member. It is a type-2 membrane protein, with a short N-terminal cytoplasmic domain which contains the hemITAM sequence, a single transmembrane domain and a C-terminal extracellular domain which is comprised of a stalk and a CTLD. The expression level of CLEC-2 varied by an order of magnitude between human and mice, with 3,700 copies present on human platelets and 41,000 copies on mouse platelets (Zeiler et al. 2014; Burkhart et al. 2012). Similar to GPVI, under resting conditions, CLEC-2 is found as a mixture of monomers and dimers, with ligand binding inducing higher order clustering (Hughes et al. 2010a; Pollitt et al. 2014). For CLEC-2, this is important for Syk binding to the hemITAM and cross-linking the dimers (Hughes et al. 2010a, 2015).

When first discovered on monocytes, dendritic cells and granulocytes, CLEC-2 was an orphan receptor, and when later found on platelets, it was as a receptor for the snake venom toxin rhodocytin (Colonna et al. 2000; Suzuki-Inoue et al. 2006). The endogenous ligand for CLEC-2 was first described the following year; podoplanin (aggrus, T1α, GP36, GP38) is expressed in some tumour cells, kidney podocytes and on the surface of lymphatic endothelial cells (Suzuki-Inoue et al. 2007; Christou et al. 2008). This expression on lymphatic rather than vascular endothelial cells underlies a major biological role for CLEC-2 in embryonic development of the vascular system. Mice lacking CLEC-2, podoplanin or several of the key downstream signalling proteins all phenocopy each other with a lack of separation between the vascular and lymphatic endothelium (Hughes et al. 2015; Finney et al. 2012; Fu et al. 2008; Ramirez et al. 2003; Schacht et al. 2003; Ichise et al. 2009; Bertozzi et al. 2010; Turner et al. 1995; Hess et al. 2014). CLEC-2 (and GPVI) has also been shown to play a role in vascular integrity during inflammation (Boulaftali et al. 2013). It is unknown whether CLEC-2 and platelets play an equivalent role in these processes in humans, although the difference in expression levels between the species may suggest a lesser role for human CLEC-2.

CLEC-2 may also be important in the more established haemostatic roles for platelets, although the picture is less well defined than for other platelet receptors. CLEC-2 mediates platelet activation by podoplanin expressing tumour cells and may therefore contribute to some forms of cancer-associated thrombosis (CAT) (Suzuki-Inoue et al. 2007). CLEC-2 contributes to thrombosis driven by inflammation in a model of salmonella infection (Hitchcock et al. 2015). It also plays a role in venous thrombosis, although there are conflicting reports about a role in arterial thrombosis which likely reflect differences in the mouse models used (Smith et al. 2024; Hughes et al. 2010b; Suzuki-Inoue et al. 2010; May et al. 2009). A role for CLEC-2 in thrombosis and haemostasis is difficult to explain as its ligand, podoplanin, is not present in blood or blood vessels. Other ligands, however, have been described in recent years. Haemin (the oxidised form of haem) is another endogenous ligand for CLEC-2, which may be released from erythrocytes at sites of damage or inflammation and may regulate some of these other processes (Oishi et al. 2021). Other exogenous ligands for CLEC-2 include katacine, fucoidan and dextran sulphate (Moran et al. 2022; Manne et al. 2013).

2.2.4 PECAM-1

Platelet endothelial cell adhesion module-1 (PECAM-1, CD31) is an Ig superfamily member, containing six extracellular Ig domains, a single transmembrane domain and a cytoplasmic domain containing an ITIM and ITSM sequence. It is expressed on both endothelial cells and on the platelet surface, with 9,400 copies on human platelets and 5,500 copies on mouse platelets, although studies using antibodies have suggested a range of expression of 5,000–17,500 per platelet in people, which may underlie an individual's platelet responsiveness and therefore thrombotic risk (Zeiler et al. 2014; Burkhart et al. 2012; Cramer et al. 1994; Mazurov et al. 1991; Metzelaar et al. 1991). Expression has also been found on other white blood cells (Albelda et al. 1990).

Activation of PECAM-1 is via a homotypic interaction, meaning that it can be activated by platelet-platelet binding or by platelet-endothelial cell binding. Activation of PECAM-1 weakly inhibits the (hem)ITAM-containing receptors in addition to other platelet activation receptors, namely the ADP and thrombin receptors (Jones et al. 2009a). Furthermore, PECAM-1 activation also inhibited thrombus formation in vitro, and its absence in knockout mice results in a more rapid thrombus growth rate in vivo (Jones et al. 2009a; Falati et al. 2006). PECAM-1 also mediates internalisation of GPIbα through αIIbβ3-dependent and AKT/protein kinase B/glycogen synthase kinase-3/dynamin-dependent mechanisms (Jones et al. 2014a). It should be noted that, compared to other platelet inhibitors such as NO or PGI_2, this inhibitory effect is small, being overcome with higher agonist concentrations. Some researchers have reported no overall effect on thrombus formation but do report effects on platelet count suggesting a role in megakaryocytes (Dhanjal et al. 2007a, b).

2.2.5 G6b-B

G6b-B is an Ig superfamily member, containing a single extracellular Ig domain, a single transmembrane domain and a cytoplasmic domain containing an ITIM and ITSM sequence. It is highly expressed on both mouse (29,600 copies) and human (13,700 copies) platelets (Zeiler et al. 2014; Burkhart et al. 2012).

Uniquely, G6b-B is tyrosine phosphorylated on its ITIM/ITSM under resting conditions, which suggests a role in the maintenance of resting conditions in the platelet (Mori et al. 2008). However, activation with antibodies is still able to inhibit platelet activation by (hem)ITAM receptors, suggesting that this level of resting phosphorylation is not maximal, or that clustering of the receptor may also be an important step (Newland et al. 2007).

G6b-B mice are macrothrombocytopenic (platelet count is reduced and platelets are larger), highlighting a role for G6b-B in platelet production (Mazharian et al. 2012). Interestingly, the authors found that the platelets from G6b-B knockout mice were hyperactive in response to a CLEC-2 (hemITAM) ligand, consistent with a negative regulatory role for G6b-B, but in response to GPVI (ITAM) ligands, the platelets were severely inhibited. This correlated with a lack of surface expression of GPVI, which was mediated by enhanced metalloproteinase levels in the megakaryocytes which led to increased GPVI shedding (Mazharian et al. 2012; Geer et al. 2018). These observations show a major role for G6b-B in maintaining appropriate levels of activation during thrombopoiesis.

Endogenous ligands for G6b-B are the glycosaminoglycans, heparin and heparan sulphate. Perlecan, a basement membrane protein with three long heparan sulphate chains, is also able to activate G6b-B (Vogtle et al. 2019). These ligands induced the higher-order clustering of G6b-B which was required to activate the downstream phosphatases, SHP-1 and SHP-2 (Vogtle et al. 2019).

2.2.6 TLT-1, CEACAM1/2 and LILRB/PIRB

TREM-like transcript-1 (TLT-1) is an Ig superfamily member, containing a single extracellular Ig domain, a single transmembrane domain and a cytoplasmic domain containing a single ITIM. It is expressed in the membrane of α-granules at high levels (14,200 copies in humans and 155,000 copies in mouse), a portion of which is brought to the plasma membrane platelet activation, with a remainder sequestered in the granulomere (central region of the platelet) (Zeiler et al. 2014; Burkhart et al. 2012; Washington et al. 2004).

TLT-1 is currently an orphan receptor, but some biological function has been observed in a knockout mouse model, where the platelets showed mildly reduced platelet aggregation and longer bleeding times, as well as increased markers of inflammation-driven thrombosis (Washington et al. 2009). This suggests a potential role in limiting the extent of platelet activity in thromboinflammation.

Leukocyte immunoglobulin-like receptor B2 (LILRB2), and the mouse orthologue, paired immunoglobulin-like receptor B (PIRB), is an Ig superfamily member containing four extracellular Ig domains, a single transmembrane domain and a cytoplasmic domain containing a single ITIM sequence. While its expression is reported in platelets, it is not detectable in proteomic databases (Zeiler et al. 2014; Burkhart et al. 2012).

There is some evidence that LILRB/PIRB can regulate platelet formation, with knockout mice having increased platelet counts, as well as increased platelet responses to ITAM and integrin ligands (Fan et al. 2014). The authors also confirmed that angiopoietin-like protein 2 (ANGPTL2) is a ligand for this receptor, although other suggested ligands include MHC class I and β-2 microglobulin (Zheng et al. 2012; Burshtyn and Morcos 2016; Borges et al. 1997).

Carcinoembryonic antigen-related cell adhesion molecule 1 (CEACAM-1) and CEACAM-2 are Ig superfamily members, each containing four extracellular Ig domains, a single transmembrane domain and a cytoplasmic domain containing an ITIM and ITSM sequence. While their expression has been reported in platelets, coverage in proteomic databases is poor and there is disagreement with RNA-seq analysis as to which forms are expressed in human versus mouse (Zeiler et al. 2014; Burkhart et al. 2012; Rowley et al. 2011). It can be assumed, however, that their expression levels are low.

Activation of CEACAM-1/2 is mostly likely a homotypic interaction, although other ligands have been suggested, including interactions with other receptors and microbes (Kim et al. 2019). Both receptors have been shown to play a small inhibitory role downstream of (hem)ITAM receptors in platelet aggregation studies, and, conversely, downstream of integrin αIIbβ3, there is evidence for an activatory role (Alshahrani et al. 2014, 2016; Yip et al. 2016; Wong et al. 2009). In in vivo models of thrombus formation, deletion of these receptors results in thrombi which are larger and more stable (Alshahrani et al. 2014; Wong et al. 2009).

2.2.7 LAIR-1

Leukocyte-associated immunoglobulin-like receptor-1 (LAIR-1) is an Ig superfamily member, containing a single extracellular Ig domain, a single transmembrane domain and a cytoplasmic domain containing an ITIM and ITSM sequence. Unlike the other ITIM receptors, it is expressed on megakaryocytes, but not detectable on platelets, suggesting a downregulation of expression during platelet genesis (Steevels et al. 2010).

LAIR-1 is a collagen receptor which appears to play a reciprocal role to GPVI. LAIR-1 expression is high in megakaryocytes while GPVI is low, which presents a mechanism for preventing collagen stimulation of the maturing megakaryocytes. During maturation and platelet production, LAIR-1 expression reduces while GPVI expression increases, producing activatable platelets. LAIR-1 knockout mice have hyperactive platelets which highlights this role for LAIR-1 in setting the resting levels of activation of platelets during their formation (Smith et al. 2017).

3 Adhesion Receptors

3.1 Integrin αIIbβ3

Integrin αIIbβ3 (GPIIb/IIIa) is abundant on the surface of platelets, with approximately 80,000 copies per platelet (Wagner et al. 1996) In resting platelets, αIIbβ3 is maintained predominantly in a closed conformation state, with a low affinity for its ligands, such as fibrinogen, fibrin, vWF, fibronectin, and vitronectin, by the interaction of α and β subunit transmembrane domains and a membrane-proximal GFFKR region and HDRxE region in the cytoplasmic tails of the α and β subunits, respectively (Lau et al. 2009; Adair and Yeager 2002; Gottschalk 2005). Following platelet activation, "inside-out" signalling results in a change in the conformation of αIIbβ3 first to an intermediate state and then to the fully activated, extended form, exposing the ligand-binding metal ion-dependent adhesion site (MIDAS), allowing the binding of ligands containing an Arg-Gly-Asp (RGD) motif or the AGDV sequence in the fibrinogen γ-chain C terminus (Sanchez-Cortes and Mrksich 2009; Litvinov et al. 2016). The binding of multivalent ligands and the clustering of αIIbβ3 promote "outside-in" signalling, propagating further platelet activation (Ginsberg et al. 2005). The combination of binding of multivalent ligands, such as fibrinogen, to αIIbβ3 and subsequent changes resulting from outside-in signalling is essential for platelet aggregation, stable thrombus formation and the transmission of force through thrombi (Coller and Shattil 2008; Durrant et al. 2017).

3.1.1 Inside-Out Signalling

The activation of αIIbβ3 ultimately results from the binding of Talin and Kindlin to the C-terminal of the β3 subunit, causing the separation of the cytoplasmic tails of αIIb and β3 (Moser et al. 2009).

Talin comprises a head domain, made up of an F0 domain and a FERM domain with three subdomains F1, F2 and F3, and a flexible rod domain (Critchley 2009). In its resting state, the rod domain of the tail both masks the F3 domain and, due to its negative charge, repels Talin from the platelet membrane (Goksoy et al. 2008; Song et al. 2012). However, upon platelet stimulation, the rapid rise in cytosolic calcium activates CalDAG-GEFI, which in turn converts Ras-related protein 1 (RAP1), a Ras subfamily member, from its inactive guanosine diphosphate (GDP) to its active guanosine triphosphate (GTP) form (Crittenden et al. 2004; Stefanini et al. 2009), RAP1-GDP binds to Talin leading to the unmasking of the phosphotyrosine-binding (PTB) subdomain F3 domain which in turn binds to the NPxY motif, and forms a salt bridge with the membrane-proximal Asp (D723), in the cytoplasmic tail of β3, resulting in a conformational change to the active form of αIIbβ3 (Ginsberg et al. 2005; Calderwood et al. 2013). In resting platelets, RAP1 is maintained in the inactive GDP form by RAP-GAP-RASA3 and can be rapidly deactivated upon activation; however, signal downstream of ADP stimulated P2Y12, inactivates RASA3 enabling sustained RAP1 activation (Stefanini et al. 2015). Platelets contain approximately 200,000 copies of both RAP1 and Talin, as no RAP1 effector has been identified with a similarly high abundance, and Rap1-guanosine triphosphate–interacting adapter molecule (RIAM), a known effector of other integrins and in other cells, appears not to play a central role in the binding of talin to β3 in platelets (Su et al. 2015; Klapproth et al. 2015; Stritt et al. 2015), the direct activation of talin by RAP1 has been proposed (Lagarrigue et al. 2020).

Kindlin also plays a crucial role in the activation of αIIbβ3 and is capable of binding the cytoplasmic tail of β3. Mouse platelets lacking Kindlin 3 show severe platelet dysfunction (Moser et al. 2008). Kindlin contains a FERM domain in which the F3 domain shares a high level of homology with Talin, and the F2 subdomain is split by a pleckstrin homology (PH) domain (Kloeker et al. 2004) and binds predominantly to the membrane distal NxxY motif of β3 (Moser et al. 2008, 2009; Yates et al. 2012). Kindlin, unlike Talin, maybe incapable of activating αIIbβ3 on its own, suggesting a role as a co-activator enhancing Talin mediation in integrin activation, possibly through an interaction with the flexible rod domain of Talin and Paxillin to promote integrin clustering (Calderwood et al. 2013; Yates et al. 2012; Lu et al. 2022).

3.1.2 Outside-In Signalling

Around the cytoplasmic tail of αIIbβ3, dynamic clusters of more than 30 molecules interact to enable the transmission of force and to translate external stimuli into internal signals that regulate platelet activation (Ginsberg et al. 2005; Durrant et al. 2017). αIIbβ3 is linked to the platelet cytoskeleton through the cytoplasmic tail of β3, binding to talin, the rod domain of which contains binding sites for vinculin and actin (Ziegler et al. 2008; Carisey et al. 2013; Fong et al. 2021), and potentially through the filamin binding to the cytoplasmic tail of the αIIb subunit (Liu et al. 2023). This is an important axis through which force can be transmitted from platelet to platelet in a forming thrombus. It facilitates firm adhesion to the site of vascular damage, enabling platelets to resist the forces on a forming thrombus; preventing embolisation and providing the mechanism through which platelt coordinate contractile forces throughout a thrombus (Fong et al. 2021; Oshinowo et al. 2023; Stalker et al. 2014).

αIIbβ3 outside-in signalling involves an enormous array of signalling molecules (such as c-Src, Lyn, Syk) and adaptors (such as paxillin, ILK) that regulate signal transmission and maintain the integrity of the signalling cluster (Durrant et al. 2017; Xin et al. 2023; Jones et al. 2014b). Briefly, upon ligand binding to αIIbβ3 and integrin clustering, the Src family of kinases (SFKs) is activated, in part via $G\alpha_{13}$ bound to the β3 cytoplasmic tail (Arias-Salgado et al. 2003; Gong et al. 2010), leading to the activation of the tyrosine kinase Syk and the phosphorylation of downstream targets SLP-76 and Vav-family RhoGEFs (Obergfell et al. 2001, 2002; Pearce et al. 2007).; The tyrosine phosphorylation of the β3-integrin tail at Tyr 747 and Tyr 759, also provides docking sites for adaptor molecules such as growth factor receptor-bound protein 2 (Grb2) and SH2 domain-containing-transforming protein C1 (Shc) (Jenkins et al. 1998; Law et al. 1996). The autophosphorylation and the activation of FAK occurs through a PKC and actin polymerisation dependent mechanism (Guidetti et al. 2019); and the phosphorylation of PLCγ2 leading to the formation of DAG and IP_3, PKC activation, and further increases in cytosolic calcium providing a positive feedback to cause the activation of more αIIbβ3 (Wonerow et al. 2003).

3.2 Other Platelet Integrins

Platelets also express three β1-containing integrin, α2β1 (a collagen receptor, also known as GPIa-IIa), α5β1 (a fibronectin receptor) and α6β1 (a laminin receptor), and one other β3-containing integrin αvβ3 (primarily a vitronectin receptor) (Janus-Bell and Mangin 2023). Of these, α2β1 is the most abundant (3,000–5,000 copies per platelet) and the most studied (Janus-Bell and Mangin 2023). Whilst α2β1 is not essential for platelet binding to collagen, variation in the copy number of α2β1 on the surface of platelets leads to significant variation in platelet adhesion to collagen in human, and mice with platelet deficiency in α2β1 showed reduced thrombus formation under shear conditions (Kunicki et al. 1993; He et al. 2003; Nieswandt et al. 2001; Gruner et al. 2003). Like αIIbβ3, conformational change of α2β1 is required for efficient ligand binding, which is dependent on the binding of talin and kindlin, without which platelet binding to collagen is defective (Moser et al. 2008; Harburger et al. 2009); however, initial interaction between collagen and α2β1 can occur prior to activation (Nissinen et al. 2012). Furthermore, inside-out signalling leading to full activation of α2β1 is dependent on outside-in signalling following ligand binging to αIIbβ3 (Van de Walle et al. 2007).

As with other integrins, α2β1 can also regulate platelet response through outside-in signalling. Src, Syk, SLP-76, Rac1, PLCγ2, FAK and plasma membrane calcium ATPase (PMCA) are all involved in signalling down stream of α2β1, leading to calcium mobilisation, Rap1 activation and Pyk2-mediated PI3Kβ activation (Inoue et al. 2003; Guidetti et al. 2009; Consonni et al. 2012).

3.3 GPIb-IX-V Complex

Present at approximately 25,000 copies per platelet, the physiological importance of GPIb-IX-V has long been known through the study of patients with the bleeding disorder Bernard-Soulier platelets who lack or have functionally compromised GPIb-IX-V (Nurden et al. 1981). The GPIbα and GPIbβ subunits are covalently connected in a ratio of 1:2; this complex associates non-covalently with another subunit, GPIX, in a 1:1 ratio (Berndt et al. 1985). Each subunit is a transmembrane protein containing leucine-rich motifs in their extracellular domains and a short cytoplasmic tail (Bendas and Schlesinger 2022). GPV, a further glycoprotein containing a leucine-rich motif, also associates weakly with this complex and has been shown to be important in the efficient expression of GPIb-IX on the platelet surface (Meyer and Fox 1995; Modderman et al. 1992).

3.3.1 GPIb-IX-V Ligands

Principally known for its binding to vWF, which tethers platelets to the site of vascular injury, the GPIB-IX-V complex, through GPIbα, can bind an array of proteins that regulate platelet adhesion, activation and coagulation; these include VWF, thrombospondin-1, P-selectin, thrombin, the heavy chain of high-molecular-weight kininogen and the coagulation factors XI and XII (Romo et al. 1999; Baglia et al. 2004; Bradford et al. 2000; Joseph et al. 1999; Jurk et al. 2003; Ruggeri et al. 1999; Zhang et al. 2022).

3.3.2 GPIb-IX-V Signalling

The cytoplasmic tail of GPIbα binds to filamin, which links it to the actin cytoskeleton enabling the transmission of force during platelet tethering and adhesion, and signalling via Syk, Cdc42 and RhoA (Zhang et al. 2022; Andrews and Fox 1991; Dutting et al. 2017). This mechanical force has been shown to alter the juxta membrane, mechanosensory domain, of GPIbα and altered calcium signalling (Zhang et al. 2015; Ju et al. 2016; Mazzucato et al. 2002). The binding of 14–3-3 to the cytoplasmic tail of GPIbα has been shown to be essential for GPIb-IX-V mediated integrin activation following vWF binding and for the cooperative signalling between PAR receptors and GPIb-IX-V during thrombi activation of platelets, in part through the formation of a complex with phosphoinositide 3-kinase (PI3K) (Zhang et al. 2022; Munday et al. 2000; Yin et al. 2008; Estevez et al. 2016).

3.4 P-selectin

P-selectin (CD62p) is expressed on the surface of platelets following α-granule secretion (Liu et al. 2010). Upon surface expression P-selectin, does not cause platelet signalling, but can bind P-selectin glycoprotein ligand-1 (PSGL-1) promoting leukocyte rolling, activation, and neutrophil extracellular traps (NETs) formation (Yang et al. 1999; Li et al. 2024; Cappenberg et al. 2022).

4 G-Protein Coupled Receptors (GPCRs)

The human genome encodes for approximately 950 different GPCRs (Takeda et al. 2002). Associated with a wide range of physiological functions, approximately 35% of approved drugs target this family of receptors (Salon et al. 2011; Sriram and Insel 2018). Platelets express several GPCRs that regulate platelet activation, aggregation and their interaction with other cells of the blood vasculature. These receptors respond to various soluble ligands, including thrombin, adenosine diphosphate (ADP) and prostaglandins. Heterozygous loss of function variations in GPCRs have been shown to affect platelet agonist responses, with some variations associated with patients with inherited platelet function disorders (Jones et al. 2015).

GPCRs are integral membrane cell surface proteins that span the membrane seven times with three extracellular loops and three intracellular loops. The C terminus is associated with guanine nucleotide binding proteins (G-proteins) (Rosenbaum et al. 2009). G-proteins are heterotrimers with α, β and γ subunits. In the inactive state, the Gα is associated with GDP and tightly associates with the βγ subunit. Upon activation, GDP is exchanged with GTP. This releases the α and βγ subunits for interactions with downstream effectors. A single GPCR can be associated with multiple G-proteins which mediate different intracellular signalling pathways. This coupling of GPCRs with multiple G-proteins may support the fine-tuning of platelet responses. However, redundancy between G-proteins may be one of the reasons why the targeting of the receptor has had more success in the development of anti-platelet therapies than targeting the G-proteins and downstream signalling pathways.

Serine/threonine phosphorylation of GPCRs by kinases at the C terminus enhances the affinity for adapter proteins known as arrestins. Arrestins fine-tune platelet responses and play a critical role in platelet GPCR signalling by regulating receptor desensitisation, internalisation and downstream signalling pathways. Arrestins bind to the phosphorylated GPCR and prevent further G-protein activation and attenuate the initial signal (Hutchinson et al. 2020). Arrestins also facilitate receptor endocytosis via clathrin-coated pits, modulating receptor recycling (Shenoy and Lefkowitz 2011). Based on proteomic data, human platelets express both β-arrestin-1 (arrestin-2) and β-arrestin-2 (arrestin-3), with β-arrestin-1 being the predominant form (Burkhart et al. 2012). Platelet studies in mice deficient in arrestins support the regulatory role of arrestins by having enhanced responses to multiple agonists (Hutchinson et al. 2020; Chaudhary et al. 2021). However, arrestin-3 deficiency additionally had impaired responses to thromboxane A_2 receptor (TP) receptor activation, suggesting that arrestin-3 may differentially regulate GPCR signalling by having both activatory and inhibitory actions in platelets (Hutchinson et al. 2020).

4.1 Protease-Activated Receptors (PARs)

Protease-activated receptors (PARs) play a crucial role in thrombin-mediated platelet activation. Thrombin is a key protease in the coagulation system generated when tissue factor exposure, following vascular endothelial damage, triggers the activation of coagulation factors in the plasma. Species-specific differences exist with respect to PAR expression. Human platelets express PAR1 and PAR4, whereas mouse platelets express PAR3 and PAR4 (Kahn et al. 1999). The way the mouse PAR3 and PAR4 interact with each other differs to how human PAR1 and PAR4 facilitate thrombin-induced platelet activation. PAR-1 is a high-affinity thrombin receptor that triggers rapid platelet activation while PAR4 responds more slowly to thrombin but sustains the response (Kahn et al. 1999). Both PAR1 and PAR4 are capable of functioning in the absence of the other. In contrast, mouse PAR3 has been suggested to act as an essential co-receptor for PAR4 activation with loss of PAR3 rendering PAR4 unable to signal (Nakanishi-Matsui et al. 2000). Similarly, mouse platelets deficient in PAR4 are also not responsive to thrombin (Lee et al. 2022). Even though PAR1 may not be an essential co-receptor for PAR4, PAR1 and PAR4 have been demonstrated to form heterodimers where PAR1 has helper functionality in assisting PAR4 activation by thrombin (Leger et al. 2006).

Activation of the PARs occurs by proteolytic cleavage of the extracellular N-terminus which unmasks the cryptic tethered ligand of the receptor. This unmasking results in PAR activation by binding of the tethered ligand to the receptor's own ligand-binding pocket. Activation of the intracellular G-proteins, G_q and G_{12}/G_{13}, follows (Vu et al. 1991). G_q activates PLC-β which hydrolyses phosphatidylinositol 4,5-bisphosphate (PIP_2) to produce inositol 1,4,5-trisphosphate (IP_3) and diacylglycerol (DAG). This leads to calcium mobilisation and PKC activation. G_{12}/G_{13} activates RhoA which promotes cytoskeletal rearrangement and platelet shape change.

The sequence of the hexapeptide ligand of PAR1, SFLLRN, has been developed as a synthetic PAR1 peptide agonist called TRAP-6. TRAP-6 can activate PAR1 independently of receptor cleavage by thrombin, providing an experimental tool to study thrombin-mediated PAR1 platelet activation without causing fibrin formation in the presence of plasma (Vu et al. 1991; Hung et al. 1992).

4.2 Purinergic Receptors $P2Y_{12}$ and $P2Y_1$

Platelets express three purinergic receptors, two of which are GPCRs. Platelet purinergic GPCR signalling is mediated by $P2Y_{12}$ and $P2Y_1$ receptors and are activated by the purine nucleotide ADP. Platelet-dense granules contain high concentrations of ADP, which is released upon platelet activation. Additionally, damaged cells at sites of vascular injury also release ADP. This extracellular ADP acts in both an autocrine and paracrine manner to activate platelets, amplifying the recruitment and aggregation process essential for thrombus formation. The full platelet aggregation response to ADP requires the combined activation of $P2Y_1$ and $P2Y_{12}$ receptors. However, $P2Y_{12}$ activation also plays an important role in the potentiation of platelet secretion induced by several other platelet agonists (Dorsam and Kunapuli 2004).

The expression of $P2Y_{12}$ is largely limited to platelets with some expression in the nervous system. This limited tissue distribution is one of the reasons why antiplatelet drugs that target $P2Y_{12}$, such as Clopidogrel, Prasugrel and Ticagrelor, have been developed and used in the treatment and prevention of arterial thrombosis (Angiolillo et al. 2017). However, while $P2Y_{12}$ inhibitor therapies have been demonstrated to reduce major cardiovascular events in acute coronary syndrome patients, these drugs are associated with an increased bleeding risk (Porto et al. 2009).

In contrast, $P2Y_1$ has a broad tissue distribution and there are currently no clinically approved anti-platelet drugs that target this receptor. One reason for the lack of approved drugs may be the potential for unforeseen side effects in targeting $P2Y_1$. However, despite the broad tissue expression, mice deficient in $P2Y_1$ are viable and appear normal. These mice have an increased bleeding time but have reduced thrombosis when challenged (Fabre et al. 1999; Lenain et al. 2003). $P2Y_1$ small molecule inhibitors have also been shown to have anti-thrombotic activities in mouse models with only a moderate increase in bleeding time (Hechler et al. 2006).

The $P2Y_1$ receptor is coupled to G_q. Activation of the receptor results in activation of PLC-β leading to calcium mobilisation and PKC activation (Jin et al. 1998). This signalling pathway mediates ADP-induced platelet shape change and an initial wave of rapidly reversible aggregation. $P2Y_{12}$, however, is negatively coupled to adenylyl cyclase through G_i and mediates a sustained ADP-induced aggregation by the resultant decrease in cyclic adenosine monophosphate (cAMP) (Soulet et al. 2004). The positive response of decreased cAMP in platelets is in contrast to most other cells where decreased cAMP drives negative responses in cellular function.

Patients with homozygous frame shift mutations that result in truncated forms of $P2Y_{12}$ display clinical bleeding. The expression of suspected function causing mutations in patients have also been identified by their expression in cell lines. Point mutations, particularly in transmembrane 6 and extracellular loop 3, have been shown to impair $P2Y_{12}$-mediated signalling using this approach (Cattaneo 2011). Dysregulated ADP-mediated signalling has also been associated with disease with constitutively active $P2Y_{12}$ observed in diabetic patients (Hu et al. 2017).

4.3 Thromboxane A_2 Receptor (TP)

The thromboxane A_2 receptor (TP) is another important GPCR expressed on platelets. The TP receptor is important for promoting the amplification of platelet aggregation (Habib et al. 1999). This GPCR is activated by the prostanoid family member thromboxane A_2 (TXA_2) which is generated from arachidonic acid via the enzyme cyclooxygenase-1 (COX-1). TXA_2 has localised effects due to its short, approximately 30 s, half-life (Bhagwat et al. 1985; Murray and FitzGerald 1989). Mice deficient in the TP receptor are viable and appear normal. When challenged, these mice have prolonged bleeding times and reduced thrombosis (Cheng et al. 2002).

Aspirin, the most prescribed antiplatelet drug, is widely used alongside $P2Y_{12}$ inhibitors in dual antiplatelet therapy to reduce major cardiovascular events in high-risk patients (Kirkby et al. 2011). It indirectly inhibits TP receptor activation by blocking COX-1-mediated thromboxane A_2 (TXA_2) production. Of the two TP isoforms, the alpha, shorter isoform (TPαR), is expressed in human platelets (Habib et al. 1999). The receptor is coupled to G_q, which results in calcium mobilisation and PKC activation, and G_{12}/G_{13} proteins, which leads to RhoA-mediated cytoskeletal rearrangement and shape change (Knezevic et al. 1993; Djellas et al. 1999).

4.4 Inhibitory Prostaglandin Receptors

Not all signalling through platelet GPCRs results in platelet activation. The prostacyclin receptor (IP) acts as a counterbalance to pro-thrombotic signalling and is activated by prostacyclin (PGI_2), a prostanoid primarily released by the endothelium (Dutta-Roy and Sinha 1987). The IP receptor is coupled to G_s and when activated stimulates adenylyl cyclase, generating cAMP (Gorman et al. 1977). In platelets, elevated cAMP maintains platelets in a resting and non-aggregated state, in contrast to other cells where elevated cAMP results in positive effects. Elevated cAMP activates protein kinase A (PKA) which phosphorylates key platelet proteins involved in calcium release, integrin activation and granule release, resulting in inhibited platelet responsiveness. Mice deficient in the IP receptor have enhanced platelet activation, supporting its role in inhibiting platelet function (Cheng et al. 2002). The prostaglandin PGE2, via the prostaglandin E2 receptor subtype EP4, has also been shown to have inhibitory effects on human platelets. Activation of this GPCR leads to increased cAMP levels, resulting in inhibited platelet responsiveness (Philipose et al. 2010).

4.5 Other GPCRs Expressed in Platelets

In addition to GPCRs that have established roles in the regulation of platelet function, there are other less well-understood GPCRs expressed on platelets. These include GPCRs that respond to hormones, chemical messengers and lipids.

The hormone adrenaline, also known as epinephrin, signals through the α2A-adrenergic receptor and can potentiate collagen-mediated platelet activation (Golaszewska et al. 2021). It has been proposed that synergy between receptors may contribute to a prothrombotic state. The α2A-adrenergic receptor is coupled to G_i, and activation of the receptor enhances platelet activation and aggregation.

Serotonin, also known as 5-hydroxytryptamine (5-HT), is a chemical messenger that is taken up by platelets and stored in dense granules. Following platelet activation, serotonin is released and activates the platelet $5\text{-}HT_{2A}$ receptor. Activation of this Gq-coupled GPCR by serotonin promotes platelet aggregation (Berger et al. 2009). Mouse models that have impaired serotonin uptake or mice that lack peripheral serotonin have impaired aggregation and also have reduced recruitment of neutrophils at sites of inflammation (Duerschmied et al. 2013; Carneiro et al. 2008).

Platelet release various chemokines from their alpha-granules and platelets have been demonstrated to express functional chemokine receptors (Clemetson et al. 2000). One example is the chemokine receptor CXCR4 which allows platelets to respond to the chemokine SDF-1 (Wang et al. 1998). SDF-1 has been suggested to activate platelets via phosphatidylinositol 3-kinase and tyrosine kinase mediated mechanisms. It has been proposed that SDF-1 produced from atherosclerotic plaques acts as a platelet agonist contributing to the pathogenesis of atherosclerosis (Abi-Younes et al. 2000). Chemokine receptors couple to G_i proteins and have been shown to potentiate the impact of other platelet stimuli.

There is evidence to suggest that platelets may express lysophosphatidic acid (LPA) receptors at the mRNA level (Motohashi et al. 2000). The expression of LPA receptors at the protein level has been hindered due to lack of effective antibodies. However, experimental evidence using megakaryocyte cell lines suggests that LPA receptors have the potential to mediated function responses (Khandoga et al. 2011).

Several sphingosine-1-phosphate receptor (S1PR) subtypes have been suggested to be expressed on platelets. These are receptors for the bioactive signalling sphingolipid sphingosine 1-phosphate (S1P), levels of which are increased in obesity and diabetes (Liu et al. 2021).

Platelets express the VPAC1 receptor, which is activated by the peptides, pituitary adenylyl cyclase-activating polypeptide (PACAP) and vasointestinal peptide (VIP). Patients with increased plasma levels of PACAP present with a multi-organ disorder which includes bleeding and mild thrombocytopenia. VPAC1 is coupled to G_s which results in increased cAMP and reduced platelet responsiveness. Patients with increased plasma levels of PACAP have elevated cAMP which provides an explanation for their reduced platelet functionality (Freson et al. 2004).

4.6 Emerging Research Areas

It has been demonstrated that GPCRs have synergistic and inhibitory interactions with other GPCR family members. For example, PAR-1-mediated platelet aggregation is transient unless strengthened by P2Y12 or PAR4 signalling (Trumel et al. 1999; Covic et al. 2000). These interactions between GPCRs also extend to less well-understood GPCRs such as the S1PR receptors which have been demonstrated to modulate PAR1-mediated platelet activation (Liu et al. 2021). These actions may be regulated by the spatial distribution of GPCRs and how this changes following activation. Indeed, many platelet GPCRs can assemble into dimers and oligomers. These distributions have been suggested to play roles in regulating the strength of GPCR signalling, for example, by protecting the receptors from arrestin-mediated internalisation (Hardy et al. 2005).

Non-classical functions of platelet GPCRs have been identified. For example, there is some evidence to suggest that GPCRs can regulate platelet formation. Patients and mouse models with elevated levels of the activatory peptide, the agonist for VPAC1, present with thrombocytopenia. Additionally, the addition of VPAC1 agonists to CD34 positive cells inhibits megakaryocyte differentiation (Freson et al. 2008).

Innovative therapeutic agents known as pepducins have been developed to modulate GPCR activity. These small, lipidated cell-permeant peptides are derived from the intracellular loops of GPCRs and can allosterically modulate GPCR activity. One example is pepducin, PZ-128, that reversibly targets the third intracellular loop of the PAR1 receptor. PZ-128 was able to inhibit PAR1-mediated platelet aggregation and inhibit arterial thrombosis in preclinical models and has been taken forward to a Phase 2 trial (Zhang et al. 2012; Kuliopulos et al. 2020).

4.6.1 Other Significant Platelet Receptors

CD36, a scavenger receptor, is a multifunctional glycoprotein expressed on a variety of cell types, including platelets. It is highly expressed in human platelets with 16,700 copies per platelet detected by proteomics and increased CD36 levels have been associated with increased platelet function (Burkhart et al. 2012; Bye et al. 2025). CD36 can bind to multiple ligands, including oxidised low-density lipoprotein (oxLDL) and thrombospondin-1, resulting in platelet activation and platelet aggregation through the inhibition of cyclic nucleotide signalling (Magwenzi et al. 2015; Roberts et al. 2010). The heightened platelet activation under conditions of dyslipidaemia has been implicated in atherothrombosis and contributes to pro-inflammatory and pro-coagulant responses. The interaction of thrombospondin-1 and CD36 likely supports thrombus formation in a paracrine manner (Kuijpers et al. 2014). Multiple CD36 polymorphisms have been associated with an increased cardiovascular disease risk (Shu et al. 2022).

Platelet endothelial aggregation receptor 1 (PEAR1) is a surface receptor protein found on both platelets and endothelial cells. Human platelets express 1,800 copies and mouse platelets express approximately 3,200 copies (Zeiler et al. 2014; Burkhart et al. 2012). PEAR1 was highlighted in genome-wide association studies as being closely associated with cardiovascular disease, although the mechanisms linking polymorphisms to function are currently unknown (Jones et al. 2009b; Herrera-Galeano et al. 2008; Faraday et al. 2011; Pi et al. 2019; Stimpfle et al. 2018). PEAR1 has a large extracellular domain comprising 15 epidermal growth factor (EGF)-like domain repeats, a single transmembrane domain and a cytoplasmic tail. It was identified in platelets as a protein which, upon platelet aggregation, is tyrosine phosphorylated on its cytoplasmic YxxM motif – a binding site for the SH2 domain of the p110 subunit of PI3K (Nanda et al. 2005). The first ligand identified for PEAR1 was Fc receptor ε Iα (FcεRIα), suggesting a cell-cell interaction, but FcεRIα alone does not induce platelet aggregation, instead synergising with other platelet agonists (Sun et al. 2015). Since this report, other ligands have been described, all of which are negatively charged proteoglycans and sulphated polysaccharides (Kardeby et al. 2019, 2023; Vandenbriele et al. 2016). Amongst these are heparin and heparin proteoglycan-mimetics, suggesting interesting parallels with G6b-B, which has also been reported to be stimulated by similar proteins (see above). As these proposed PEAR1 ligands can all be found in mast cells, it has been proposed that PEAR1 plays a more important role in inflammation rather than thrombosis, which is also supported by the finding that PEAR1 knockout mice have normal platelet function (Criel et al. 2016).

5 Conclusion

This chapter explores platelet receptors, their associated signalling pathways and their diverse roles in the pathophysiological regulation of platelet function. Activatory and inhibitory pathways work together to maintain a balance between haemostasis and thrombosis. These enable platelets to respond to stimuli, activating in a rapid and coordinated manner in response to vascular damage while preventing inappropriate and excessive activation, which is essential for maintaining platelets in a resting state and preventing vessel occlusion. This balance maintains vascular integrity while preventing both excessive bleeding and pathological thrombosis.

It is also becoming increasingly clear that platelet receptors do not function in isolation and cannot be viewed as completely independent pathways. The spatial and temporal regulation of multiple receptors works in concert to regulate platelet activation and responses to different stimuli, and understanding this complexity is essential for designing new treatments. The current arsenal of anti-platelet therapies targets only a small number of the receptors and signalling proteins discussed in this chapter. But as we present here, there is a rich vein of potential targets for novel anti-platelet therapies and the development of targeted or personalised approaches for the treatment of thrombotic and cardiovascular diseases.

References

Abi-Younes S, Sauty A, Mach F, Sukhova GK, Libby P, Luster AD (2000) The stromal cell-derived factor-1 chemokine is a potent platelet agonist highly expressed in atherosclerotic plaques. Circ Res 86(2):131–138

Adair BD, Yeager M (2002) Three-dimensional model of the human platelet integrin alpha IIbbeta 3 based on electron cryomicroscopy and x-ray crystallography. Proc Natl Acad Sci USA 99(22): 14059–14064

Albelda SM, Oliver PD, Romer LH, Buck CA (1990) EndoCAM: a novel endothelial cell-cell adhesion molecule. J Cell Biol 110(4):1227–1237

Alevriadou BR, Moake JL, Turner NA, Ruggeri ZM, Folie BJ, Phillips MD et al (1993) Real-time analysis of shear-dependent thrombus formation and its blockade by inhibitors of von Willebrand factor binding to platelets. Blood 81(5):1263–1276

Alshahrani MM, Yang E, Yip J, Ghanem SS, Abdallah SL, deAngelis AM et al (2014) CEACAM2 negatively regulates hemi (ITAM-bearing) GPVI and CLEC-2 pathways and thrombus growth in vitro and in vivo. Blood 124(15):2431–2441

Alshahrani MM, Kyriacou RP, O'Malley CJ, Heinrich G, Najjar SM, Jackson DE (2016) CEACAM2 positively regulates integrin alpha(IIb)beta(3)-mediated platelet functions. Platelets 27(8):743–750

Alshehri OM, Hughes CE, Montague S, Watson SK, Frampton J, Bender M et al (2015a) Fibrin activates GPVI in human and mouse platelets. Blood 126(13):1601–1608

Alshehri OM, Montague S, Watson S, Carter P, Sarker N, Manne BK et al (2015b) Activation of glycoprotein VI (GPVI) and C-type lectin-like receptor-2 (CLEC-2) underlies platelet activation by diesel exhaust particles and other charged/hydrophobic ligands. Biochem J 468(3):459–473

Andrews RK, Fox JE (1991) Interaction of purified actin-binding protein with the platelet membrane glycoprotein Ib-IX complex. J Biol Chem 266(11):7144–7147

Andrews RK, Suzuki-Inoue K, Shen Y, Tulasne D, Watson SP, Berndt MC (2002) Interaction of calmodulin with the cytoplasmic domain of platelet glycoprotein VI. Blood 99(11):4219–4221

Angiolillo DJ, Rollini F, Storey RF, Bhatt DL, James S, Schneider DJ et al (2017) International Expert Consensus on Switching Platelet P2Y12 Receptor–Inhibiting Therapies. Circulation 136(20):1955–1975

Arias-Palomo E, Recuero-Checa MA, Bustelo XR, Llorca O (2007) 3D structure of Syk kinase determined by single-particle electron microscopy. Biochim Biophys Acta 1774(12): 1493–1499

Arias-Salgado EG, Lizano S, Sarkar S, Brugge JS, Ginsberg MH, Shattil SJ (2003) Src kinase activation by direct interaction with the integrin beta cytoplasmic domain. Proc Natl Acad Sci USA 100(23):13298–13302

Asselin J, Gibbins JM, Achison M, Lee YH, Morton LF, Farndale RW et al (1997) A collagen-like peptide stimulates tyrosine phosphorylation of syk and phospholipase C gamma2 in platelets independent of the integrin alpha2beta1. Blood 89(4):1235–1242

Atkinson BT, Ellmeier W, Watson SP (2003) Tec regulates platelet activation by GPVI in the absence of Btk. Blood 102(10):3592–3599

Baglia FA, Shrimpton CN, Emsley J, Kitagawa K, Ruggeri ZM, Lopez JA et al (2004) Factor XI interacts with the leucine-rich repeats of glycoprotein Ibalpha on the activated platelet. J Biol Chem 279(47):49323–49329

Bendas G, Schlesinger M (2022) The GPIb-IX complex on platelets: insight into its novel physiological functions affecting immune surveillance, hepatic thrombopoietin generation, platelet clearance and its relevance for cancer development and metastasis. Exp Hematol Oncol 11(1):19

Bennett JS (2001) Platelet-fibrinogen interactions. Ann N Y Acad Sci 936:340–354

Berger M, Gray JA, Roth BL (2009) The expanded biology of serotonin. Annu Rev Med 60:355–366

Berlanga O, Bori-Sanz T, James JR, Frampton J, Davis SJ, Tomlinson MG et al (2007) Glycoprotein VI oligomerization in cell lines and platelets. J Thromb Haemost 5(5):1026–1033

Berndt MC, Gregory C, Kabral A, Zola H, Fournier D, Castaldi PA (1985) Purification and preliminary characterization of the glycoprotein Ib complex in the human platelet membrane. Eur J Biochem 151(3):637–649

Berrou E, Soukaseum C, Favier R, Adam F, Elaib Z, Kauskot A et al (2018) A mutation of the human EPHB2 gene leads to a major platelet functional defect. Blood 132(19):2067–2077

Bertozzi CC, Schmaier AA, Mericko P, Hess PR, Zou Z, Chen M et al (2010) Platelets regulate lymphatic vascular development through CLEC-2-SLP-76 signaling. Blood 116(4):661–670

Best D, Senis YA, Jarvis GE, Eagleton HJ, Roberts DJ, Saito T et al (2003) GPVI levels in platelets: relationship to platelet function at high shear. Blood 102(8):2811–2818

Bevers EM, Comfurius P, van Rijn JL, Hemker HC, Zwaal RF (1982) Generation of prothrombin-converting activity and the exposure of phosphatidylserine at the outer surface of platelets. Eur J Biochem 122(2):429–436

Bhagwat SS, Hamann PR, Still WC, Bunting S, Fitzpatrick FA (1985) Synthesis and structure of the platelet aggregation factor thromboxane A2. Nature 315(6019):511–513

Billadeau DD, Leibson PJ (2002) ITAMs versus ITIMs: striking a balance during cell regulation. J Clin Invest 109(2):161–168

Borges L, Hsu ML, Fanger N, Kubin M, Cosman D (1997) A family of human lymphoid and myeloid Ig-like receptors, some of which bind to MHC class I molecules. J Immunol 159(11): 5192–5196

Bori-Sanz T, Inoue KS, Berndt MC, Watson SP, Tulasne D (2003) Delineation of the region in the glycoprotein VI tail required for association with the Fc receptor gamma-chain. J Biol Chem 278(38):35914–35922
Boulaftali Y, Hess PR, Getz TM, Cholka A, Stolla M, Mackman N et al (2013) Platelet ITAM signaling is critical for vascular integrity in inflammation. J Clin Invest 123(2):908–916
Boylan B, Gao C, Rathore V, Gill JC, Newman DK, Newman PJ (2008) Identification of FcgammaRIIa as the ITAM-bearing receptor mediating alphaIIbbeta3 outside-in integrin signaling in human platelets. Blood 112(7):2780–2786
Bradford HN, Pixley RA, Colman RW (2000) Human factor XII binding to the glycoprotein Ib-IX-V complex inhibits thrombin-induced platelet aggregation. J Biol Chem 275(30):22756–22763
Brdicka T, Kadlecek TA, Roose JP, Pastuszak AW, Weiss A (2005) Intramolecular regulatory switch in ZAP-70: analogy with receptor tyrosine kinases. Mol Cell Biol 25(12):4924–4933
Burkhart JM, Vaudel M, Gambaryan S, Radau S, Walter U, Martens L et al (2012) The first comprehensive and quantitative analysis of human platelet protein composition allows the comparative analysis of structural and functional pathways. Blood 120(15):e73–e82
Burshtyn DN, Morcos C (2016) The expanding spectrum of ligands for leukocyte Ig-like receptors. J Immunol 196(3):947–955
Bye AP, Hoepel W, Mitchell JL, Jegouic S, Loureiro S, Sage T et al (2021) Aberrant glycosylation of anti-SARS-CoV-2 spike IgG is a prothrombotic stimulus for platelets. Blood 138(16): 1481–1489
Bye AP, Kriek N, Kempster C, Dunster JL, Mitchell JL, Sage T et al (2025) TRIPLE score: GPVI and CD36 expression predict a prothrombotic platelet function phenotype. Circ Res 136(4): 439–441
Calderwood DA, Campbell ID, Critchley DR (2013) Talins and kindlins: partners in integrin-mediated adhesion. Nat Rev Mol Cell Biol 14(8):503–517
Cappenberg A, Kardell M, Zarbock A (2022) Selectin-mediated signaling-shedding light on the regulation of integrin activity in neutrophils. Cells 11(8):1310
Carisey A, Tsang R, Greiner AM, Nijenhuis N, Heath N, Nazgiewicz A et al (2013) Vinculin regulates the recruitment and release of core focal adhesion proteins in a force-dependent manner. Curr Biol 23(4):271–281
Carneiro AM, Cook EH, Murphy DL, Blakely RD (2008) Interactions between integrin alphaIIbbeta3 and the serotonin transporter regulate serotonin transport and platelet aggregation in mice and humans. J Clin Invest 118(4):1544–1552
Cattaneo M (2011) Molecular defects of the platelet P2 receptors. Purinergic Signal 7(3):333–339
Chaudhary PK, Kim S, Kim S (2021) The predominant role of arrestin3 in general GPCR desensitization in platelets. J Clin Med 10(20):4743
Cheng Y, Austin SC, Rocca B, Koller BH, Coffman TM, Grosser T et al (2002) Role of prostacyclin in the cardiovascular response to thromboxane A2. Science 296(5567):539–541
Christou CM, Pearce AC, Watson AA, Mistry AR, Pollitt AY, Fenton-May AE et al (2008) Renal cells activate the platelet receptor CLEC-2 through podoplanin. Biochem J 411(1):133–140
Clark EA, Shattil SJ, Ginsberg MH, Bolen J, Brugge JS (1994) Regulation of the protein tyrosine kinase pp72syk by platelet agonists and the integrin alpha IIb beta 3. J Biol Chem 269(46): 28859–28864
Clark JC, Neagoe RAI, Zuidscherwoude M, Kavanagh DM, Slater A, Martin EM et al (2021) Evidence that GPVI is expressed as a mixture of monomers and dimers, and that the D2 domain is not essential for GPVI activation. Thromb Haemost 121(11):1435–1447
Clemetson JM, Polgar J, Magnenat E, Wells TN, Clemetson KJ (1999) The platelet collagen receptor glycoprotein VI is a member of the immunoglobulin superfamily closely related to FcalphaR and the natural killer receptors. J Biol Chem 274(41):29019–29024
Clemetson KJ, Clemetson JM, Proudfoot AE, Power CA, Baggiolini M, Wells TN (2000) Functional expression of CCR1, CCR3, CCR4, and CXCR4 chemokine receptors on human platelets. Blood 96(13):4046–4054

Coller BS, Shattil SJ (2008) The GPIIb/IIIa (integrin alphaIIbbeta3) odyssey: a technology-driven saga of a receptor with twists, turns, and even a bend. Blood 112(8):3011–3025
Colonna M, Samaridis J, Angman L (2000) Molecular characterization of two novel C-type lectin-like receptors, one of which is selectively expressed in human dendritic cells. Eur J Immunol 30(2):697–704
Consonni A, Cipolla L, Guidetti G, Canobbio I, Ciraolo E, Hirsch E et al (2012) Role and regulation of phosphatidylinositol 3-kinase beta in platelet integrin alpha2beta1 signaling. Blood 119(3): 847–856
Coppinger JA, Cagney G, Toomey S, Kislinger T, Belton O, McRedmond JP et al (2004) Characterization of the proteins released from activated platelets leads to localization of novel platelet proteins in human atherosclerotic lesions. Blood 103(6):2096–2104
Coughlin SR (2000) Thrombin signalling and protease-activated receptors. Nature 407(6801): 258–264
Covic L, Gresser AL, Kuliopulos A (2000) Biphasic kinetics of activation and signaling for PAR1 and PAR4 thrombin receptors in platelets. Biochemistry 39(18):5458–5467
Cramer EM, Berger G, Berndt MC (1994) Platelet alpha-granule and plasma membrane share two new components: CD9 and PECAM-1. Blood 84(6):1722–1730
Criel M, Izzi B, Vandenbriele C, Liesenborghs L, Van Kerckhoven S, Lox M et al (2016) Absence of Pear1 does not affect murine platelet function in vivo. Thromb Res 146:76–83
Critchley DR (2009) Biochemical and structural properties of the integrin-associated cytoskeletal protein talin. Annu Rev Biophys 38:235–254
Crittenden JR, Bergmeier W, Zhang Y, Piffath CL, Liang Y, Wagner DD et al (2004) CalDAG-GEFI integrates signaling for platelet aggregation and thrombus formation. Nat Med 10(9): 982–986
Daeron M (1995) Intracytoplasmic sequences involved in the biological properties of low-affinity receptors for IgG expressed by murine macrophages. Braz J Med Biol Res 28(3):263–274
D'Ambrosio D, Hippen KL, Minskoff SA, Mellman I, Pani G, Siminovitch KA et al (1995) Recruitment and activation of PTP1C in negative regulation of antigen receptor signaling by Fc gamma RIIB1. Science 268(5208):293–297
Deindl S, Kadlecek TA, Brdicka T, Cao X, Weiss A, Kuriyan J (2007) Structural basis for the inhibition of tyrosine kinase activity of ZAP-70. Cell 129(4):735–746
Dhanjal TS, Ross EA, Auger JM, McCarty OJ, Hughes CE, Senis YA et al (2007a) Minimal regulation of platelet activity by PECAM-1. Platelets 18(1):56–67
Dhanjal TS, Pendaries C, Ross EA, Larson MK, Protty MB, Buckley CD et al (2007b) A novel role for PECAM-1 in megakaryocytokinesis and recovery of platelet counts in thrombocytopenic mice. Blood 109(10):4237–4244
Dinh M, Grunberger D, Ho H, Tsing SY, Shaw D, Lee S et al (2007) Activation mechanism and steady state kinetics of Bruton's tyrosine kinase. J Biol Chem 282(12):8768–8776
Djellas Y, Manganello JM, Antonakis K, Le Breton GC (1999) Identification of Galpha13 as one of the G-proteins that couple to human platelet thromboxane A2 receptors. J Biol Chem 274(20): 14325–14330
Dorsam RT, Kunapuli SP (2004) Central role of the P2Y12 receptor in platelet activation. J Clin Invest 113(3):340–345
Duerschmied D, Suidan GL, Demers M, Herr N, Carbo C, Brill A et al (2013) Platelet serotonin promotes the recruitment of neutrophils to sites of acute inflammation in mice. Blood 121(6): 1008–1015
Dunster JL, Unsworth AJ, Bye AP, Haining EJ, Sowa MA, Di Y et al (2020) Interspecies differences in protein expression do not impact the spatiotemporal regulation of glycoprotein VI mediated activation. J Thromb Haemost 18(2):485–496
Durrant TN, van den Bosch MT, Hers I (2017) Integrin alpha(IIb)beta(3) outside-in signaling. Blood 130(14):1607–1619
Dutta-Roy AK, Sinha AK (1987) Purification and properties of prostaglandin E1/prostacyclin receptor of human blood platelets. J Biol Chem 262(26):12685–12691

Dutting S, Vogtle T, Morowski M, Schiessl S, Schafer CM, Watson SK et al (2014) Growth factor receptor-bound protein 2 contributes to (hem)immunoreceptor tyrosine-based activation motif-mediated signaling in platelets. Circ Res 114(3):444–453

Dutting S, Gaits-Iacovoni F, Stegner D, Popp M, Antkowiak A, van Eeuwijk JMM et al (2017) A Cdc42/RhoA regulatory circuit downstream of glycoprotein Ib guides transendothelial platelet biogenesis. Nat Commun 8:15838

Estevez B, Kim K, Delaney MK, Stojanovic-Terpo A, Shen B, Ruan C et al (2016) Signaling-mediated cooperativity between glycoprotein Ib-IX and protease-activated receptors in thrombin-induced platelet activation. Blood 127(5):626–636

Ezumi Y, Shindoh K, Tsuji M, Takayama H (1998) Physical and functional association of the Src family kinases Fyn and Lyn with the collagen receptor glycoprotein VI-Fc receptor gamma chain complex on human platelets. J Exp Med 188(2):267–276

Fabre J-E, Nguyen M, Latour A, Keifer JA, Audoly LP, Coffman TM et al (1999) Decreased platelet aggregation, increased bleeding time and resistance to thromboembolism in P2Y1-deficient mice. Nat Med 5(10):1199–1202

Falati S, Patil S, Gross PL, Stapleton M, Merrill-Skoloff G, Barrett NE et al (2006) Platelet PECAM-1 inhibits thrombus formation in vivo. Blood 107(2):535–541

Fan X, Shi P, Dai J, Lu Y, Chen X, Liu X et al (2014) Paired immunoglobulin-like receptor B regulates platelet activation. Blood 124(15):2421–2430

Faraday N, Yanek LR, Yang XP, Mathias R, Herrera-Galeano JE, Suktitipat B et al (2011) Identification of a specific intronic PEAR1 gene variant associated with greater platelet aggregability and protein expression. Blood 118(12):3367–3375

Favaloro EJ, Pasalic L, Lippi G (2022) Antibodies against platelet factor 4 and their associated pathologies: from HIT/HITT to spontaneous HIT-like syndrome, to COVID-19, to VITT/TTS. Antibodies (Basel) 11(1):7

Finney BA, Schweighoffer E, Navarro-Nunez L, Benezech C, Barone F, Hughes CE et al (2012) CLEC-2 and Syk in the megakaryocytic/platelet lineage are essential for development. Blood 119(7):1747–1756

Fong KP, Molnar KS, Agard N, Litvinov RI, Kim OV, Wells JA et al (2021) Cleavage of talin by calpain promotes platelet-mediated fibrin clot contraction. Blood Adv 5(23):4901–4909

Freson K, Hashimoto H, Thys C, Wittevrongel C, Danloy S, Morita Y et al (2004) The pituitary adenylate cyclase-activating polypeptide is a physiological inhibitor of platelet activation. J Clin Invest 113(6):905–912

Freson K, Peeters K, De Vos R, Wittevrongel C, Thys C, Hoylaerts MF et al (2008) PACAP and its receptor VPAC1 regulate megakaryocyte maturation: therapeutic implications. Blood 111(4): 1885–1893

Fu J, Gerhardt H, McDaniel JM, Xia B, Liu X, Ivanciu L et al (2008) Endothelial cell O-glycan deficiency causes blood/lymphatic misconnections and consequent fatty liver disease in mice. J Clin Invest 118(11):3725–3737

Fuller GL, Williams JA, Tomlinson MG, Eble JA, Hanna SL, Pohlmann S et al (2007) The C-type lectin receptors CLEC-2 and Dectin-1, but not DC-SIGN, signal via a novel YXXL-dependent signaling cascade. J Biol Chem 282(17):12397–12409

Furihata K, Clemetson KJ, Deguchi H, Kunicki TJ (2001) Variation in human platelet glycoprotein VI content modulates glycoprotein VI-specific prothrombinase activity. Arterioscler Thromb Vasc Biol 21(11):1857–1863

Futterer K, Wong J, Grucza RA, Chan AC, Waksman G (1998) Structural basis for Syk tyrosine kinase ubiquity in signal transduction pathways revealed by the crystal structure of its regulatory SH2 domains bound to a dually phosphorylated ITAM peptide. J Mol Biol 281(3):523–537

Gachet C, Hechler B, Leon C, Vial C, Leray C, Ohlmann P et al (1997) Activation of ADP receptors and platelet function. Thromb Haemost 78(1):271–275

Gao J, Zoller KE, Ginsberg MH, Brugge JS, Shattil SJ (1997) Regulation of the pp72syk protein tyrosine kinase by platelet integrin alpha IIb beta 3. EMBO J 16(21):6414–6425

Geer MJ, van Geffen JP, Gopalasingam P, Vogtle T, Smith CW, Heising S et al (2018) Uncoupling ITIM receptor G6b-B from tyrosine phosphatases Shp1 and Shp2 disrupts murine platelet homeostasis. Blood 132(13):1413–1425

Gibbins JM, Briddon S, Shutes A, van Vugt MJ, van de Winkel JG, Saito T et al (1998) The p85 subunit of phosphatidylinositol 3-kinase associates with the Fc receptor gamma-chain and linker for activitor of T cells (LAT) in platelets stimulated by collagen and convulxin. J Biol Chem 273(51):34437–34443

Ginsberg MH, Partridge A, Shattil SJ (2005) Integrin regulation. Curr Opin Cell Biol 17(5): 509–516

Goksoy E, Ma YQ, Wang X, Kong X, Perera D, Plow EF et al (2008) Structural basis for the autoinhibition of talin in regulating integrin activation. Mol Cell 31(1):124–133

Golaszewska A, Misztal T, Marcinczyk N, Chabielska E, Rusak T (2021) Adrenaline may contribute to prothrombotic condition via augmentation of platelet procoagulant response, enhancement of fibrin formation, and attenuation of fibrinolysis. Front Physiol 12:657881

Gong H, Shen B, Flevaris P, Chow C, Lam SC, Voyno-Yasenetskaya TA et al (2010) G protein subunit Galpha13 binds to integrin alphaIIbbeta3 and mediates integrin "outside-in" signaling. Science 327(5963):340–343

Gorman RR, Bunting S, Miller OV (1977) Modulation of human platelet adenylate cyclase by prostacyclin (PGX). Prostaglandins 13(3):377–388

Gottschalk KE (2005) A coiled-coil structure of the alphaIIbbeta3 integrin transmembrane and cytoplasmic domains in its resting state. Structure 13(5):703–712

Greinacher A, Selleng K, Mayerle J, Palankar R, Wesche J, Reiche S et al (2021) Anti-platelet factor 4 antibodies causing VITT do not cross-react with SARS-CoV-2 spike protein. Blood 138(14):1269–1277

Gross BS, Lee JR, Clements JL, Turner M, Tybulewicz VL, Findell PR et al (1999a) Tyrosine phosphorylation of SLP-76 is downstream of Syk following stimulation of the collagen receptor in platelets. J Biol Chem 274(9):5963–5971

Gross BS, Melford SK, Watson SP (1999b) Evidence that phospholipase C-gamma2 interacts with SLP-76, Syk, Lyn, LAT and the Fc receptor gamma-chain after stimulation of the collagen receptor glycoprotein VI in human platelets. Eur J Biochem 263(3):612–623

Grucza RA, Futterer K, Chan AC, Waksman G (1999) Thermodynamic study of the binding of the tandem-SH2 domain of the Syk kinase to a dually phosphorylated ITAM peptide: evidence for two conformers. Biochemistry 38(16):5024–5033

Gruner S, Prostredna M, Schulte V, Krieg T, Eckes B, Brakebusch C et al (2003) Multiple integrin-ligand interactions synergize in shear-resistant platelet adhesion at sites of arterial injury in vivo. Blood 102(12):4021–4027

Guidetti GF, Bernardi B, Consonni A, Rizzo P, Gruppi C, Balduini C et al (2009) Integrin alpha2beta1 induces phosphorylation-dependent and phosphorylation-independent activation of phospholipase Cgamma2 in platelets: role of Src kinase and Rac GTPase. J Thromb Haemost 7(7):1200–1206

Guidetti GF, Torti M, Canobbio I (2019) Focal adhesion kinases in platelet function and thrombosis. Arterioscler Thromb Vasc Biol 39(5):857–868

Habib A, FitzGerald GA, Maclouf J (1999) Phosphorylation of the thromboxane receptor α the predominant isoform expressed in human platelets*. J Biol Chem 274(5):2645–2651

Harburger DS, Bouaouina M, Calderwood DA (2009) Kindlin-1 and -2 directly bind the C-terminal region of beta integrin cytoplasmic tails and exert integrin-specific activation effects. J Biol Chem 284(17):11485–11497

Hardy AR, Conley PB, Luo J, Benovic JL, Poole AW, Mundell SJ (2005) P2Y1 and P2Y12 receptors for ADP desensitize by distinct kinase-dependent mechanisms. Blood 105(9): 3552–3560

Hartwig JH (2006) The platelet: form and function. Semin Hematol 43(1 Suppl 1):S94–S100

He L, Pappan LK, Grenache DG, Li Z, Tollefsen DM, Santoro SA et al (2003) The contributions of the alpha 2 beta 1 integrin to vascular thrombosis in vivo. Blood 102(10):3652–3657

Hechler B, Nonne C, Roh EJ, Cattaneo M, Cazenave J-P, Lanza F et al (2006) MRS2500 [2-iodo-N6-methyl-(N)-methanocarba-2'-deoxyadenosine-3',5'-bisphosphate], a potent, selective, and stable antagonist of the platelet P2Y1 receptor with strong antithrombotic activity in mice. J Pharmacol Exp Ther 316(2):556–563

Herrera-Galeano JE, Becker DM, Wilson AF, Yanek LR, Bray P, Vaidya D et al (2008) A novel variant in the platelet endothelial aggregation receptor-1 gene is associated with increased platelet aggregability. Arterioscler Thromb Vasc Biol 28(8):1484–1490

Hess PR, Rawnsley DR, Jakus Z, Yang Y, Sweet DT, Fu J et al (2014) Platelets mediate lymphovenous hemostasis to maintain blood-lymphatic separation throughout life. J Clin Invest 124(1):273–284

Hitchcock JR, Cook CN, Bobat S, Ross EA, Flores-Langarica A, Lowe KL et al (2015) Inflammation drives thrombosis after Salmonella infection via CLEC-2 on platelets. J Clin Invest 125(12): 4429–4446

Honda Z, Suzuki T, Kono H, Okada M, Yamamoto T, Ra C et al (2000) Sequential requirements of the N-terminal palmitoylation site and SH2 domain of Src family kinases in the initiation and progression of FcepsilonRI signaling. Mol Cell Biol 20(5):1759–1771

Horii K, Kahn ML, Herr AB (2006) Structural basis for platelet collagen responses by the immune-type receptor glycoprotein VI. Blood 108(3):936–942

Hu L, Chang L, Zhang Y, Zhai L, Zhang S, Qi Z et al (2017) Platelets express activated P2Y12 receptor in patients with diabetes mellitus. Circulation 136(9):817–833

Hughes CE, Auger JM, McGlade J, Eble JA, Pearce AC, Watson SP (2008) Differential roles for the adapters Gads and LAT in platelet activation by GPVI and CLEC-2. J Thromb Haemost 6(12): 2152–2159

Hughes CE, Pollitt AY, Mori J, Eble JA, Tomlinson MG, Hartwig JH et al (2010a) CLEC-2 activates Syk through dimerization. Blood 115(14):2947–2955

Hughes CE, Navarro-Nunez L, Finney BA, Mourao-Sa D, Pollitt AY, Watson SP (2010b) CLEC-2 is not required for platelet aggregation at arteriolar shear. J Thromb Haemost 8(10):2328–2332

Hughes CE, Sinha U, Pandey A, Eble JA, O'Callaghan CA, Watson SP (2013) Critical role for an acidic amino acid region in platelet signaling by the HemITAM (hemi-immunoreceptor tyrosine-based activation motif) containing receptor CLEC-2 (C-type lectin receptor-2). J Biol Chem 288(7):5127–5135

Hughes CE, Finney BA, Koentgen F, Lowe KL, Watson SP (2015) The N-terminal SH2 domain of Syk is required for (hem)ITAM, but not integrin, signaling in mouse platelets. Blood 125(1): 144–154

Hung DT, Vu TH, Nelken NA, Coughlin SR (1992) Thrombin-induced events in non-platelet cells are mediated by the unique proteolytic mechanism established for the cloned platelet thrombin receptor. J Cell Biol 116(3):827–832

Hutchinson JL, Zhao X, Hill R, Mundell SJ (2020) Arrestin-3 differentially regulates platelet GPCR subsets. Platelets 31(5):641–645

Ichise H, Ichise T, Ohtani O, Yoshida N (2009) Phospholipase Cgamma2 is necessary for separation of blood and lymphatic vasculature in mice. Development 136(2):191–195

Inoue O, Suzuki-Inoue K, Dean WL, Frampton J, Watson SP (2003) Integrin alpha2beta1 mediates outside-in regulation of platelet spreading on collagen through activation of Src kinases and PLCgamma2. J Cell Biol 160(5):769–780

Inoue O, Suzuki-Inoue K, McCarty OJ, Moroi M, Ruggeri ZM, Kunicki TJ et al (2006) Laminin stimulates spreading of platelets through integrin alpha6beta1-dependent activation of GPVI. Blood 107(4):1405–1412

Italiano JE Jr, Richardson JL, Patel-Hett S, Battinelli E, Zaslavsky A, Short S et al (2008) Angiogenesis is regulated by a novel mechanism: pro- and antiangiogenic proteins are organized into separate platelet alpha granules and differentially released. Blood 111(3): 1227–1233

Janus-Bell E, Mangin PH (2023) The relative importance of platelet integrins in hemostasis, thrombosis and beyond. Haematologica 108(7):1734–1747

Jarvis GE, Bihan D, Hamaia S, Pugh N, Ghevaert CJ, Pearce AC et al (2012) A role for adhesion and degranulation-promoting adapter protein in collagen-induced platelet activation mediated via integrin alpha(2) beta(1). J Thromb Haemost 10(2):268–277

Jenkins AL, Nannizzi-Alaimo L, Silver D, Sellers JR, Ginsberg MH, Law DA et al (1998) Tyrosine phosphorylation of the beta3 cytoplasmic domain mediates integrin-cytoskeletal interactions. J Biol Chem 273(22):13878–13885

Jin J, Daniel JL, Kunapuli SP (1998) Molecular basis for ADP-induced platelet activation: II. The P2Y1 receptor mediates ADP-induced intracellular calcium mobilization and shape change in platelets*. J Biol Chem 273(4):2030–2034

Jones CI, Garner SF, Moraes LA, Kaiser WJ, Rankin A, Bloodomics C et al (2009a) PECAM-1 expression and activity negatively regulate multiple platelet signaling pathways. FEBS Lett 583(22):3618–3624

Jones CI, Bray S, Garner SF, Stephens J, de Bono B, Angenent WG et al (2009b) A functional genomics approach reveals novel quantitative trait loci associated with platelet signaling pathways. Blood 114(7):1405–1416

Jones CI, Barrett NE, Moraes LA, Gibbins JM, Jackson DE (2012) Endogenous inhibitory mechanisms and the regulation of platelet function. Methods Mol Biol 788:341–366

Jones CI, Sage T, Moraes LA, Vaiyapuri S, Hussain U, Tucker KL et al (2014a) Platelet endothelial cell adhesion molecule-1 inhibits platelet response to thrombin and von Willebrand factor by regulating the internalization of glycoprotein Ib via AKT/glycogen synthase kinase-3/dynamin and integrin alphaIIbbeta3. Arterioscler Thromb Vasc Biol 34(9):1968–1976

Jones CI, Tucker KL, Sasikumar P, Sage T, Kaiser WJ, Moore C et al (2014b) Integrin-linked kinase regulates the rate of platelet activation and is essential for the formation of stable thrombi. J Thromb Haemost 12(8):1342–1352

Jones ML, Norman JE, Morgan NV, Mundell SJ, Lordkipanidzé M, Lowe GC et al (2015) Diversity and impact of rare variants in genes encoding the platelet G protein-coupled receptors. Thromb Haemost 113(4):826–837

Jooss NJ, Smith CW, Pike JA, Farndale RW, Henskens YMC, Watson SP et al (2023) Platelet glycoprotein VI cluster size is related to thrombus formation and phosphatidylserine exposure in collagen-adherent platelets under arterial shear. J Thromb Haemost 21(8):2260–2267

Joseph K, Nakazawa Y, Bahou WF, Ghebrehiwet B, Kaplan AP (1999) Platelet glycoprotein Ib: a zinc-dependent binding protein for the heavy chain of high-molecular-weight kininogen. Mol Med 5(8):555–563

Joseph RE, Fulton DB, Andreotti AH (2007) Mechanism and functional significance of Itk autophosphorylation. J Mol Biol 373(5):1281–1292

Joseph RE, Severin A, Min L, Fulton DB, Andreotti AH (2009) SH2-dependent autophosphorylation within the Tec family kinase Itk. J Mol Biol 391(1):164–177

Ju L, Chen Y, Xue L, Du X, Zhu C (2016) Cooperative unfolding of distinctive mechanoreceptor domains transduces force into signals. elife 5:e15447

Jung SM, Moroi M, Soejima K, Nakagaki T, Miura Y, Berndt MC et al (2012) Constitutive dimerization of glycoprotein VI (GPVI) in resting platelets is essential for binding to collagen and activation in flowing blood. J Biol Chem 287(35):30000–30013

Jurk K, Clemetson KJ, de Groot PG, Brodde MF, Steiner M, Savion N et al (2003) Thrombospondin-1 mediates platelet adhesion at high shear via glycoprotein Ib (GPIb): an alternative/backup mechanism to von Willebrand factor. FASEB J 17(11):1490–1492

Kahn ML, Nakanishi-Matsui M, Shapiro MJ, Ishihara H, Coughlin SR (1999) Protease-activated receptors 1 and 4 mediate activation of human platelets by thrombin. J Clin Invest 103(6): 879–887

Kardeby C, Falker K, Haining EJ, Criel M, Lindkvist M, Barroso R et al (2019) Synthetic glycopolymers and natural fucoidans cause human platelet aggregation via PEAR1 and GPIbalpha. Blood Adv 3(3):275–287

Kardeby C, Evans A, Campos J, Al-Wahaibi AM, Smith CW, Slater A et al (2023) Heparin and heparin proteoglycan-mimetics activate platelets via PEAR1 and PI3Kbeta. J Thromb Haemost 21(1):101–116

Khandoga AL, Pandey D, Welsch U, Brandl R, Siess W (2011) GPR92/LPA5 lysophosphatidate receptor mediates megakaryocytic cell shape change induced by human atherosclerotic plaques. Cardiovasc Res 90(1):157–164

Kim WM, Huang YH, Gandhi A, Blumberg RS (2019) CEACAM1 structure and function in immunity and its therapeutic implications. Semin Immunol 42:101296

Kirkby NS, Leadbeater PD, Chan MV, Nylander S, Mitchell JA, Warner TD (2011) Antiplatelet effects of aspirin vary with level of $P2Y_{12}$ receptor blockade supplied by either ticagrelor or prasugrel. J Thromb Haemost 9(10):2103–2105

Klapproth S, Sperandio M, Pinheiro EM, Prunster M, Soehnlein O, Gertler FB et al (2015) Loss of the Rap1 effector RIAM results in leukocyte adhesion deficiency due to impaired beta2 integrin function in mice. Blood 126(25):2704–2712

Kloeker S, Major MB, Calderwood DA, Ginsberg MH, Jones DA, Beckerle MC (2004) The Kindler syndrome protein is regulated by transforming growth factor-beta and involved in integrin-mediated adhesion. J Biol Chem 279(8):6824–6833

Knezevic I, Borg C, Le Breton GC (1993) Identification of Gq as one of the G-proteins which copurify with human platelet thromboxane A2/prostaglandin H2 receptors. J Biol Chem 268(34):26011–26017

Knight CG, Morton LF, Onley DJ, Peachey AR, Ichinohe T, Okuma M et al (1999) Collagen-platelet interaction: Gly-Pro-Hyp is uniquely specific for platelet Gp VI and mediates platelet activation by collagen. Cardiovasc Res 41(2):450–457

Koegl M, Zlatkine P, Ley SC, Courtneidge SA, Magee AI (1994) Palmitoylation of multiple Src-family kinases at a homologous N-terminal motif. Biochem J 303(Pt 3):749–753

Krueger I, Gremer L, Mangels L, Klier M, Jurk K, Willbold D et al (2020) Reelin amplifies glycoprotein VI activation and AlphaIIb Beta3 integrin outside-in signaling via PLC gamma 2 and Rho GTPases. Arterioscler Thromb Vasc Biol 40(10):2391–2403

Kuijpers MJ, de Witt S, Nergiz-Unal R, van Kruchten R, Korporaal SJ, Verhamme P et al (2014) Supporting roles of platelet thrombospondin-1 and CD36 in thrombus formation on collagen. Arterioscler Thromb Vasc Biol 34(6):1187–1192

Kuliopulos A, Gurbel PA, Rade JJ, Kimmelstiel CD, Turner SE, Bliden KP et al (2020) PAR1 (protease-activated receptor 1) pepducin therapy targeting myocardial necrosis in coronary artery disease and acute coronary syndrome patients undergoing cardiac catheterization. Arterioscler Thromb Vasc Biol 40(12):2990–3003

Kunicki TJ, Orchekowski R, Annis D, Honda Y (1993) Variability of integrin alpha 2 beta 1 activity on human platelets. Blood 82(9):2693–2703

Lagarrigue F, Paul DS, Gingras AR, Valadez AJ, Sun H, Lin J et al (2020) Talin-1 is the principal platelet Rap1 effector of integrin activation. Blood 136(10):1180–1190

Lau TL, Kim C, Ginsberg MH, Ulmer TS (2009) The structure of the integrin alphaIIbbeta3 transmembrane complex explains integrin transmembrane signalling. EMBO J 28(9): 1351–1361

Law DA, Nannizzi-Alaimo L, Phillips DR (1996) Outside-in integrin signal transduction. Alpha IIb beta 3-(GP IIb IIIa) tyrosine phosphorylation induced by platelet aggregation. J Biol Chem 271(18):10811–10815

Law DA, DeGuzman FR, Heiser P, Ministri-Madrid K, Killeen N, Phillips DR (1999) Integrin cytoplasmic tyrosine motif is required for outside-in alphaIIbbeta3 signalling and platelet function. Nature 401(6755):808–811

Lee RH, Kawano T, Grover SP, Bharathi V, Martinez D, Cowley DO et al (2022) Genetic deletion of platelet PAR4 results in reduced thrombosis and impaired hemostatic plug stability. J Thromb Haemost 20(2):422–433

Leger AJ, Jacques SL, Badar J, Kaneider NC, Derian CK, Andrade-Gordon P et al (2006) Blocking the protease-activated receptor 1-4 heterodimer in platelet-mediated thrombosis. Circulation 113(9):1244–1254

Lenain N, Freund M, Léon C, Cazenave JP, Gachet C (2003) Inhibition of localized thrombosis in P2Y1-deficient mice and rodents treated with MRS2179, a P2Y1 receptor antagonist. J Thromb Haemost 1(6):1144–1149

Li X, Ma Y, Wang D (2024) The role of P-selectin/PSGL-1 in regulating NETs as a novel mechanism in cerebral ischemic injury. Front Neurol 15:1442613

Lin L, Czerwinski R, Kelleher K, Siegel MM, Wu P, Kriz R et al (2009) Activation loop phosphorylation modulates Bruton's tyrosine kinase (Btk) kinase domain activity. Biochemistry 48(9):2021–2032

Litvinov RI, Farrell DH, Weisel JW, Bennett JS (2016) The platelet integrin alphaIIbbeta3 differentially interacts with fibrin versus fibrinogen. J Biol Chem 291(15):7858–7867

Liu Z, Miner JJ, Yago T, Yao L, Lupu F, Xia L et al (2010) Differential regulation of human and murine P-selectin expression and function in vivo. J Exp Med 207(13):2975–2987

Liu H, Jackson ML, Goudswaard LJ, Moore SF, Hutchinson JL, Hers I (2021) Sphingosine-1-phosphate modulates PAR1-mediated human platelet activation in a concentration-dependent biphasic manner. Sci Rep 11(1):15308

Liu J, Lu F, Ithychanda SS, Apostol M, Das M, Deshpande G et al (2023) A mechanism of platelet integrin alphaIIbbeta3 outside-in signaling through a novel integrin alphaIIb subunit-filamin-actin linkage. Blood 141(21):2629–2641

Locke D, Liu C, Peng X, Chen H, Kahn ML (2003) Fc Rgamma -independent signaling by the platelet collagen receptor glycoprotein VI. J Biol Chem 278(17):15441–15448

Lu F, Zhu L, Bromberger T, Yang J, Yang Q, Liu J et al (2022) Mechanism of integrin activation by talin and its cooperation with kindlin. Nat Commun 13(1):2362

Ma YQ, Qin J, Plow EF (2007) Platelet integrin alpha(IIb)beta(3): activation mechanisms. J Thromb Haemost 5(7):1345–1352

Magwenzi S, Woodward C, Wraith KS, Aburima A, Raslan Z, Jones H et al (2015) Oxidized LDL activates blood platelets through CD36/NOX2-mediated inhibition of the cGMP/protein kinase G signaling cascade. Blood 125(17):2693–2703

Mammadova-Bach E, Ollivier V, Loyau S, Schaff M, Dumont B, Favier R et al (2015) Platelet glycoprotein VI binds to polymerized fibrin and promotes thrombin generation. Blood 126(5): 683–691

Mangin PH, Onselaer MB, Receveur N, Le Lay N, Hardy AT, Wilson C et al (2018) Immobilized fibrinogen activates human platelets through glycoprotein VI. Haematologica 103(5):898–907

Mangin PH, Gardiner EE, Ariens RAS, Jandrot-Perrus M (2023) Glycoprotein VI interplay with fibrin(ogen) in thrombosis. J Thromb Haemost 21(7):1703–1713

Manne BK, Getz TM, Hughes CE, Alshehri O, Dangelmaier C, Naik UP et al (2013) Fucoidan is a novel platelet agonist for the C-type lectin-like receptor 2 (CLEC-2). J Biol Chem 288(11): 7717–7726

Manne BK, Badolia R, Dangelmaier C, Eble JA, Ellmeier W, Kahn M et al (2015) Distinct pathways regulate Syk protein activation downstream of immune tyrosine activation motif (ITAM) and hemITAM receptors in platelets. J Biol Chem 290(18):11557–11568

Maxwell MJ, Yuan Y, Anderson KE, Hibbs ML, Salem HH, Jackson SP (2004) SHIP1 and Lyn kinase negatively regulate integrin alpha IIb beta 3 signaling in platelets. J Biol Chem 279(31): 32196–32204

May F, Hagedorn I, Pleines I, Bender M, Vogtle T, Eble J et al (2009) CLEC-2 is an essential platelet-activating receptor in hemostasis and thrombosis. Blood 114(16):3464–3472

Mazharian A, Wang YJ, Mori J, Bem D, Finney B, Heising S et al (2012) Mice lacking the ITIM-containing receptor G6b-B exhibit macrothrombocytopenia and aberrant platelet function. Sci Signal 5(248):ra78

Mazharian A, Mori J, Wang YJ, Heising S, Neel BG, Watson SP et al (2013) Megakaryocyte-specific deletion of the protein-tyrosine phosphatases Shp1 and Shp2 causes abnormal megakaryocyte development, platelet production, and function. Blood 121(20):4205–4220

Mazurov AV, Vinogradov DV, Kabaeva NV, Antonova GN, Romanov YA, Vlasik TN et al (1991) A monoclonal antibody, VM64, reacts with a 130 kDa glycoprotein common to platelets and endothelial cells: heterogeneity in antibody binding to human aortic endothelial cells. Thromb Haemost 66(4):494–499

Mazzucato M, Pradella P, Cozzi MR, De Marco L, Ruggeri ZM (2002) Sequential cytoplasmic calcium signals in a 2-stage platelet activation process induced by the glycoprotein Ibalpha mechanoreceptor. Blood 100(8):2793–2800

McKenzie SE, Reilly MP (2004) Heparin-induced thrombocytopenia and other immune thrombocytopenias: lessons from mouse models. Semin Thromb Hemost 30(5):559–568

Meier RT, Porcelijn L, Hofstede-van Egmond S, Caram-Deelder C, Coutinho JM, Henskens YMC et al (2024) Antibodies against platelet glycoproteins in clinically suspected VITT patients. Antibodies (Basel) 13(2):35

Metzelaar MJ, Korteweg J, Sixma JJ, Nieuwenhuis HK (1991) Biochemical characterization of PECAM-1 (CD31 antigen) on human platelets. Thromb Haemost 66(6):700–707

Meyer SC, Fox JE (1995) Interaction of platelet glycoprotein V with glycoprotein Ib-IX regulates expression of the glycoproteins and binding of von Willebrand factor to glycoprotein Ib-IX in transfected cells. J Biol Chem 270(24):14693–14699

Modderman PW, Admiraal LG, Sonnenberg A, von dem Borne AE (1992) Glycoproteins V and Ib-IX form a noncovalent complex in the platelet membrane. J Biol Chem 267(1):364–369

Moran LA, Di Y, Sowa MA, Hermida-Nogueira L, Barrachina MN, Martin E et al (2022) Katacine is a new ligand of CLEC-2 that acts as a platelet agonist. Thromb Haemost 122(8):1361–1368

Mori J, Pearce AC, Spalton JC, Grygielska B, Eble JA, Tomlinson MG et al (2008) G6b-B inhibits constitutive and agonist-induced signaling by glycoprotein VI and CLEC-2. J Biol Chem 283(51):35419–35427

Morton LF, Hargreaves PG, Farndale RW, Young RD, Barnes MJ (1995) Integrin alpha 2 beta 1-independent activation of platelets by simple collagen-like peptides: collagen tertiary (triple-helical) and quaternary (polymeric) structures are sufficient alone for alpha 2 beta 1-independent platelet reactivity. Biochem J 306(Pt 2):337–344

Moser M, Nieswandt B, Ussar S, Pozgajova M, Fassler R (2008) Kindlin-3 is essential for integrin activation and platelet aggregation. Nat Med 14(3):325–330

Moser M, Legate KR, Zent R, Fassler R (2009) The tail of integrins, talin, and kindlins. Science 324(5929):895–899

Motohashi K, Shibata S, Ozaki Y, Yatomi Y, Igarashi Y (2000) Identification of lysophospholipid receptors in human platelets: the relation of two agonists, lysophosphatidic acid and sphingosine 1-phosphate. FEBS Lett 468(2–3):189–193

Munday AD, Berndt MC, Mitchell CA (2000) Phosphoinositide 3-kinase forms a complex with platelet membrane glycoprotein Ib-IX-V complex and 14-3-3zeta. Blood 96(2):577–584

Murray R, FitzGerald GA (1989) Regulation of thromboxane receptor activation in human platelets. Proc Natl Acad Sci 86(1):124–128

Nakanishi-Matsui M, Zheng YW, Sulciner DJ, Weiss EJ, Ludeman MJ, Coughlin SR (2000) PAR3 is a cofactor for PAR4 activation by thrombin. Nature 404(6778):609–613

Nanda N, Bao M, Lin H, Clauser K, Komuves L, Quertermous T et al (2005) Platelet endothelial aggregation receptor 1 (PEAR1), a novel epidermal growth factor repeat-containing transmembrane receptor, participates in platelet contact-induced activation. J Biol Chem 280(26): 24680–24689

Nesbitt WS, Westein E, Tovar-Lopez FJ, Tolouei E, Mitchell A, Fu J et al (2009) A shear gradient-dependent platelet aggregation mechanism drives thrombus formation. Nat Med 15(6):665–673

Newland SA, Macaulay IC, Floto AR, de Vet EC, Ouwehand WH, Watkins NA et al (2007) The novel inhibitory receptor G6B is expressed on the surface of platelets and attenuates platelet function in vitro. Blood 109(11):4806–4809

Nicolson PLR, Hughes CE, Watson S, Nock SH, Hardy AT, Watson CN et al (2018) Inhibition of Btk by Btk-specific concentrations of ibrutinib and acalabrutinib delays but does not block platelet aggregation mediated by glycoprotein VI. Haematologica 103(12):2097–2108
Nicolson PLR, Nock SH, Hinds J, Garcia-Quintanilla L, Smith CW, Campos J et al (2021) Low-dose Btk inhibitors selectively block platelet activation by CLEC-2. Haematologica 106(1):208–219
Nieswandt B, Bergmeier W, Schulte V, Rackebrandt K, Gessner JE, Zirngibl H (2000) Expression and function of the mouse collagen receptor glycoprotein VI is strictly dependent on its association with the FcRgamma chain. J Biol Chem 275(31):23998–24002
Nieswandt B, Brakebusch C, Bergmeier W, Schulte V, Bouvard D, Mokhtari-Nejad R et al (2001) Glycoprotein VI but not alpha2beta1 integrin is essential for platelet interaction with collagen. EMBO J 20(9):2120–2130
Nissinen L, Koivunen J, Kapyla J, Salmela M, Nieminen J, Jokinen J et al (2012) Novel alpha2beta1 integrin inhibitors reveal that integrin binding to collagen under shear stress conditions does not require receptor preactivation. J Biol Chem 287(53):44694–44702
Nurden AT, Dupuis D, Kunicki TJ, Caen JP (1981) Analysis of the glycoprotein and protein composition of Bernard-Soulier platelets by single and two-dimensional sodium dodecyl sulfate-polyacrylamide gel electrophoresis. J Clin Invest 67(5):1431–1440
Obergfell A, Judd BA, del Pozo MA, Schwartz MA, Koretzky GA, Shattil SJ (2001) The molecular adapter SLP-76 relays signals from platelet integrin alphaIIbbeta3 to the actin cytoskeleton. J Biol Chem 276(8):5916–5923
Obergfell A, Eto K, Mocsai A, Buensuceso C, Moores SL, Brugge JS et al (2002) Coordinate interactions of Csk, Src, and Syk kinases with [alpha]IIb[beta]3 initiate integrin signaling to the cytoskeleton. J Cell Biol 157(2):265–275
Oishi S, Tsukiji N, Otake S, Oishi N, Sasaki T, Shirai T et al (2021) Heme activates platelets and exacerbates rhabdomyolysis-induced acute kidney injury via CLEC-2 and GPVI/FcRgamma. Blood Adv 5(7):2017–2026
Oshinowo O, Azer SS, Lin J, Lam WA (2023) Why platelet mechanotransduction matters for hemostasis and thrombosis. J Thromb Haemost 21(9):2339–2353
Pallini C, Pike JA, O'Shea C, Andrews RK, Gardiner EE, Watson SP et al (2021) Immobilized collagen prevents shedding and induces sustained GPVI clustering and signaling in platelets. Platelets 32(1):59–73
Pasquet JM, Gross B, Quek L, Asazuma N, Zhang W, Sommers CL et al (1999) LAT is required for tyrosine phosphorylation of phospholipase cgamma2 and platelet activation by the collagen receptor GPVI. Mol Cell Biol 19(12):8326–8334
Pearce AC, Wilde JI, Doody GM, Best D, Inoue O, Vigorito E et al (2002) Vav1, but not Vav2, contributes to platelet aggregation by CRP and thrombin, but neither is required for regulation of phospholipase C. Blood 100(10):3561–3569
Pearce AC, Senis YA, Billadeau DD, Turner M, Watson SP, Vigorito E (2004) Vav1 and vav3 have critical but redundant roles in mediating platelet activation by collagen. J Biol Chem 279(52): 53955–53962
Pearce AC, McCarty OJ, Calaminus SD, Vigorito E, Turner M, Watson SP (2007) Vav family proteins are required for optimal regulation of PLCgamma2 by integrin alphaIIbbeta3. Biochem J 401(3):753–761
Philipose S, Konya V, Sreckovic I, Marsche G, Lippe IT, Peskar BA et al (2010) The prostaglandin E2 receptor EP4 is expressed by human platelets and potently inhibits platelet aggregation and thrombus formation*. Arterioscler Thromb Vasc Biol 30(12):2416–2423
Pi L, Xu Y, Fu L, Zhang L, Liu Y, Zhou H et al (2019) A PEAR1 polymorphism (rs12041331) is associated with risk of coronary artery aneurysm in Kawasaki disease. Ann Hum Genet 83(1): 54–62
Pollitt AY, Poulter NS, Gitz E, Navarro-Nunez L, Wang YJ, Hughes CE et al (2014) Syk and Src family kinases regulate C-type lectin receptor 2 (CLEC-2)-mediated clustering of podoplanin and platelet adhesion to lymphatic endothelial cells. J Biol Chem 289(52):35695–35710

Poole A, Gibbins JM, Turner M, van Vugt MJ, van de Winkel JG, Saito T et al (1997) The Fc receptor gamma-chain and the tyrosine kinase Syk are essential for activation of mouse platelets by collagen. EMBO J 16(9):2333–2341

Porto I, Giubilato S, De Maria GL, Biasucci LM, Crea F (2009) Platelet P2Y12 receptor inhibition by thienopyridines: status and future. Expert Opin Investig Drugs 18(9):1317–1332

Poulter NS, Pollitt AY, Owen DM, Gardiner EE, Andrews RK, Shimizu H et al (2017) Clustering of glycoprotein VI (GPVI) dimers upon adhesion to collagen as a mechanism to regulate GPVI signaling in platelets. J Thromb Haemost 15(3):549–564

Prevost N, Woulfe D, Tanaka T, Brass LF (2002) Interactions between Eph kinases and ephrins provide a mechanism to support platelet aggregation once cell-to-cell contact has occurred. Proc Natl Acad Sci USA 99(14):9219–9224

Prevost N, Woulfe DS, Tognolini M, Tanaka T, Jian W, Fortna RR et al (2004) Signaling by ephrinB1 and Eph kinases in platelets promotes Rap1 activation, platelet adhesion, and aggregation via effector pathways that do not require phosphorylation of ephrinB1. Blood 103(4): 1348–1355

Prevost N, Woulfe DS, Jiang H, Stalker TJ, Marchese P, Ruggeri ZM et al (2005) Eph kinases and ephrins support thrombus growth and stability by regulating integrin outside-in signaling in platelets. Proc Natl Acad Sci USA 102(28):9820–9825

Pytela R, Pierschbacher MD, Ginsberg MH, Plow EF, Ruoslahti E (1986) Platelet membrane glycoprotein IIb/IIIa: member of a family of Arg-Gly-Asp--specific adhesion receptors. Science 231(4745):1559–1562

Quek LS, Bolen J, Watson SP (1998) A role for Bruton's tyrosine kinase (Btk) in platelet activation by collagen. Curr Biol 8(20):1137–1140

Quek LS, Pasquet JM, Hers I, Cornall R, Knight G, Barnes M et al (2000) Fyn and Lyn phosphorylate the Fc receptor gamma chain downstream of glycoprotein VI in murine platelets, and Lyn regulates a novel feedback pathway. Blood 96(13):4246–4253

Ramirez MI, Millien G, Hinds A, Cao Y, Seldin DC, Williams MC (2003) T1alpha, a lung type I cell differentiation gene, is required for normal lung cell proliferation and alveolus formation at birth. Dev Biol 256(1):61–72

Reilly MP, Taylor SM, Hartman NK, Arepally GM, Sachais BS, Cines DB et al (2001) Heparin-induced thrombocytopenia/thrombosis in a transgenic mouse model requires human platelet factor 4 and platelet activation through FcgammaRIIA. Blood 98(8):2442–2447

Riba R, Hughes CE, Graham A, Watson SP, Naseem KM (2008) Globular adiponectin induces platelet activation through the collagen receptor GPVI-Fc receptor gamma chain complex. J Thromb Haemost 6(6):1012–1020

Roberts W, Magwenzi S, Aburima A, Naseem KM (2010) Thrombospondin-1 induces platelet activation through CD36-dependent inhibition of the cAMP/protein kinase A signaling cascade. Blood 116(20):4297–4306

Romo GM, Dong JF, Schade AJ, Gardiner EE, Kansas GS, Li CQ et al (1999) The glycoprotein Ib-IX-V complex is a platelet counterreceptor for P-selectin. J Exp Med 190(6):803–814

Rosenbaum DM, Rasmussen SG, Kobilka BK (2009) The structure and function of G-protein-coupled receptors. Nature 459(7245):356–363

Rowley JW, Oler AJ, Tolley ND, Hunter BN, Low EN, Nix DA et al (2011) Genome-wide RNA-seq analysis of human and mouse platelet transcriptomes. Blood 118(14):e101–e111

Ruggeri ZM (2003) Von Willebrand factor, platelets and endothelial cell interactions. J Thromb Haemost 1(7):1335–1342

Ruggeri ZM, Dent JA, Saldivar E (1999) Contribution of distinct adhesive interactions to platelet aggregation in flowing blood. Blood 94(1):172–178

Saito K, Tolias KF, Saci A, Koon HB, Humphries LA, Scharenberg A et al (2003) BTK regulates PtdIns-4,5-P2 synthesis: importance for calcium signaling and PI3K activity. Immunity 19(5): 669–678

Salon JA, Lodowski DT, Palczewski K (2011) The significance of G protein-coupled receptor crystallography for drug discovery. Pharmacol Rev 63(4):901–937

Samaha FF, Hibbard C, Sacks J, Chen H, Varello MA, George T et al (2004) Measurement of platelet collagen receptor density in human subjects. Arterioscler Thromb Vasc Biol 24(11): e181–e182

Sanchez-Cortes J, Mrksich M (2009) The platelet integrin alphaIIbbeta3 binds to the RGD and AGD motifs in fibrinogen. Chem Biol 16(9):990–1000

Schacht V, Ramirez MI, Hong YK, Hirakawa S, Feng D, Harvey N et al (2003) T1alpha/podoplanin deficiency disrupts normal lymphatic vasculature formation and causes lymphedema. EMBO J 22(14):3546–3556

Schmaier AA, Zou Z, Kazlauskas A, Emert-Sedlak L, Fong KP, Neeves KB et al (2009) Molecular priming of Lyn by GPVI enables an immune receptor to adopt a hemostatic role. Proc Natl Acad Sci USA 106(50):21167–21172

Senis YA, Tomlinson MG, Ellison S, Mazharian A, Lim J, Zhao Y et al (2009) The tyrosine phosphatase CD148 is an essential positive regulator of platelet activation and thrombosis. Blood 113(20):4942–4954

Senis YA, Mazharian A, Mori J (2014) Src family kinases: at the forefront of platelet activation. Blood 124(13):2013–2024

Severin S, Nash CA, Mori J, Zhao Y, Abram C, Lowell CA et al (2012) Distinct and overlapping functional roles of Src family kinases in mouse platelets. J Thromb Haemost 10(8):1631–1645

Shattil SJ, Newman PJ (2004) Integrins: dynamic scaffolds for adhesion and signaling in platelets. Blood 104(6):1606–1615

Shenoy SK, Lefkowitz RJ (2011) β-Arrestin-mediated receptor trafficking and signal transduction. Trends Pharmacol Sci 32(9):521–533

Shu H, Peng Y, Hang W, Nie J, Zhou N, Wang DW (2022) The role of CD36 in cardiovascular disease. Cardiovasc Res 118(1):115–129

Sidorenko SP, Clark EA (2003) The dual-function CD150 receptor subfamily: the viral attraction. Nat Immunol 4(1):19–24

Siess W, Cuatrecasas P, Lapetina EG (1983a) A role for cyclooxygenase products in the formation of phosphatidic acid in stimulated human platelets. Differential mechanisms of action of thrombin and collagen. J Biol Chem 258(8):4683–4686

Siess W, Siegel FL, Lapetina EG (1983b) Arachidonic acid stimulates the formation of 1,2-diacylglycerol and phosphatidic acid in human platelets. Degree of phospholipase C activation correlates with protein phosphorylation, platelet shape change, serotonin release, and aggregation. J Biol Chem 258(18):11236–11242

Siljander PR, Munnix IC, Smethurst PA, Deckmyn H, Lindhout T, Ouwehand WH et al (2004) Platelet receptor interplay regulates collagen-induced thrombus formation in flowing human blood. Blood 103(4):1333–1341

Smith CW, Thomas SG, Raslan Z, Patel P, Byrne M, Lordkipanidze M et al (2017) Mice lacking the inhibitory collagen receptor LAIR-1 exhibit a mild thrombocytosis and hyperactive platelets. Arterioscler Thromb Vasc Biol 37(5):823–835

Smith CW, Montague SJ, Kardeby C, Di Y, Lowe GC, Lester WA et al (2021) Antiplatelet drugs block platelet activation by VITT patient serum. Blood 138(25):2733–2740

Smith CW, Campos J, Brown HC, Jooss NJ, Ivanova VS, Harbi M et al (2024) Selective Btk inhibition by PRN1008/PRN473 blocks human CLEC-2, and PRN473 reduces venous thrombosis formation in mice. Blood Adv 8(21):5557–5570

Song X, Yang J, Hirbawi J, Ye S, Perera HD, Goksoy E et al (2012) A novel membrane-dependent on/off switch mechanism of talin FERM domain at sites of cell adhesion. Cell Res 22(11): 1533–1545

Soulet C, Sauzeau V, Plantavid M, Herbert JM, Pacaud P, Payrastre B et al (2004) Gi-dependent and -independent mechanisms downstream of the P2Y12 ADP-receptor. J Thromb Haemost 2(1):135–146

Spalton JC, Mori J, Pollitt AY, Hughes CE, Eble JA, Watson SP (2009) The novel Syk inhibitor R406 reveals mechanistic differences in the initiation of GPVI and CLEC-2 signaling in platelets. J Thromb Haemost 7(7):1192–1199

Sriram K, Insel PA (2018) G protein-coupled receptors as targets for approved drugs: how many targets and how many drugs? Mol Pharmacol 93(4):251–258

Stalker TJ, Welsh JD, Tomaiuolo M, Wu J, Colace TV, Diamond SL et al (2014) A systems approach to hemostasis: 3. Thrombus consolidation regulates intrathrombus solute transport and local thrombin activity. Blood 124(11):1824–1831

Steevels TA, Westerlaken GH, Tijssen MR, Coffer PJ, Lenting PJ, Akkerman JW et al (2010) Co-expression of the collagen receptors leukocyte-associated immunoglobulin-like receptor-1 and glycoprotein VI on a subset of megakaryoblasts. Haematologica 95(12):2005–2012

Stefanini L, Roden RC, Bergmeier W (2009) CalDAG-GEFI is at the nexus of calcium-dependent platelet activation. Blood 114(12):2506–2514

Stefanini L, Paul DS, Robledo RF, Chan ER, Getz TM, Campbell RA et al (2015) RASA3 is a critical inhibitor of RAP1-dependent platelet activation. J Clin Invest 125(4):1419–1432

Stimpfle F, Bauer M, Rath D, Schaeffeler E, Schwab M, Gawaz M et al (2018) Variants of PEAR1 are associated with outcome in patients with ACS and stable CAD undergoing PCI. Front Pharmacol 9:490

Stritt S, Wolf K, Lorenz V, Vogtle T, Gupta S, Bosl MR et al (2015) Rap1-GTP-interacting adaptor molecule (RIAM) is dispensable for platelet integrin activation and function in mice. Blood 125(2):219–222

Su W, Wynne J, Pinheiro EM, Strazza M, Mor A, Montenont E et al (2015) Rap1 and its effector RIAM are required for lymphocyte trafficking. Blood 126(25):2695–2703

Sun Y, Vandenbriele C, Kauskot A, Verhamme P, Hoylaerts MF, Wright GJ (2015) A human platelet receptor protein microarray identifies the high affinity immunoglobulin E receptor subunit alpha (FcepsilonR1alpha) as an activating platelet endothelium aggregation receptor 1 (PEAR1) ligand. Mol Cell Proteomics 14(5):1265–1274

Suzuki-Inoue K, Tulasne D, Shen Y, Bori-Sanz T, Inoue O, Jung SM et al (2002) Association of Fyn and Lyn with the proline-rich domain of glycoprotein VI regulates intracellular signaling. J Biol Chem 277(24):21561–21566

Suzuki-Inoue K, Fuller GL, Garcia A, Eble JA, Pohlmann S, Inoue O et al (2006) A novel Syk-dependent mechanism of platelet activation by the C-type lectin receptor CLEC-2. Blood 107(2):542–549

Suzuki-Inoue K, Kato Y, Inoue O, Kaneko MK, Mishima K, Yatomi Y et al (2007) Involvement of the snake toxin receptor CLEC-2, in podoplanin-mediated platelet activation, by cancer cells. J Biol Chem 282(36):25993–26001

Suzuki-Inoue K, Inoue O, Ding G, Nishimura S, Hokamura K, Eto K et al (2010) Essential in vivo roles of the C-type lectin receptor CLEC-2: embryonic/neonatal lethality of CLEC-2-deficient mice by blood/lymphatic misconnections and impaired thrombus formation of CLEC-2-deficient platelets. J Biol Chem 285(32):24494–24507

Takeda S, Kadowaki S, Haga T, Takaesu H, Mitaku S (2002) Identification of G protein-coupled receptor genes from the human genome sequence. FEBS Lett 520(1–3):97–101

Tomlinson MG, Woods DB, McMahon M, Wahl MI, Witte ON, Kurosaki T et al (2001) A conditional form of Bruton's tyrosine kinase is sufficient to activate multiple downstream signaling pathways via PLC Gamma 2 in B cells. BMC Immunol 2:4

Trumel C, Payrastre B, Plantavid M, Hechler B, Viala C, Presek P et al (1999) A key role of adenosine diphosphate in the irreversible platelet aggregation induced by the PAR1-activating peptide through the late activation of phosphoinositide 3-kinase. Blood 94(12):4156–4165

Tsang E, Giannetti AM, Shaw D, Dinh M, Tse JK, Gandhi S et al (2008) Molecular mechanism of the Syk activation switch. J Biol Chem 283(47):32650–32659

Turner M, Mee PJ, Costello PS, Williams O, Price AA, Duddy LP et al (1995) Perinatal lethality and blocked B-cell development in mice lacking the tyrosine kinase Syk. Nature 378(6554): 298–302

Vaiyapuri S, Sage T, Rana RH, Schenk MP, Ali MS, Unsworth AJ et al (2015) EphB2 regulates contact-dependent and contact-independent signaling to control platelet function. Blood 125(4): 720–730

Van de Walle GR, Schoolmeester A, Iserbyt BF, Cosemans JM, Heemskerk JW, Hoylaerts MF et al (2007) Activation of alphaIIbbeta3 is a sufficient but also an imperative prerequisite for activation of alpha2beta1 on platelets. Blood 109(2):595–602

Vandenbriele C, Sun Y, Criel M, Cludts K, Van Kerckhoven S, Izzi B et al (2016) Dextran sulfate triggers platelet aggregation via direct activation of PEAR1. Platelets 27(4):365–372

Varga-Szabo D, Braun A, Nieswandt B (2009) Calcium signaling in platelets. J Thromb Haemost 7(7):1057–1066

Vogtle T, Sharma S, Mori J, Nagy Z, Semeniak D, Scandola C et al (2019) Heparan sulfates are critical regulators of the inhibitory megakaryocyte-platelet receptor G6b-B. elife 8:e46840

Vu T-KH, Hung DT, Wheaton VI, Coughlin SR (1991) Molecular cloning of a functional thrombin receptor reveals a novel proteolytic mechanism of receptor activation. Cell 64(6):1057–1068

Wagner CL, Mascelli MA, Neblock DS, Weisman HF, Coller BS, Jordan RE (1996) Analysis of GPIIb/IIIa receptor number by quantification of 7E3 binding to human platelets. Blood 88(3): 907–914

Wang JF, Liu ZY, Groopman JE (1998) The alpha-chemokine receptor CXCR4 is expressed on the megakaryocytic lineage from progenitor to platelets and modulates migration and adhesion. Blood 92(3):756–764

Washington AV, Schubert RL, Quigley L, Disipio T, Feltz R, Cho EH et al (2004) A TREM family member, TLT-1, is found exclusively in the alpha-granules of megakaryocytes and platelets. Blood 104(4):1042–1047

Washington AV, Gibot S, Acevedo I, Gattis J, Quigley L, Feltz R et al (2009) TREM-like transcript-1 protects against inflammation-associated hemorrhage by facilitating platelet aggregation in mice and humans. J Clin Invest 119(6):1489–1501

Watson AA, Christou CM, James JR, Fenton-May AE, Moncayo GE, Mistry AR et al (2009) The platelet receptor CLEC-2 is active as a dimer. Biochemistry 48(46):10988–10996

Wee JL, Jackson DE (2005) The Ig-ITIM superfamily member PECAM-1 regulates the "outside-in" signaling properties of integrin alpha(IIb)beta3 in platelets. Blood 106(12):3816–3823

Wonerow P, Pearce AC, Vaux DJ, Watson SP (2003) A critical role for phospholipase Cgamma2 in alphaIIbbeta3-mediated platelet spreading. J Biol Chem 278(39):37520–37529

Wong C, Liu Y, Yip J, Chand R, Wee JL, Oates L et al (2009) CEACAM1 negatively regulates platelet-collagen interactions and thrombus growth in vitro and in vivo. Blood 113(8): 1818–1828

Woodside DG, Obergfell A, Leng L, Wilsbacher JL, Miranti CK, Brugge JS et al (2001) Activation of Syk protein tyrosine kinase through interaction with integrin beta cytoplasmic domains. Curr Biol 11(22):1799–1804

Woodside DG, Obergfell A, Talapatra A, Calderwood DA, Shattil SJ, Ginsberg MH (2002) The N-terminal SH2 domains of Syk and ZAP-70 mediate phosphotyrosine-independent binding to integrin beta cytoplasmic domains. J Biol Chem 277(42):39401–39408

Wu YP, Vink T, Schiphorst M, van Zanten GH, IJsseldijk MJ, de Groot PG et al (2000) Platelet thrombus formation on collagen at high shear rates is mediated by von Willebrand factor-glycoprotein Ib interaction and inhibited by von Willebrand factor-glycoprotein IIb/IIIa interaction. Arterioscler Thromb Vasc Biol 20(6):1661–1667

Xin H, Huang J, Song Z, Mao J, Xi X, Shi X (2023) Structure, signal transduction, activation, and inhibition of integrin alphaIIbbeta3. Thromb J 21(1):18

Yang J, Furie BC, Furie B (1999) The biology of P-selectin glycoprotein ligand-1: its role as a selectin counterreceptor in leukocyte-endothelial and leukocyte-platelet interaction. Thromb Haemost 81(1):1–7

Yates LA, Fuzery AK, Bonet R, Campbell ID, Gilbert RJ (2012) Biophysical analysis of Kindlin-3 reveals an elongated conformation and maps integrin binding to the membrane-distal beta-subunit NPXY motif. J Biol Chem 287(45):37715–37731

Yin H, Stojanovic A, Hay N, Du X (2008) The role of Akt in the signaling pathway of the glycoprotein Ib-IX induced platelet activation. Blood 111(2):658–665

Yip J, Alshahrani M, Beauchemin N, Jackson DE (2016) CEACAM1 regulates integrin alphaIIbbeta3-mediated functions in platelets. Platelets 27(2):168–177

Zeiler M, Moser M, Mann M (2014) Copy number analysis of the murine platelet proteome spanning the complete abundance range. Mol Cell Proteomics 13(12):3435–3445

Zhang P, Gruber A, Kasuda S, Kimmelstiel C, O'Callaghan K, Cox DH et al (2012) Suppression of arterial thrombosis without affecting hemostatic parameters with a cell-penetrating PAR1 pepducin. Circulation 126(1):83–91

Zhang W, Deng W, Zhou L, Xu Y, Yang W, Liang X et al (2015) Identification of a juxtamembrane mechanosensitive domain in the platelet mechanosensor glycoprotein Ib-IX complex. Blood 125(3):562–569

Zhang Y, Ehrlich SM, Zhu C, Du X (2022) Signaling mechanisms of the platelet glycoprotein Ib-IX complex. Platelets 33(6):823–832

Zheng J, Umikawa M, Cui C, Li J, Chen X, Zhang C et al (2012) Inhibitory receptors bind ANGPTLs and support blood stem cells and leukaemia development. Nature 485(7400): 656–660

Zhi H, Rauova L, Hayes V, Gao C, Boylan B, Newman DK et al (2013) Cooperative integrin/ITAM signaling in platelets enhances thrombus formation in vitro and in vivo. Blood 121(10): 1858 1867

Zhi Z, Jooss NJ, Sun Y, Colicchia M, Slater A, Moran LA et al (2022) Galectin-9 activates platelet ITAM receptors glycoprotein VI and C-type lectin-like receptor-2. J Thromb Haemost 20(4): 936–950

Ziegler WH, Gingras AR, Critchley DR, Emsley J (2008) Integrin connections to the cytoskeleton through talin and vinculin. Biochem Soc Trans 36(Pt 2):235–239

Antiplatelet Therapy

Richard T. Amison and Simon C. Pitchford

Contents

Abstract

Platelets are a crucial component in the maintenance of normal haemostasis. In response to vascular damage, activated platelets adhere to the damaged endothelium leading to both aggregation and coagulation. Under healthy conditions, these processes prevent excessive vascular haemorrhage and promote vascular repair and regeneration. However, in cardiovascular diseases, hyperactive platelet activation leads to acute coronary syndrome characterised by occlusive thrombus

R. T. Amison (✉) · S. C. Pitchford
Unit of Pulmonary Pharmacology, Institute of Pharmaceutical Sciences, School of Cancer & Pharmaceutical Science, King's College London, London, UK
e-mail: richard.amison@kcl.ac.uk

E. Gray, J. Hogwood (eds.), *Antithrombotic and Antiplatelet Agents*, Handbook of Experimental Pharmacology 291, https://doi.org/10.1007/164_2025_784

formation, myocardial infarction and stroke. Targeted platelet therapy has been used extensively in the inhibition of inappropriate platelet activation for the treatment of cardiovascular diseases including cyclooxygenase inhibitors, purinergic antagonists, thrombin inhibitors, PAR receptor antagonists, and phosphodiesterase inhibitors. In this review, we discuss the current clinical portfolio of antiplatelet therapies whilst also discussing promising new antiplatelet targets for the treatment of cardiovascular disorders.

Keywords

COX inhibitors · GPIIbIIIa antagonists · Phosphodiesterase inhibitors · Platelet aggregation · Protease-activated receptor antagonists · Purinergic antagonists · Thrombosis & Hemostasis

1 Introduction

Platelets are a requisite cellular component of haemostasis. Platelets adhere to the site of vessel damage and become activated, causing the recruitment of additional platelets. This results in platelet aggregation and the production of a soft clot which acts as a platform for a fibrin mesh to be created in concert with activation of the clotting cascade. These actions prevent excessive haemorrhage after vessel injury. Platelets finally act to regenerate the damaged vasculature through the release of proliferative growth factors and mediators. Unfortunately, the inappropriate activation of platelets also propagates arterial thrombosis in atherosclerotic individuals suffering from coronary heart disease. This thrombotic event can cause myocardial infarctions and strokes. Therefore, suppression of platelet activation is the therapeutic mainstay in the prevention of these life-threatening events occurring. A consequence to suppressing thrombosis is that all current antiplatelet drugs target platelet activation pathways involved in the normal processes of haemostasis. Thus, a side effect of our pharmacopoeia is increased likelihood of bleeding, and this can be life-threatening in certain individuals. On a population basis, it is very difficult to determine which individuals might have their first, or primary cardiovascular event in the future, and who might be at risk of excessive bleeding.

Because this fulcrum of efficacy versus safety is difficult to balance based on the on-target effects as opposed to off-target effects of drugs, the use of antiplatelet drugs at inhibiting cardiovascular events means that a risk-benefit analysis is undertaken, and on a population scale the benefit of inhibiting a cardiovascular event outweighs the risk of bleeding in individuals who have already had a primary event. Thus, antiplatelets are used for secondary prevention (unless a patient's particular medical history shows them to be at high risk of a primary event) (Zheng and Roddick 2019). Another aspect of the use of anti-platelet agents is that they often are used together (dual antiplatelet therapy DAPT) in order to increase clinical efficacy compared to the inhibition of one pathway alone, such combinations tend to be aspirin combined with a $P2Y_{12}R$ antagonist. The mechanisms of action,

Table 1 Summary of clinically approved antiplatelet agents

Drug Class	Drug Name	Target	Indication	Dose	Route of Administration
Cycoloxygenase Inhibitor	Asprin	COX	Secondary Prevention of Cardiovascula Disease, Management of STEMI, Management of NSTEMI	75mg once daily	Oral
			Transient Ischaemic Attack, Ischaemic Stoke, Post Coronoary By-pass surgery	75-300mg once daily	Oral
Purinergic Antagonists	Clopidogrel	P2Y12	Transient Ischaemic Attack, Minor Ischaemic Stoke	75mg once daily as adjunct to aspirin	Oral
			Prevention of antithrombotic events in PAD, ACS, Acute MI	75mg once daily	Oral
	Prasugrel	P2Y12	Unstable Angina/NSTEMI during angiograpgy	5-10mg once daily	Oral
			Prevention of atherothrombotic events in PCI	5-10mg once daily	Oral
	Ticagrelor	P2Y12	Prevention of atherothrombotic events in ACS and history of MI	60-90mg twice daily	Oral
	Cangrelor	P2Y12	Reducing thrombotic events priot to PCI where oral P2Y12 therapy is not viable	4μg/kg/min for upto 4 hours	IV infusion
αIIbβ3 antagonists	Abciximab	αIIbβ3	Prevention of ischaemic complications in patients undergoing PTCI	10μg/kg for upto 18 hours as adjunct to aspirin	IV infusion
	Eptifibatide	αIIbβ3	Prevention of MI in non-STEMI	180μg/kg for upto 96 hours as adjunt to aspirin/heparin	IV infusion
	Tirofiban	αIIbβ3	Prevention of MI in non-STEMI	100ng/kg/min for upto 48 hours as adjunct to aspirin/heparin/Clopidogrel	IV infusion
PAR Antagonists	Varopaxar	PAR4	Reducing thrombotic events in patients with MI/Stroke/PAD	2mg once daily as adjunct to aspirin/Clopidogrel	Oral
Phosphodiesterase Inhibitors	Cilostazol	PDE3	Intermittent Claudication in PAD	100mg twice daily	Oral
	Dipyridamole	PDE3	Treatment of Ischaemic Stroke and transient ischaemic attacks	200mg twice daily (with or without aspirin)	Oral

clinical uses, and side effects of common antiplatelet drugs are provided below and summarised in Table 1, before discussion on strategies to improve antiplatelet therapy for the future.

2 Traditional Targets for Antiplatelet Therapy

2.1 COX Inhibitors

Low-dose aspirin (acetylsalicylic acid, 75 mg/once per day) is the most prevalent drug prescribed in the secondary prevention of cardiovascular disease. The first clinical trials to evaluate the effectiveness of aspirin in the secondary prevention of cardiovascular events were reported in 1974 (Elwood et al. 1974), culminating in meta-analyses confirming the effectiveness of this approach above primary prevention (Zheng and Roddick 2019). Aspirin is classed as a non-steroidal anti-inflammatory drug (NSAID) due to its mechanism of action. However, the dose used in the context described here is lower than the 300 mg/ three to four times a day regimen used for analgesia (e.g. headaches, toothache, period pains). Aspirin acts as an irreversible cyclo-oxygenase enzyme (COX) inhibitor, an enzyme that converts arachidonic acid (a product of membrane-bound phospholipids metabolised by phospholipases) into prostaglandin H2 (PGH_2) (Vane 1971; Pedersen and FitzGerald 1984). PGH_2 is a precursor that is then converted via specific isomerases to biologically active prostaglandins released by many cell types, such as PGD_2 (released by mast cells, brain, airways), PGE_2 (platelets, brain, vascular smooth muscle), and PGF_2 (uterus, eyes, vascular smooth muscle, airways) (Smyth et al. 2009).

Platelets express the COX-1 isoform (as opposed to COX-2) and it is the production of the platelet-specific prostaglandin thromboxane A2 (TXA_2) that is the clinical target of aspirin therapy in the prevention of cardiovascular disease (Patrono et al. 1985). The production and release of TXA_2 by activated platelets is a potent platelet agonist, inducing platelet aggregation, vasoconstriction, and mitogenesis of smooth muscle by activating a G protein-coupled receptor (GPCR) known as the thromboxane receptor (TP) (Habib et al. 1999; Narumiya and FitzGerald 2001). Other COX isoforms exist, notably COX-2, that is expressed by endothelial cells to produce Prostacyclin (PGI2), a prostaglandin that in contrast to TXA_2, inhibits platelet activation induced by other agonists and stress via the prostacyclin receptor (IP) (Cheng et al. 2002). Aspirin is relatively more selective for COX-1 over COX-2, and is considered to be cardioprotective because low-dose aspirin suppresses platelet COX-1 activity irreversibly as a result of aspirin acetylation (conversion to salicylic acid) of a hydroxyl group on serine 529 within the catalytic site of the enzyme, inhibiting arachidonic acid entry (Pedersen and FitzGerald 1984). Because platelets are anuclear, and are unable to reverse the inhibition caused by aspirin through de novo synthesis of COX-1 (Patrignani et al. 1982), and in contrast endothelial cells have the capacity to synthesise new COX-2 to overcome the irreversible inhibition caused by aspirin (Patrono et al. 1985), the inhibition of TXA_2 production over PGI_2 production predominates, to provide a cardioprotective effect (Patrignani et al. 1982; FitzGerald et al. 1983). It is noticeable that all other NSAIDs cause reversible inhibition of COX (irrespective of COX-1 or COX-2 selectivity) and therefore do not confer cardio-protection, despite the half-life of aspirin being short within the circulation (20-30 min). Aspirin is readily absorbed from the gut and undergoes first-pass metabolism in the liver resulting in partial deacetylation of acetylsalicylic acid to salicylic acid. Interestingly, it is this portal circulation that has twice the level of aspirin compared to systemic circulation as a whole, and is an important pre-systemic site for platelet exposure (Patrignani et al. 2014). This perhaps also provides a 'organ'-specific mechanism for platelet inactivation above the vascular endothelium. The relatively slow turn-over of the platelet population (platelet lifespan is 8–10 days) means that a once a day administration of aspirin is sufficient to provide day-long protection, and the pharmacodynamics of platelet inactivation by aspirin can be assessed through the urinary excretion of a stable metabolite of TXA_2, 11-dehydro-TXB_2 (Kumlin and Granström 1986).

Despite the effectiveness of aspirin as an antiplatelet drug, there are some limitations with its use. Notably, an incomplete inhibition of platelet activation is observed in some patients who have type 2 diabetes, obesity, or myeloproliferative neoplasms, and this is perhaps due to non-TXA_2-dependent platelet activation pathways (Patrono and Rocca 2017). The phenomenon of 'aspirin resistance' has also been debated, where some patients appear not to respond to aspirin therapy. The reason for this is unknown, but has been explained as some patients possess differing pharmacokinetics from the population norm and therefore inadequate bioavailability, or that different aspirin capsule formulations will affect pharmacokinetics after absorption from the gut (Rocca and Patrono 2005), or the competition by other traditional NSAIDs for the catalytic site of COX-1 (Catella-Lawson et al. 2001; Renda et al. 2006).

Notable side effects of aspirin are the incidence of major bleeding events caused through platelet inhibition (Patrono and Rocca 2017) and gastrointestinal ulcers due to aspirin suppression of PCI_2 and PGE_2-induced production of mucus and bicarbonate that would otherwise protect the gut (Sostres and Lanas 2011; Nwose and Yee 2016). Therefore, as an extension of aspirin ultimately suppressing TXA_2, attempts have been made to develop more selective inhibitors of TXA_2 production, and antagonists of the TP receptor. Dazoxiben was created as an orally available TXA_2 synthase inhibitor, with the expectation that this might lead to an improved safety profile to reduce gastrointestinal ulcers and bleeding. However, negative clinical trial results in patients with Raynaud's syndrome, with recognised platelet activation status, suggest targeted suppression of TXA_2 synthase reduces efficacy (Tyler et al. 1981; Belch et al. 1983). A pharmacological explanation was proposed that the precursor PGH_2 instead accumulates and is able to act as an agonist on the same TP receptor (FitzGerald et al. 1983). As an alternative approach, TP antagonists have been created, which were expected to have an advantage over aspirin by inhibiting all endoperoxides/prostanoids, isoprostanes that can also activate the TP receptor and that are synthesised via COX-independent pathways (Capra et al. 2014), but still preserve PGI_2. Interestingly, many TP antagonists (ridogrel, terutroban and picotamide) have an additive quality of having TXA_2 synthase inhibition and ridogrel has been shown to have dual inhibition and therefore a stronger inhibition of platelet aggregation. However, ridogrel was reported to have no benefit over aspirin in patients with acute MI used as an adjunct therapy for thrombolysis (van der Wicken et al. 1995). Furthermore, terutroban and picotamide did not improve outcomes compared to aspirin in patients experiencing a cerebral ischaemic event or peripheral artery disease (Bousser et al. 2011; Neri Serneri et al. 2004). It is not known whether these drugs would improve patient outcomes compared to aspirin in longer term secondary prevention studies.

3 Purinergic Antagonists

A key mediator of thrombosis and haemostasis are the purine and pyrimidine nucleotides ADP and ATP. The receptors activated by these agonists are termed the P2 receptors and are defined by their molecular structure. P2Y receptors are GPCRS that are stimulated by ADP, whilst the P2X receptors are ligand-gated ion channels that mediate rapid changes in membrane permeability to both mono- and divalent cations including Na^+, K^+ and Ca^{2+}. Whilst thrombin is considered a 'strong' platelet agonist, ADP is a weak platelet agonist capable of inducing platelet shape change and reversible platelet aggregation. However, whilst it is itself only a weak platelet agonist, ADP is considered crucial in thrombosis and haemostasis due to its amplification of platelet responses induced by other platelet agonists following its release from intracellular platelet granules.

Human platelets have been shown to express 4 P2 receptors including the ADP receptors $P2Y_1$ and $P2Y_{12}$, the ATP receptor $P2X_1$ and the UDP receptor $P2Y_{14}$. Whilst the $P2Y_1$, $P2Y_{12}$ and $P2X_1$ receptors have been demonstrated to play significant roles in platelet activation and aggregation, the $P2Y_{14}$ receptor appears to be redundant in platelet aggregation and rather is implicated in the inflammatory functions of platelets (Dovlatova et al. 2008; Moore et al. 2003; Amison et al. 2017; Hossain et al. 2025). ATP-mediated activation of the $P2X_1$ receptor generates significant elevations in intracellular Ca^{2+} leading to shape change, and whilst stimulation of $P2X_1$ receptors alone appear to be capable of only inducing reversible shape change without subsequent platelet aggregation (Rolf et al. 2001), $P2X_1$ receptor activation has been shown to contribute to platelet aggregation in response to other platelet agonists including ADP, collagen, adrenaline, TXA_2 and thrombin (Fung et al. 2007; Rolf et al. 2001; Braun et al. 2001; Hechler et al. 2005; Kassack et al. 2004), potentially through $P2X_1$ contributions to shape change and granule secretion contributing to a positive feedback of additional platelet agonists inducing subsequent aggregation (Gachet 2008; Mahaut-Smith et al. 2011). In contrast, co-stimulation of both $P2Y_1$ and $P2Y_{12}$ receptors is necessary for full ADP-induced platelet aggregation (Cattaneo 2005, 2011; Jin and Kunapuli 1998). ADP stimulation of the primarily Gq-coupled P2Y1 receptor facilitates PLC activation, subsequent PKC activation and mobilisation of intracellular Ca^{2+} (Stefanini et al. 2009, 2012). This initiates platelet shape change, granule release, thromboxane production and initial aggregation via the activation of CalDAG GEF, which converts RAP1 GDP to RAP1 GTP, necessary for transient GPIIb/IIIa conformational change and activation. As part of this initial aggregation, further ADP is released from dense granules leading to positive feedback stimulation of the Gi-coupled $P2Y_{12}$ receptor. Through the alpha subunit, this activation leads to inhibition of adenylyl cyclase, reduced cAMP levels thereby reducing PKA activation (Yang et al. 2002). Concurrently, the β/γ subunits of Gi promote PI3K activation and increased Akt and Rap1b signalling via the inhibition of RAP-GTPase activating protein RASA3 which otherwise acts as a constitutive molecular brake to CalDAG GEF that converts RAP1 GDP to RAP1 GTP. This combined signalling via the α and β/γ subunits of Gi promotes sustained GPIIb/IIIa activation, amplification of activation and the stabilisation of platelet aggregation (Jantzen et al. 2001; Gratacap et al. 2000; Dangelmaier et al. 2001; Woulfe et al. 2002; Lova et al. 2002; Larson et al. 2003).

P2X1 receptors have been shown to potentiate the platelet activation responses to a range of haemostatic agents. Significantly antagonism of the P2X1 receptor showed a reduction in maximal platelet aggregation to ADP (69%), collagen (18%), TXA2 (34%) and thrombin (69%) (Fung et al. 2007). Furthermore, additional studies have demonstrated a significant role for P2X1 receptors in thrombus generation under shear conditions on collagen-coated services using P2X1 knockout mice whilst only mildly increasing bleeding times (Rolf et al. 2001). This therefore highlights a potential role for P2X1 antagonists in reducing thrombus formation and size in areas exhibiting high shear stress for example sites of severe arterial stenosis, whilst limiting the impact on the formation of haemostatic plugs therefore reducing the risk of associated increased bleeding. However, development of antagonists of the P2X1 receptor has been limited by rapid desensitisation of the P2X1 receptor making it harder to study the functional impact of novel P2X1 receptor antagonists (Rolf et al. 2001). The primary limitation has been a failure to develop drugs with the appropriate affinity and selectivity for the P2X1 receptor over other P2 receptor subtypes. Currently, the only P2X1 antagonists available for study are the suramin analogues NF449 and NF864 (Braun et al. 2001; Hechler et al. 2005). Both of these drugs show favourable selectivity for P2X1 over L2X3, P2X7, P2Y1, P2Y2 and P2Y12 and have demonstrated significant reduction in both intravascular aggregation in a model of systemic thromboembolism, alongside a dose-dependent reduction in thrombus size following laser-induced injury of mesenteric arterioles (Braun et al. 2001; Hechler et al. 2005; Kassack et al. 2004). However, currently, there has been no clinical evaluation of putative P2X1 receptor antagonists for antiplatelet therapy.

4 P2Y12 Receptor Antagonists

The main platelet expressed ADP receptor involved in platelet aggregation is the P2Y12 receptor which demonstrates significantly higher levels of expression compared to the P2Y1 receptor with individual platelets expressing greater than 1,000 receptors compared to the much smaller 100–150 P2Y1 receptors expressed per individual platelet (Baurand et al. 2001; Burnstock 2007). Furthermore, the P2Y12 receptor has limited systemic expression, with P2Y12 receptor expression largely restricted to platelets and glial cells (Burnstock 2007). Combined with the extensively described role of platelets in platelet aggregation and thrombosis its limited systemic tissue distribution, the P2Y12 receptor has been an attractive target for antithrombotic therapies for a number of decades.

4.1 Clopidogrel and Ticlopidine

The first FDA-approved P2Y12 selective antagonist was the thienopyridine ticlopidine in 1991 which reduced the risk of myocardial infarction and stroke through its potent inhibition of platelet aggregation. However, the use of ticlopidine was limited by frequent adverse events including major bleeding events and this has therefore largely been replaced with the second-generation thienopyridine clopidogrel which received FDA approval in 1997 due to its more favourable safety profile (Bertrand et al. 2000; Love et al. 1998). Clopidogrel is an orally administered prodrug which requires metabolic transformation by the hepatic CYP450 enzymes CYP2C19 and CYP3A4 to elicit its pharmacological effects (Lopez et al. 2023). The active metabolite of clopidogrel interacts with the P2Y12 receptor in a competitive but irreversible manner, therefore the pharmacodynamic effects of clopidogrel on platelet aggregation last for the duration of the platelet lifespan, approximately 8–10 days (Savi and Herbert 2005). Clinically, due to its high activity against the P2Y12 receptor, clopidogrel remains the most widely used P2Y12 receptor antagonist for the treatment of patients with stable coronary artery disease undergoing PCI, or in those with STEMI treated with thrombolytic agents (O'Gara et al. 2013; Levine et al. 2011; Byrne et al. 2023; Montalescot et al. 2013).

Significantly, despite the proven clinical efficacy of clopidogrel, a wide range of interpatient variability towards the drug is observed. Some of this can be attributed to clinical factors such as poor absorption, drug-drug interactions, acute coronary syndrome (ACS), chronic kidney disease, cellular factors such as accelerated platelet turnover, reduced CYP3A4 metabolic activity, and upregulation of the P2Y12 receptor pathway (Patrignani et al. 2014; Kumlin and Granström 1986; Patrono and Rocca 2017; Rocca and Patrono 2005). However, the requirement for metabolic transformation has been associated with a number of factors associated with clopidogrel use. The formation of the active metabolite is consistent with the delay in observed maximal inhibition of ADP-induced platelet aggregation observed with clopidogrel (2–5 h post 400 mg dose (Savcic et al. 1999)). However, more significant is the fact that patients with polymorphisms in the relevant CYP450 enzymes such as CYP2C10 and CYP3A4 can also experience a decrease in efficacy of clopidogrel due to reduced formation of the active metabolite (Lopez et al. 2023). Whilst screening processes for the presence of clinically relevant polymorphisms exist, they are cumbersome and are only typically used in high-risk patients. However, the clinical implications of these polymorphisms are highlighted by pharmacodynamic studies revealing that 30–40% of patients retaining high platelet reactivity despite clopidogrel treatment correlate with poor clinical outcomes (Angiolillo et al. 2007; Stone et al. 2013; Tantry et al. 2013; Brar et al. 2011). Combined with large-scale clinical trials revealing that increasing dosages of clopidogrel failed to improve clinical outcome (Price et al. 2011; Collet et al. 2012), further research has led to the development and approval of more potent third-generation P2Y12 antagonists including prasugrel, ticagrelor and cangrelor.

4.2 Prasugrel

Whilst prasugrel also requires metabolic transformation to elicit its pharmacological effects, it is more readily converted into its active form when compared to clopidogrel (Hagihara et al. 2010). Furthermore, preclinical studies revealed that compared to clopidogrel and ticlopidine, prasugrel demonstrated significantly improved potency with a dose-dependent inhibition of ADP-induced platelet aggregation observed at doses 10–100 fold lower than those of clopidogrel and ticlopidine (Niitsu et al. 2005). Phase II clinical trials (JUMBO-TIMI 26) also revealed that prasugrel was superior (10 mg/kg/day) to clopidogrel (150 mg/kg/day) in inhibiting P2Y12-dependent platelet function (Jakubowski et al. 2012), which was further supported by Phase III clinical trials (TRITON TIMI-38). These showed that prasugrel significantly reduced the rate of cardiovascular death, nonfatal MI or nonfatal stroke compared to clopidogrel (Wiviott 2007). Crucially, unlike clopidogrel, clinical outcomes associated with prasugrel treatment were not affected by polymorphisms in CYP450 enzyme systems (Mega et al. 2009). However, whilst these studies revealed higher potency, prasugrel was also associated with a significant increase in the incidence of life-threatening and fatal bleeding complications as well as thrombolysis in MI (Jakubowski et al. 2012; Antman et al. 2008). Accordingly, whilst prasugrel received FDA approval, Clopidogrel continues to be preferred in most situations except for recommendations of prasugrel treatment in high-risk patients or for shorter treatment periods (Ajani and Lefkovits 2008).

4.3 Ticagrelor

The remaining clinically approved direct P2Y12 antagonists are ticagrelor and cangrelor. Unlike clopidogrel and prasugrel, both ticagrelor and cangrelor are both pharmacologically active and do not require prior metabolism for therapeutic activity, although studies have demonstrated that approximately 30–40% of inhibition of platelet aggregation can be attributed to the formation of a further active metabolite of ticagrelor by CYP3A4 and CYP3A5 enzymes (Wallentin et al. 2009). Phase II clinical trials (DISPERSE-1, DISPERSE-2) revealed that compared to clopidogrel, ticagrelor demonstrates more rapid and effective platelet inhibition with significantly reduced variability, which is likely due to reduced dependence on enzyme-mediated activation (Husted et al. 2006; Cannon et al. 2007). Importantly, unlike prasugrel, ticagrelor showed no statistically significant difference in the incidence of major bleeding events compared to clopidogrel. Subsequent Phase III clinical trials including PLATO demonstrated that in patients with major adverse cardiovascular events (MACE), ticagrelor demonstrated significantly greater reductions in the incidence of cardiovascular death, MI or stroke compared to clopidogrel (Wallentin et al. 2009). Whilst ticagrelor has demonstrated improved inhibition of platelet activation combined with reduced major bleeding events compared to clopidogrel, Phase II and Phase III clinical trials did reveal an increased incidence of dyspnoea following ticagrelor therapy, believed to be due to inhibition of P2Y12 receptors in the central nervous system (Husted et al. 2006; Cannon et al. 2007; Cattaneo and Faioni 2012). However, despite the reported increase in dyspnoea, ticagrelor is now widely used for the management of acute coronary syndrome (ACS), in patients managed medically and those who undergo percutaneous coronary intervention (PCI).

4.4 Cangrelor

Cangrelor is an analogue of ATP and is the only intravenous P2Y12 antagonist, with clopidogrel, prasugrel and ticagrelor all being orally available P2Y12 antagonists (Alexopoulos et al. 2012; Parodi et al. 2013). Cangrelor possesses potent inhibition of ADP-induced platelet aggregation and like ticagrelor does not require metabolism into its active form. Phase II clinical trials evaluated the safety and efficacy of cangrelor in patients undergoing PCI. No significant difference in bleeding events was observed between cangrelor and the GPIIb/IIIa antagonist abciximab. Whilst the mean inhibition of platelet aggregation was no different between cangrelor and abciximab, platelet aggregation returned to baseline levels much more quickly following cangrelor treatment (Greenbaum et al. 2006). Phase III studies including CHAMPION PCI, CHAMPION PLATFORM and CHAMPION-PHOENIX sought to compare cangrelor to clopidogrel therapy in patients with PCI (Bhatt et al. 2009; Harrington et al. 2009; Bhatt et al. 2013). Initial reports from CHAMPION-PHOENIX demonstrated that cangrelor significantly reduced the rate of ischemic events, including stent thrombosis during PCI with no significant increase in severe bleeding (Bhatt et al. 2013). However, it is important to note that both CHAMPION PCI and CHAMPION PLATFORM studies were prematurely terminated due to insufficient evidence of clinical activity (Bhatt et al. 2009; Harrington et al. 2009). More recent research showed a reduced risk of MACE and all-cause mortality for patients with cardiogenic shock following treatment with cangrelor during PCI (Emilsson et al. 2025).

A range of additional studies have now evaluated the benefit of cangrelor as an adjunct to standard antitherapy agents. As previously discussed, traditional oral P2Y12 antagonists including ticagrelor and clopidogrel have a delay onset of action, especially in patients with ST-segment elevation myocardial infarction (STEMI). Due to the rapid onset of action of cangrelor, the combination of cangrelor with ticagrelor demonstrated a reduction in cardiac damage and improved platelet inhibition during PCI compared with ticagrelor alone (Mohammad et al. 2017; Abo-Aly et al. 2021). Furthermore, a number of other clinical studies have demonstrated therapeutic benefits of combining cangrelor with standard P2Y12 therapies such as clopidogrel and ticagrelor alongside attenuation of platelet activation by other antithrombotic therapies such as tissue plasminogen activation (tPA) (Greenbaum et al. 2007).

The benefits of the improved pharmacokinetic/pharmacodynamic relationship exhibited by cangrelor has informed the use of cangrelor in antiplatelet therapy. Due to cangrelor being the only IV P2Y12 antagonist approved for clinical use, it is the primary therapy for the 5–6% of patients with STEMI who experience resuscitated cardiac arrest and are unconscious on clinical presentation, and >80% platelet inhibition can be achieved within minutes of reaching steady-state plasma concentrations (Angiolillo et al. 2012). Ongoing research continues to evaluate the therapeutic benefit of cangrelor as adjunct therapies for the treatment of a range of cardiovascular disorders.

4.5 Selatogrel

Selatogrel is a novel non-thienopyridine, potent, reversible and selective P2Y12 receptor antagonist. Originally synthesised in 2015 (Caroff et al. 2015), selatogrel demonstrated improved antithrombotic activity compared to clopidogrel in a rat $FeCl_3$-induced thrombosis model, whilst significantly less bleeding was observed compared to clopidogrel in a rat model of blood loss (Caroff et al. 2015). Clinically, Phase I analysis revealed that selatogrel induced a concentration-dependent inhibition of ADP-induced platelet aggregation ex vivo, however this study also identified poor oral bioavailability of the prodrug (Baldoni et al. 2014). Following subcutaneous delivery, selatogrel demonstrated a dose-dependent reduction in impendence platelet aggregation (IPA), and a VerifyNow™ assay of platelet aggregation (Juif et al. 2019). Additional Phase II clinical trials demonstrated significant inhibition of platelet aggregation in patients with chronic coronary syndromes (Storey et al. 2020) and acute myocardial infarction (Sinnaeve et al. 2020). The promising early clinical evaluation of selatogrel has led Phase III evaluation in patients with a confirmed diagnosis of type 1 acute MI due to be completed in Autumn 2025 (https://clinicaltrials.gov/study/NCT04957719).

5 Integrin αIIbβ3 (GPIIbIIIa) Antagonists

The integrin αIIbβ3 (otherwise known as the glycoprotein GPIIbIIIa) is highly expressed on platelets. Upon platelet activation, αIIbβ3 undergoes a conformational change that results in increased avidity and adhesion to fibrinogen (and vWF) to cause crosslinking bridges between platelets and the formation of soft platelet plugs during the initiation of clotting. This process is the final pathway of platelet aggregation and is therefore non-redundant. Such a pathway leads to a compelling target which will provide high potency of drugs that inhibit the pathway (Scarborough et al. 1999). αIIbβ3 antagonists therefore prevent platelet aggregation by selectively blocking αIIbβ3 engagement with fibrinogen. αIIbβ3 antagonists include the antibody chimera abciximab; and smaller molecule antagonists that are derived from peptide sequences that mimic RGD (eptifibatide and tirofiban). These are administered intravenously and provide fast-acting and potent antiplatelet effects during percutaneous coronary interventions (PCI) to inhibit restenosis because of reactive thrombosis during and after the surgical procedure, in patients with high-risk unstable angina and non-ST elevation myocardial infarction (nSTEMI). However, αIIbβ3 antagonists come with a high risk of severe bleeding and thrombocytopaenia, and their use is becoming restricted to patients with a high thrombotic burden, slow coronary flow and other thrombotic complications (Gresele and Momi 2022; Ibanez et al. 2018; Hunt et al. 2001). Therefore, despite these drugs having very potent antiplatelet affects and being fast-acting, their use is now limited owing to high rates of bleeding complications and the development of alternative treatment strategies with improved safety profiles.

Oral αIIbβ3 antagonists were developed for long-term prevention of cardiovascular events. However, these were associated with increased mortality due to pro-thrombotic effects and were therefore not introduced into clinical practice (Chew et al. 2001; Cox 2005). The reasons for this are not fully understood, but possibilities include that the drugs acted as partial agonists, in the absence of vWF or low fibrinogen plasma concentrations; or due to differences in the pharmacokinetics of acute infusions that automatically have high concentrations of the drug circulating, compared to oral formulations that had low bioavailability and were plagued with a high peak-to-trough difference, leading to incomplete platelet suppression. Other problems encountered included drug-induced conformational changes to the αIIbβ3 binding site (Cox 2005). Awareness of these issues has however led to renewed interest in the development of drugs acting on αIIbβ3 and is discussed in novel approaches below.

6 Thrombin Inhibitors and PAR Receptor Antagonists

Protease-activated receptors (PAR) expressed on platelets are key receptors involved in thrombosis and haemostasis. Whilst the PAR receptor family includes PAR1–4, human platelets only express PAR1 and PAR4 (Xu et al. 1998; Kahn et al. 1999a; Vu et al. 1991). Unlike other subfamilies of GPCRs, PAR receptors are unique in that they do not have physiologically soluble ligands but are activated by N-terminal proteolytic cleavage. The serine protease thrombin cleaves a site in the extracellular N-terminal domain of the PAR receptor (the Arg41-Ser42 peptide bond in PAR1 and the Arg47-Gly48 peptide bond in PAR4) (Xu et al. 1998; Vu et al. 1991), this cleavage exposes a new N-terminus which functions as a 'tethered ligand' which interacts with the extracellular loop 2 domain initiating receptor signalling. Whilst it is widely accepted that thrombin serves as one of the primary endogenous proteases of platelet PAR receptors with regard to thrombosis, numerous other proteinases have also been identified that possess the ability to cleave and subsequently activate PAR1 and PAR4 including but not limited to Factor Xa, Plasmin, activated protein C (APC), matrix metalloproteinase-1 (MMP1), neutrophil elastase (NE), and neutrophil proteinase-3 (PR3) (Gieseler et al. 2013). As a GPCR, PAR1 couples to different G protein subfamilies including G_i, G_q and $G_{12/13}$ (Flaumenhaft and De Ceunynck 2017), with signalling pathways determined by the endogenous cleaving proteinase. With regard to thrombin-mediated activation, PAR1 triggers downstream RhoGEF, RhoA and NFkB signalling via the $G_{a12/13}$ subunit (Goggs et al. 2015; Huang et al. 2007; Moers et al. 2003), PLC, CA2+, RAS and ERK1/2 signalling via G_{aq} (Hung et al. 1992; Offermanns et al. 1997), and PI3K, PLCβ and Rac1 signalling via the $\beta\gamma$ subunits of G_i (Jantzen et al. 2001; Voss et al. 2007; Kim et al. 2002; Shankar et al. 2006). These lead to a variety of thrombin-mediated effects on platelets including TXA_2 production, ADP release, 5-HT/adrenaline release, P-selectin and CD40L mobilisation and integrin activation particularly GPIIb/IIIa (Vu et al. 1991; Jin et al. 2009; Kahn et al. 1999b; Faruqi et al. 2000). Furthermore, PAR-1 activation also stimulates procoagulant activity, leading to an amplification of thrombin production and the conversion of fibrinogen to fibrin (Duvernay et al. 2013; French et al. 2016a; Vretenbrant et al. 2007). The net result of these interactions is subsequent thrombus formation mediated by platelet/platelet interactions mediated by fibrin-GPIIb/IIIa interactions.

Similarly to PAR-1, thrombin-mediated cleavage of the PAR4 receptor at the Arg47-Gly48 peptide bond in the extracellular N-terminus exposes a tethered ligand triggering receptor activation (Xu et al. 1998). Like PAR-1, PAR4 receptors also initiate signalling through coupling to G_i and $G_{12/13}$ pathways. However, unlike PAR1 signalling which is typically transient in nature, activation of PAR4 mediates prolonged receptor signalling and sustained platelet activation.

Whilst both PAR1 and PAR4 receptors are most widely understood for their potent response to thrombin, there exists variable affinity of thrombin for each of PAR1 and PAR4 receptors. The PAR1 receptor is activated transiently by thrombin at around 50 pmol/L whilst the affinity of thrombin for the PAR4 receptor is approximately 100-fold less at around 5 nmol/L. Alongside the difference in affinity of thrombin for PAR1 and PAR4, the most dramatic difference between the signalling of these two receptors are the kinetics and duration of activation associated Ca^{2+} signalling. Whilst the specific individual roles of PAR1 and PAR4 receptors in thrombus generation have been reviewed elsewhere, when PAR1 is stimulated there is an initial burst of intracellular Ca^{2+} which rapidly dissipates. However, in contrast, stimulation of PAR4 results in a prolonged Ca^{2+} signal (Shapiro et al. 2000; Covic et al. 2002a; Mazharian et al. 2007). Research has indicated that this sustained Ca^{2+} signal contributes to platelet microparticle release, increased procoagulant activity and thrombin generation (Duvernay et al. 2013; French et al. 2016a; Vretenbrant et al. 2007). This prolonged and sustained platelet activation is therefore widely considered necessary for stable thrombus formation and full platelet spreading on fibrinogen in a p38 and ERK1/2-dependent manner (Covic et al. 2002a; Mazharian et al. 2007). Ultimately, dual-stimulation of both PAR1 and PAR4 is required for full thrombin-induced platelet activation. The nature of this dual-receptor mechanism for thrombin stimulation and the varying contribution of each PAR receptor due to the kinetics of receptor activation with regard to thrombus generation and stability provides a unique opportunity to fine-tune thrombin signalling to optimise platelet responses.

As PAR receptors are not activated by a classical soluble agonist, there are 3 main strategies that can be applied for the blocking of PAR signalling, these include (i) preventing protease engagement and cleavage using blocking antibodies, (ii) blocking the tethered ligand binding site on the extracellular loop (ECLs) 2 of the GPCR using peptide mimetics and small molecules, and (iii) Using pepducins targeting intracellular loops (ICLs) of GPCRs to function as decoy sequestering

G-proteins from the activated receptors thereby disconnecting the receptor from downstream signalling cascades. Here, we will discuss the different approaches currently being evaluated for targeted PAR receptor inhibition to treat a range of cardiovascular diseases associated with inappropriate platelet aggregation and thrombus generation.

The first therapeutic drug targeting PAR receptor signalling was the orthosteric antagonist vorapaxar which received FDA approval in 2014 as a first-in-class PAR1 antagonist (Tricoci et al. 2012; Morrow et al. 2012; Gryka et al. 2017; Goto et al. 2010a). Vorapaxar specifically targets PAR1 receptor signalling through competitive high-affinity binding to the tethered ligand binding site on ECLs 2-3 of PAR1 (Zhang et al. 2012a). Phase III trials including TRACER (thrombin receptor antagonist clinical event reduction in acute coronary syndrome), and TRA-2P-TIMI 50 (thrombin receptor antagonist in secondary prevention of atherothrombotic ischaemic events-TIMI059) revealed that vorapaxar reduced the risk of MI, stroke, or cardiovascular death in patients with history of MI and peripheral arterial disease (PAD) (Tricoci et al. 2012; Morrow et al. 2012). However, whilst both the TRACER and TRA-2P-TIMI 50 trials also revealed these clinical benefits by targeting platelet PAR1, the very same inhibition of PAR1 signalling in the vasculature also led to significant increases in moderate/severe GUSTO bleeding scores (Tricoci et al. 2012) leading to contraindication in patients with a prior history of stroke, transient ischaemic attack, intracranial haemorrhage, or bodyweight less than 60 kg due to alterations in the risk:benefit ratio between therapeutic benefit and increased risk of bleeding (Xu et al. 2021).

Atopaxar (E5555) is another low molecular weight competitive antagonist of PAR-1 competing for the tethered ligand binding site on ECLs 2-3 (Serebruany et al. 2009; Kogushi et al. 2011). Phase II studies revealed that atopaxar demonstrated significant levels of platelet inhibition alongside no evidence of clinically significant bleeding. However, despite evidence of potential benefits, Phase III investigations were not pursued due to identification of significant dose-dependent increases in liver function abnormalities and QTc prolongation (Goto et al. 2010b).

High-throughput screening has also identified a series of allosteric modulators of PAR-1 called parmodulins (parmodulin 1and parmodulin 2) which bind to the C-terminal eighth helix of the PAR1 receptor. Unlike the orthosteric antagonists vorapaxar and atopaxar, parmodulin 1 (JF5) and parmodulin 2 (ML161) selectively inhibit G_q-associated signalling whilst leaving $G_{12/13}$ pathways unaltered (Dowal et al. 2011; Aisiku et al. 2015). This has reduced the overall potency of these compounds with impaired activity for example, inhibition of platelet aggregation at 10uM is maintained, but failing to inhibit platelet shape change at these concentrations (Dowal et al. 2011). Other small molecule antagonists of PAR1 include F-16618, F-16357, ML-161, SCH-79797 and RWJ-58259 which have demonstrated inhibition of platelet aggregation in vitro and antithrombotic activity using in vivo models including the rat arteriovenous shunt model, guinea pig arteriovenous shunt model, guinea pig model of carotoid artery injury and thrombosis and electrolytic injury-induced carotid thrombosis model in cynomolgus monkeys but these have not been taken forward into clinical trials (Perez et al. 2009; Dockendorff et al. 2012; Ahn et al. 2000; Damiano et al. 2003).

The only remaining novel PAR1 targeted therapy that has been explored in clinical trials is the pepducin PZ-128 (Covic et al. 2002a; Zhang et al. 2012b; O'Callaghan et al. 2012). PZ-128 functions as an antagonist through interactions with intracellular loop 3 of PAR1 and modulating corresponding G-protein activity resulting in the inhibition of signalling through PAR1 to the G proteins following stimulation by endogenous agonists. PZ-128 completely inhibits human platelet activation stimulated by the thrombin-receptor activating peptide (TRAP) and SFLLRN, whilst also inhibiting PAR1-dependent platelet aggregation in the baboon (Zhang et al. 2012b). This promising preclinical data has led to PZ-128 being evaluated in Phase II clinical trials which whilst well tolerated with no clear increases in bleeding events, PZ-128 treatment did not significantly change major adverse coronary events at 30 or 90 days (Kuliopulos et al. 2020). Therefore, through a combination of limited efficacy and the incidence of significant adverse bleeding events, there has been limited further clinical development of PAR1 antagonists. This has resulted in an increased focus on PAR4-targeted therapies. Indeed, selective targeting of PAR4 provides a potential opportunity to fine-tune thrombin signalling to optimise platelet responses. Blocking the sustained signalling from PAR4 receptors may limit thrombus stability and vessel occlusion through inhibiting late-stage platelet activation whilst leaving transient PAR1 signalling unaffected sparing the initial response to thrombin and reducing the risk of bleeding complications observed with PAR1 antagonists such as vorapaxar and atopaxar (Han and Nieman 2018). Experimentally, the treatment of isolated platelets with a rabbit polyclonal antibody against the thrombin cleavage site of PAR4 selectively inhibited platelet procoagulant activity whilst a PAR1 receptor antagonist could not (French et al. 2016b). Furthermore, a novel PAR4 antagonist BMS-986120 exhibited efficacious antithrombotic activity in a cynomolgus monkey arterial thrombosis model and demonstrated a low bleeding phenotype compared to P2Y12 and PAR1 antagonists in the same model (Wong et al. 2017). Whilst there are currently no PAR4 antagonists approved for antiplatelet therapy, like PAR1 therapeutics, potential drugs currently under preclinical and clinical investigation also include blocking antibodies, orthosteric antagonists, allosteric antagonists, and pepducins.

Two small-molecule antagonists which exhibit high selectivity for PAR4 over PAR1 include BMS-986120 and BMS-986141 (Wong et al. 2017; Wilson et al. 2018; Priestley et al. 2022). Both of these compounds have completed Phase 1 clinical trials and have shown significant inhibition of PAR4 agonist peptide (PAR4-AP)-induced platelet aggregation with no evidence of significant bleeding impairments (Merali et al. 2022, 2023). Significantly, studies comparing BMS-986120 to current standard-of-care therapeutics such as the P2Y12 antagonist clopidogrel revealed that at equivalent doses that achieved a 80% reduction in thrombus size in cynomolgus monkeys BMS-986120 demonstrated nearly a tenfold reduction in bleeding compared to clopidogrel (Wong et al. 2017; Wilson et al. 2018), a finding further supported by Phase I clinical trial data showing reduced incidence of bleeding compared to standard antiplatelet care (Merali et al. 2022,

2023). The promising activity of these PAR4 antagonists has led to progress further into Phase II clinical trials. In addition to the small molecule compounds described above, anti-PAR4 therapies also include function-blocking antibodies (French et al. 2018; Mumaw et al. 2014), peptidomimetics (Hollenberg et al. 2004) and pepducins (Wielders et al. 2007; Covic et al. 2002b; Rudinga et al. 2018). The PAR4 blocking antibody CAN12 has been shown to inhibit both thrombin and PAR4-AP mediated aggregation of human platelets, however its inhibition of ADP and collagen induced aggregation suggests poor selectivity for the PAR4 receptor (Mumaw et al. 2014). Subsequent development of a new series of monoclonal antibodies targeting the anionic region or the thrombin cleavage site on PAR4 has shown promising reduction of thrombin and PAR4-AP-mediated platelet aggregation and coagulation (French et al. 2018). A peptide antagonist of the PAR4 receptor tc-YPGKF-NH2 has also shown a capacity to inhibit PAR4-AP and thrombin-induced platelet aggregation in murine and human platelets through blocking of the peptide binding site on extracellular loops 2–3 (Hollenberg et al. 2004).

Whilst research has evaluated small molecule antagonists, blocking antibodies, and peptide antagonists to modulate PAR4 signalling, pepducins have also been investigated. Pepducins are small-lipidated peptides which penetrate the lipid bilayer allowing for allosteric modulation of the activity of GPCRs (Xu and Tilley 2022). Depending on the peptide sequence, pepducins can act as either agonists, antagonists or modulators of GPCR activity. The pepducins P4pal-10 and P4pal-il completely inhibited PAR4 agonist-induced platelet aggregation in vitro (Hollenberg et al. 2004) whilst P4pal-10 also delayed thrombin generation and platelet accumulation in the carotoid artery, whilst also protecting against PAR4 agonist-induced systemic thrombus formation (Wielders et al. 2007; Covic et al. 2002b; Rudinga et al. 2018). However, at the current time of publication, no PAR4-specific pepducins have been taken into clinical trials.

7 Phosphodiesterase Inhibitors

Platelets contain three phosphodiesterase (PDE) enzyme classes: PDE2, PDE3, and PDE5. These cytosolic enzymes reduce platelet activity and secretion by increasing cytosolic levels of cAMP (PDE2, and PDE3), and cGMP (PDE5), thus interfering with many signalling pathways that occur upon platelet activation (Gresele and Momi 2022). Cilostazol is a PDE3 inhibitor and has demonstrated efficacy both compared to aspirin (PICASSO clinical trial), and as a DAPT in combination with aspirin or clopidogrel where the combination reduced the incidence of stroke by half compared to the monotherapies alone (Toyoda et al. 2019; Kim et al. 2020). Interestingly, dipyridamole exhibits polypharmacology in that it inhibits both PDE3 and PDE5, and also increases circulating levels of the nucleoside adenosine, which inhibits platelet activation via A_{2A} and A_{2B} receptors. Currently, dipyridamole is used in combination with aspirin for the secondary prevention of stroke (Gresele and Momi 2022; Halkes et al. 2006).

8 Novel Targets for Antiplatelet Therapy

It can be argued that improvements in antiplatelet medication are obtainable, considering the use of current drugs (notably aspirin and clopidogrel) was based entirely on clinical observations, and thus their establishment in cardiovascular disease was not initially based on preclinical laboratory design, and that despite the benefits of DAPT, thrombotic events are still prevalent in patients (Angiolillo et al. 2007). Nevertheless, previous preclinical testing and strategies have failed to predict lack of efficacy (TP receptor antagonists, 5-HT2A antagonists) or safety concerns (oral αIIbβ3 inhibitors) that were based on rational target identification strategies. To improve on current medications, preclinical research might therefore require (1) Identification for a target to be important in the activation of a panel of potent platelet agonists, both in vitro (aggregation) and in vivo (since platelet activation is heavily influenced by external factors from the endothelium); (2) A requirement to recapitulate models of disease, potentially combining conditions of atherosclerosis (e.g. use of ApoE mice) with thrombosis and MI (combined) via intra-vital/laser, ferric chloride, Rose Bengal, or mechanical injury, where components of thrombotic clot are dependent on inducing agent; (3) To develop a more accurate extrapolation of bleeding risk pertinent to trauma; and (4) Continued development of laboratory responses to individual patients (to personalise effective antiplatelet medication). It is hoped that within this strategy, platelet targets that are pertinent to thrombosis induced by atherosclerosis can be identified that are qualitatively different from processes required for healthy haemostasis. Novel approaches are focused on inference of platelet adhesion (targeting glycoprotein GPIb as part of the GPIb-V-IX complex, glycoprotein GPVI, integrin α2β1, P-selectin); interference to platelet activation pathways and amplification processes (prostaglandin EP3 receptor, protease receptor PAR1/4, combined $P2Y_1R$-$P2Y_{12}R$ antagonism), and direct interference of aggregation (targeting selective integrin αIIbβ3 epitopes).

The rationale for interference of platelet adhesion is due to initial adhesion events with the damaged vasculature being critical to the formation of a thrombus, a perception of little redundancy, that adhesion events do not target the venous circulation (so less risk of haemorrhage), decreased adhesion leading to reduced platelet activation and secretion, and lastly the discovery that platelets are involved in the inflammatory processes during atherosclerosis which also requires adhesion events for the inflammatory response to occur.

Glycoprotein GPIb adhesion leads to the arrest of platelets during fast blood flow, as it reversibly binds to vWF expressed on endothelial cells. This has made GPIb a particularly attractive target. Antagonistic peptides (aptamers, e.g. ARC545C, BT200), monoclonal antibodies and Fab fragments (e.g.AJW200, h6B4-Fab) have been developed that are directed against the binding site of vWF on the GPIb receptor (Gresele and Momi 2022). As an example, h6B4-Fab has been shown to inhibit aggregation, and delay thrombus formation, with only minor bleeding in preclinical in vivo models (Fontayne et al. 2008), and some inhibitors of GPIb (e.g. anfibatide, a modified snake C-type lectin) have progressed through to small-scale clinical trials (Zheng et al. 2021). Thrombocytopaenia can occur with the administration of the full antibodies, but this detrimental effect has been engineered out with the design of Fab fragments or non-antibody molecules.

P-selectin is stored in platelet α granules, as well as the Weibel-Palade bodies of endothelial cells. P-selectin is necessary for the adhesion of platelets to inflamed vessels and during thrombosis, and also platelet-dependent leukocyte recruitment (Pitchford et al. 2005). Both small molecule antagonists (e.g. PSI-697, ML355) and monoclonal antibodies have been developed (inclacumab, crizanlizumab) which showed a reduction in thrombus size in vivo, without an increase in bleeding time. Some of these compounds have progressed through to phase II clinical trials (SELECT-ACS Trial: inclacumab) in patients with non-STEMI, with reduced myocardial damage and no significant bleeding events (Tardif et al. 2013; Stähli et al. 2016). Crizanlizumab and inclacumab are now indicated for (Ataga et al. 2017), or in phase I clinical trial (inclacumab) reducing thrombo-occlusive crises in patients with sickle cell anaemia (Mayer et al. 2023). A potential advantage of blocking P-selectin includes an anti-inflammatory effect and therefore may provide a treatment option for the reduction in myocardial damage after PCI, due to the acute inflammation associated with thrombosis. Whilst the incidence of adverse events was not reduced in the SELECT-ACS Trial (Tardif et al. 2013; Stähli et al. 2016), P-selectin and pan-selectin antagonists are being developed preclinically as a treatment for atherosclerosis in mind (Wagner et al. 2024).

The integrin $\alpha_2\beta_1$ is present on many cell types, including platelets where it acts to adhere to collagen and laminin. $\alpha_2\beta_1$ is upregulated with MI and stroke. In vitro tests of antagonists and Mabs reveal reduction in aggregate size. Patients with $\alpha_2\beta_1$ integrin deficiency suffer from only mild bleeding. Small molecule inhibitors have shown in vivo efficacy (He et al. 2003; Kuijpers et al. 2007). However, because the integrin is not platelet-specific, targeting it could result in side effects (Janus-Bell and Mangin 2023).

GPVI is a member of the Ig superfamily of receptors associated with the dimeric Fc receptor γ-chain (FcRγ) (Gibbins et al. 1997). GPVI is exclusively expressed on platelets and is a major collagen receptor that is important in primary adhesion during arterial thrombosis, which does not appear to play a role in normal haemostasis (Mangin et al. 2012). Early data reported that certain snake venom metalloproteinases (kistomin), cleaved GPVI and inhibited platelet aggregation and thrombus formation (Hsu et al. 2008), whilst GPVI-deficient mice were protected from thromboembolism (Lockyer et al. 2006; Massberg et al. 2003). Preclinical studies showed that monoclonal antibodies against GPVI inhibited thrombosis, with only minor bleeding associated (Li et al. 2007). Confidence in targeting GPVI has led to the development of glenzocimab (ACT017 Fab); and revacept (GPVI-Fc Fc fragment) that have been well tolerated in phase I clinical trials with no apparent bleeding events (Voors-Pette et al. 2019). Both compounds have now progressed through to Phase II/III clinical trials (Uphaus et al. 2022); ACTISAVE: NCT05070260). The challenge now is to create orally available small molecule inhibitors of GPVI that would potentially open up the use of anti-GPVI therapy as a preventative antiplatelet drug (Damaskinaki et al. 2021).

CLEC-2 is a type II transmembrane receptor which is highly expressed in both megakaryocytes and platelets. CLEC-2 signalling is dependent on Syk activation leading to phosphorylation of downstream adapter proteins such as SH2 and PLCγ2 thereby increasing intracellular calcium leading to platelet activation. This CLEC-2-mediated platelet activation has been reported to play a key role in the process of thrombosis, with impaired platelet aggregate formation observed in CLEC-2-deficient platelets and increased bleeding times in mice treated with the CLEC-2 inhibitor INU1 (Meng et al. 2021). Downstream of Syk is Bruton's tyrosine kinase (Btk). The Btk inhibitor ibtrutinib has recently been demonstrated to inhibit CLEC-2 mediated platelet aggregation in human platelets, a phenomenon reported with the second-generation Btk inhibitor acalabrutinib (Nicolson et al. 2021). However, both contributed to increased bleeding risk due to off-target Syk-mediated effects. Subsequent development of a reversible Btk inhibitor MK-1026 also revealed inhibition of GPVI and CLEC-2-mediated platelet aggregation. Significantly, MK-1026 showed less off-target effects and only inhibited the activation of isolated platelets (Tullemans et al. 2021). Further research is therefore required to further characterise the validity of therapeutics targeting CLEC-2 activation in the treatment of thrombosis.

Interest in prostaglandin control of platelet function has not been limited to aspirin, TXA_2 and PCI_2. The prostaglandin PGE_2 causes potent platelet aggregation through stimulation of the EP3 receptor and enhances platelet activation to other agonists (Matthews and Jones 1993; Fabre et al. 2001). PGE_2 activation of platelets increases in plaques but its physiological role appears negligible in healthy individuals. Thus, development and evaluation of EP3 receptor antagonists, for example, DG-041 has demonstrated the ability to inhibit thrombosis with no detriment to haemostasis (Heptinstall et al. 2008; Tilly et al. 2014). Whether these observations of potency and safety translate to clinical trials remains unknown.

ADP-induced platelet activation can also be targeted by the $P2Y_1$ receptor (as well as $P2Y_{12}$ antagonists used clinically). Antagonists of $P2Y_1$ such as MRS2179 and MRS2500 have efficacy at inhibiting platelet aggregation in vitro, and thromboembolism in vivo to a range of platelet agonists (Hechler et al. 2006; Léon et al. 2001), with only a moderate prolongation of bleeding time. MRS2179 and MRS2500 are however nucleotide-based structures and will have unfavourable pharmacokinetic qualities as drugs. Orally available P2Y1 antagonists therefore are being developed (Pfefferkorn et al. 2008; Qiao et al. 2013), but as yet no clinical trials have occurred. Synergistic inhibition of platelet activation occurs when antagonism of $P2Y_1$ and $P2Y_{12}$ is combined (Hechler et al. 2006). Due to this significant inhibition of platelet aggregation through combined inhibition of $P2Y_1$ and $P2Y_{12}$, recent research has reported the development of a new class of diadenosine tetraphosphate (AP_4A) compounds that demonstrate simultaneous inhibitory activity at both $P2Y_1$ and $P2Y_{12}$ receptors (Koganov et al. 2018). A lead AP_4A-derived compound GLS-409 demonstrated reversible inhibition of ADP-induced platelet aggregation in human platelets, alongside inhibition in a canine model of recurrent coronary thrombosis without altering bleeding time in these animals (Koganov et al. 2018). Whilst further research is required to characterise the preclinical activity of this novel class of dual $P2Y_1$:$P2Y_{12}$ antagonists, this research highlights the therapeutic potential of such an approach.

The adenosine A_{2A} and A_{2B} receptors have received attention because the activation of these receptors by the endogenous ligand adenosine suppresses platelet activation (Wolska and Rozalski 2019). However, adenosine has a very short half-life in the circulation (1 s), and thus various synthetic small molecule agonists have been developed, that reduce platelet aggregation in vitro. Adenosine will also activate endothelial cells expressing A_{2A} to cause vasodilation, and so this activity may make the development of adenosine agonists as antiplatelet agents unlikely (Gresele and Momi 2022).

The modulation of platelet signalling pathways has also been studied, notably phosphoinositide 3-kinase β (PI3Kβ), spleen tyrosine kinase (syk) and tyrosine kinase (TK), with selective inhibitors. Studies are at a preclinical stage, with the exception of PI3Kβ inhibitor AZD6482, which has been administered to healthy adult males resulting in greater inhibition of platelet aggregation and lower prolongation of bleeding time compared to aspirin + clopidogrel (Nylander et al. 2015). However, AZD6482 was administered via infusion, and thus the rationale for use is to prophylactically prevent cardiovascular events, and possibility for the eventual development of an orally available PI3Kβ inhibitor for long-term use remains to be tested.

9 Conclusion

Despite the effectiveness of current antiplatelet drugs in preventing thrombosis, there is clearly a requirement for more potent, and safer strategies to prevent platelet activation. These strategies may require the development of compounds against targets discussed above, or better patient management of existing drugs. Such decisions might include choosing amongst the $P2Y_{12}$R antagonists used clinically to combine with aspirin (DAPT), decisions on the duration of antiplatelet therapy and considerations to when to stop aspirin use, personalised antiplatelet therapy, or the addition of a third agent (e.g. thrombin blockade).

References

Abo-Aly M, George B, Shokri E, Chelvarajan L, El-Helw M, Smyth SS, et al (2021) Cangrelor in addition to standard therapy reduces cardiac damage and inflammatory markers in patients with ST-segment elevation myocardial infarction. J Thromb Thrombolysis [Internet] [cited 2025 Jul 17];52(3):934–940. Available from: https://pubmed.ncbi.nlm.nih.gov/33258102/

Ahn HS, Foster C, Boykow G, Stamford A, Manna M, Graziano M (2000) Inhibition of cellular action of thrombin by N3-cyclopropyl-7-{[4-(1-methylethyl)phenyl]methyl}-7H-pyrrolo[3,2-f]quinazoline-1,3-diamine (SCH 79797), a nonpeptide thrombin receptor antagonist. Biochem Pharmacol [Internet] [cited 2025 Jul 3];60(10):1425–1434. Available from: https://www.sciencedirect.com/science/article/pii/S0006295200004603?via%3Dihub

Aisiku O, Peters CG, De Ceunynck K, Ghosh CC, Dilks JR, Fustolo-Gunnink SF, et al (2015) Parmodulins inhibit thrombus formation without inducing endothelial injury caused by vorapaxar. Blood [Internet] [cited 2025 Jul 11];125(12):1976–1985. Available from: https://pubmed.ncbi.nlm.nih.gov/25587041/

Ajani AE, Lefkovits J (2008) Approaching an age of reason with antiplatelet therapy. Lancet [Internet] [cited 2025 Jul 14];371(9621):1315–1316. Available from: https://www.sciencedirect.com/science/article/abs/pii/S0140673608605735

Alexopoulos D, Xanthopoulou I, Gkizas V, Kassimis G, Theodoropoulos KC, Makris G, et al (2012) Randomized assessment of ticagrelor versus prasugrel antiplatelet effects in patients with ST-segment-elevation myocardial infarction. Circ Cardiovasc Interv [Internet] [cited 2025 Jul 17];5(6):797–804. Available from: https://pubmed.ncbi.nlm.nih.gov/23169985/

Amison RT, Arnold S, O'Shaughnessy BG, Cleary SJ, Ofoedu J, Idzko M, et al (2017) Lipopolysaccharide (LPS) induced pulmonary neutrophil recruitment and platelet activation is mediated via the P2Y 1 and P2Y 14 receptors in mice. Pulm Pharmacol Ther [Internet] [cited 2019 Aug 2];45:62–68. Available from: http://www.ncbi.nlm.nih.gov/pubmed/28487256

Angiolillo DJ, Fernandez-Ortiz A, Bernardo E, Alfonso F, Macaya C, Bass TA, et al (2007) Variability in individual responsiveness to clopidogrel. Clinical implications, management, and future perspectives. J Am Coll Cardiol [Internet] [cited 2025 Jul 17];49(14):1505–1516. Available from: https://pubmed.ncbi.nlm.nih.gov/17418288/

Angiolillo DJ, Schneider DJ, Bhatt DL, French WJ, Price MJ, Saucedo JF, et al (2012) Pharmacodynamic effects of cangrelor and clopidogrel: the platelet function substudy from the cangrelor versus standard therapy to achieve optimal management of platelet inhibition (CHAMPION) trials. J Thromb Thrombolysis [Internet] [cited 2025 Jul 17];34(1):44–55. Available from: https://pubmed.ncbi.nlm.nih.gov/22569899/

Antman EM, Wiviott SD, Murphy SA, Voitk J, Hasin Y, Widimsky P, et al (2008) Early and late benefits of prasugrel in patients with acute coronary syndromes undergoing percutaneous coronary intervention: a TRITON–TIMI 38 (TRial to Assess Improvement in Therapeutic Outcomes by Optimizing Platelet InhibitioN with Prasugrel–Thrombolysis In Myocardial Infarction) analysis J Am Coll Cardiol [Internet] [cited 2025 Jul 14];51(21):2028–2033. Available from: https://www.sciencedirect.com/science/article/pii/S0735109708012709

Ataga KI, Kutlar A, Kanter J, Liles D, Cancado R, Friedrisch J, et al (2017) Crizanlizumab for the Prevention of Pain Crises in Sickle Cell Disease. N Engl J Med [Internet] [cited 2025 Aug 26];376(5):429–439. Available from: https://www.nejm.org/doi/pdf/10.1056/NEJMoa1611770

Baldoni D, Bruderer S, Krause A, Gutierrez M, Gueret P, Astruc B, et al (2014) A new reversible and potent P2Y12 receptor antagonist (ACT-246475): tolerability, pharmacokinetics, and pharmacodynamics in a first-in-man trial. Clin Drug Investig [Internet] [cited 2025 Jul 17];34 (11):807–818. Available from: https://pubmed.ncbi.nlm.nih.gov/25331625/

Baurand A, Raboisson P, Freund M, Léon C, Cazenave JP, Bourguignon JJ et al (2001) Inhibition of platelet function by administration of MRS2179, a P2Y1 receptor antagonist. Eur J Pharmacol [Internet]. 412(3):213–221. Available from: http://www.ncbi.nlm.nih.gov/pubmed/11166284

Belch J, Cormie J, Newman P, McLaren M, Barbenel J, Capell H, et al (1983) Dazoxiben, a thromboxane synthetase inhibitor, in the treatment of Raynaud's syndrome: a double-blind trial. Br J Clin Pharmacol [Internet] [cited 2025 Aug 26];15(1 S):113S–116S. Available from: https://pubmed.ncbi.nlm.nih.gov/6337601/

Bertrand ME, Rupprecht HJ, Urban P, Gershlick AH (2000) Double-blind study of the safety of clopidogrel with and without a loading dose in combination with aspirin compared with ticlopidine in combination with aspirin after coronary stenting: The clopidogrel aspirin stent international cooperative study (CLASSICS). Circulation [Internet] [cited 2025 Jul 17];102(6): 624–629. Available from: https://pubmed.ncbi.nlm.nih.gov/10931801/

Bhatt DL, Lincoff AM, Gibson CM, Stone GW, McNulty S, Montalescot G et al (2009) Intravenous platelet blockade with cangrelor during PCI. N Engl J Med 361(24):2330–2341

Bhatt DL, Stone GW, Mahaffey KW, Michael Gibson C, Gabriel Steg P, Hamm CW, et al (2013) Effect of platelet inhibition with cangrelor during PCI on ischemic events. N Engl J Med [Internet] [cited 2025 Jul 17];368(14):1303–1313. Available from: https://www.nejm.org/doi/pdf/10.1056/NEJMoa1300815

Bousser MG, Amarenco P, Chamorro A, Fisher M, Ford I, Fox KM, et al (2011) Terutroban versus aspirin in patients with cerebral ischaemic events (PERFORM): a randomised, double-blind, parallel-group trial. Lancet [Internet] [cited 2025 Aug 26];377(9782):2013–2022. Available from: https://pubmed.ncbi.nlm.nih.gov/21616527/

Brar SS, Ten Berg J, Marcucci R, Price MJ, Valgimigli M, Kim HS, et al (2011) Impact of platelet reactivity on clinical outcomes after percutaneous coronary intervention: a collaborative meta-analysis of individual participant data. J Am Coll Cardiol [Internet] [cited 2025 Jul 17];58(19): 1945–1954. Available from: https://pubmed.ncbi.nlm.nih.gov/22032704/

Braun K, Rettinger J, Ganso M, Kassack M, Hildebrandt C, Ullmann H et al (2001) Nf449: a subnanomolar potency antagonist at recombinant rat P2X1 receptors. Naunyn Schmiedebergs Arch Pharmacol 364(3):285–290

Burnstock G (2007) Purine and pyrimidine receptors. Cell Mol Life Sci [Internet] [cited 2013 Sep 24];64(12):1471–1483. Available from: http://www.ncbi.nlm.nih.gov/pubmed/17375261

Byrne RA, Rossello X, Coughlan JJ, Barbato E, Berry C, Chieffo A et al (2023) 2023 ESC guidelines for the management of acute coronary syndromes. Eur Heart J 44(38):3720–3826

Cannon CP, Husted S, Harrington RA, Scirica BM, Emanuelsson H, Peters G, et al (2007) Safety, tolerability, and initial efficacy of AZD6140, the first reversible oral adenosine diphosphate receptor antagonist, compared with clopidogrel, in patients with non–ST-segment elevation acute coronary syndrome: primary results of the DISPERSE-2 trial. J Am Coll Cardiol [Internet] [cited 2025 Jul 17];50(19):1844–1851. Available from: https://www.sciencedirect.com/science/article/pii/S0735109707026344

Capra V, Bäck M, Angiolillo DJ, Cattaneo M, Sakariassen KS (2014) Impact of vascular thromboxane prostanoid receptor activation on hemostasis, thrombosis, oxidative stress, and inflammation. J Thromb Haemost [Internet] [cited 2025 Aug 26];12(2):126–137. Available from: https://pubmed.ncbi.nlm.nih.gov/24298905/

Caroff E, Hubler F, Meyer E, Renneberg D, Gnerre C, Treiber A, et al (2015) Methoxypyrrolidin-1-yl)-2-phenylpyrimidine-4-carbonyl]amino}-3-phosphonopropionyl)piperazine-1-carboxylic acid butyl ester (ACT-246475) and its prodrug (ACT-281959), a novel P2Y 12 receptor antagonist with a wider therapeutic window in the rat than clopidogrel. [cited 2025 Jul 10];4–6. Available from: https://pubs.acs.org/sharingguidelines

Catella-Lawson F, Reilly MP, Kapoor SC, Cucchiara AJ, DeMarco S, Tournier B, et al (2001) Cyclooxygenase inhibitors and the antiplatelet effects of aspirin. N Engl J Med [Internet] [cited 2025 Aug 26];345(25):1809–1817. Available from: https://pubmed.ncbi.nlm.nih.gov/11752357/

Cattaneo M (2005) The P2 receptors and congenital platelet function defects. Semin Thromb Hemost [Internet] [cited 2025 Jul 14];31(2):168–173. Available from: http://www.thieme-connect.de/products/ejournals/html/10.1055/s-2005-869522

Cattaneo M (2011) Resistance to anti-platelet agents. Thromb Res [Internet] [cited 2011 Oct 31];127 Suppl:S61–S63. Available from: http://www.ncbi.nlm.nih.gov/pubmed/21262444

Cattaneo M, Faioni EM (2012) Why does ticagrelor induce dyspnea? Thromb Haemost [Internet] [cited 2025 Jul 17];108(6):1031–1036. Available from: http://www.thieme-connect.de/products/ejournals/html/10.1160/TH12-08-0547

Cheng Y, Austin SC, Rocca B, Koller BH, Coffman TM, Grosser T, et al (2002) Role of prostacyclin in the cardiovascular response to thromboxane A2. Science (80-) [Internet] [cited 2025 Aug 26];296(5567):539–541. Available from: https://pubmed.ncbi.nlm.nih.gov/11964481/

Chew DP, Bhatt DL, Sapp S, Topol EJ (2001) The online version of this article, along with updated information and services, is located on the World Wide Web at: http://circ.ahajournals.org/content/103/2/201. Online. pp 201–206

Collet J-P, Cuisset T, Rangé G, Cayla G, Elhadad S, Pouillot C, et al (2012) Bedside monitoring to adjust antiplatelet therapy for coronary stenting. N Engl J Med [Internet] [cited 2025 Jul 17];367(22):2100–2109. Available from: https://pubmed.ncbi.nlm.nih.gov/23121439/

Covic L, Singh C, Smith H, Kuliopulos A (2002a) Role of the PAR4 thrombin receptor in stabilizing platelet-platelet aggregates as revealed by a patient with Hermansky-Pudlak syndrome. Thromb Haemost 87(4):722–727

Covic L, Gresser AL, Talavera J, Swift S, Kuliopulos A (2002b) Activation and inhibition of G protein-coupled receptors by cell-penetrating membrane-tethered peptides. Proc Natl Acad Sci U S A [Internet] [cited 2025 Jul 11];99(2):643–648. Available from: https://pubmed.ncbi.nlm.nih.gov/11805322/

Cox D (2005) Oral GPIIb / IIIa Antagonists: What Went Wrong? Curr Pharm Des [Internet] [cited 2025 Aug 26];10(14):1587–1596. Available from: https://pubmed.ncbi.nlm.nih.gov/15134557/

Damaskinaki FN, Moran LA, Garcia A, Kellam B, Watson SP (2021) Overcoming challenges in developing small molecule inhibitors for GPVI and CLEC-2. Platelets [Internet] [cited 2025 Aug 26];32(6):744–752. Available from: https://pubmed.ncbi.nlm.nih.gov/33406951/

Damiano BP, Derian CK, Maryanoff BE, Zhang HC, Gordon PA (2003) RWJ-58259: a selective antagonist of protease activated Receptor-1. Cardiovasc Drug Rev [Internet] [cited 2025 Jul 3];21(4):313–326. Available from: /doi/pdf/10.1111/j.1527 3466.2003 tb00124.x

Dangelmaier C, Jin J, Smith JB, Kunapuli SP (2001) Potentiation of thromboxane A2-induced platelet secretion by Gi signaling through the phosphoinositide-3 kinase pathway. Thromb Haemost 85(2):341–348

Dockendorff C, Aisiku O, Verplank L, Dilks JR, Smith DA, Gunnink SF, et al (2012) Discovery of 1,3-diaminobenzenes as selective inhibitors of platelet activation at the PAR1 receptor. ACS Med Chem Lett [Internet] [cited 2025 Jul 3];3(3):232–237. Available from: /doi/pdf/10.1021/ml2002696?ref=article_openPDF

Dovlatova N, Wijeyeratne YD, Fox SC, Manolopoulos P, Johnson AJ, White AE, et al (2008) Detection of P2Y(14) protein in platelets and investigation of the role of P2Y(14) in platelet function in comparison with the EP(3) receptor. Thromb Haemost [Internet] [cited 2016 Jan 12];100(2):261–270. Available from: http://www.ncbi.nlm.nih.gov/pubmed/18690346

Dowal L, Sim DS, Dilks JR, Blair P, Beaudry S, Denker BM, et al (2011) Identification of an antithrombotic allosteric modulator that acts through helix 8 of PAR1. Proc Natl Acad Sci U S A [Internet] [cited 2025 Jul 11];108(7):2951–2956. Available from: /doi/pdf/10.1073/pnas.1014863108?download=true

Duvernay M, Young S, Gailani D, Schoenecker J, Hamm H (2013) Protease-Activated Receptor (PAR) 1 and PAR4 differentially regulate factor V expression from human platelets. Mol Pharmacol [Internet] [cited 2025 Jul 11];83(4):781–792. Available from: https://www.sciencedirect.com/science/article/pii/S0026895X24036824

Elwood PC, Cochrane AL, Burr ML, Sweetnam PM, Williams G, Welsby E, et al (1974) A randomized controlled trial of acetyl salicylic acid in the secondary prevention of mortality from myocardial infarction. Br Med J [Internet] [cited 2025 Aug 26];1(5905):436–440. Available from: https://pubmed.ncbi.nlm.nih.gov/4593555/

Emilsson OL, Mohammad MA, Grimfjärd P, Persson J, Santos-Pardo I, Erlinge D, et al (2025) Cangrelor during percutaneous coronary intervention in patients with cardiogenic shock or cardiac arrest. JACC Cardiovasc Interv [Internet] [cited 2025 Jul 17];18(7):853–862. Available from: https://www.sciencedirect.com/science/article/pii/S1936879825007897

Fabre JE, Nguyen MT, Athirakul K, Coggins K, McNeish JD, Austin S, et al (2001) Activation of the murine EP3 receptor for PGE2 inhibits cAMP production and promotes platelet aggregation. J Clin Invest [Internet] [cited 2025 Aug 26];107(5):603–610. Available from: https://pubmed.ncbi.nlm.nih.gov/11238561/

Faruqi TR, Weiss EJ, Shapiro MJ, Huang W, Coughlin SR (2000) Structure-function analysis of protease-activated receptor 4 tethered ligand peptides: determinants of specificity and utility in assays of receptor function. J Biol Chem [Internet] [cited 2025 Jul 14];275(26):19728–19734. Available from: https://www.sciencedirect.com/science/article/pii/S0021925819800431

FitzGerald GA, Oates JA, Hawiger J, Maas RL, Roberts LJ, Lawson JA, et al (1983) Endogenous biosynthesis of prostacyclin and thromboxane and platelet function during chronic administration of aspirin in man. J Clin Invest [Internet] [cited 2025 Aug 26];71(3):676–688. Available from: https://pubmed.ncbi.nlm.nih.gov/6338043/

Flaumenhaft R, De Ceunynck K (2017) Targeting PAR1: now what? Trends Pharmacol Sci [Internet] [cited 2025 Jul 11];38(8):701. Available from: https://pmc.ncbi.nlm.nih.gov/articles/PMC5580498/

Fontayne A, Meiring M, Lamprecht S, Roodt J, Demarsin E, Barbeaux P, et al (2008) The humanized anti-glycoprotein Ib monoclonal antibody h6B4-Fab is a potent and safe antithrombotic in a high shear arterial thrombosis model in baboons. Thromb Haemost [Internet] [cited 2025 Aug 26];100(4):670–677. Available from: http://www.thieme-connect.com/products/ejournals/html/10.1160/TH08-02-0073

French SL, Arthur JF, Lee H, Nesbitt WS, Andrews RK, Gardiner EE, et al (2016a) Inhibition of protease-activated receptor 4 impairs platelet procoagulant activity during thrombus formation in human blood. J Thromb Haemost [Internet] [cited 2025 Jul 11];14(8):1642–1654. Available from: https://www.sciencedirect.com/science/article/pii/S1538783622035231

French SL, Arthur JF, Lee H, Nesbitt WS, Andrews RK, Gardiner EE, et al (2016b) Inhibition of protease-activated receptor 4 impairs platelet procoagulant activity during thrombus formation in human blood. J Thromb Haemost [Internet] [cited 2025 Jul 14];14(8):1642–1654. Available from: https://pubmed.ncbi.nlm.nih.gov/26878340/

French SL, Thalmann C, Bray PF, Macdonald LE, Murphy AJ, Sleeman MW, et al (2018) A function-blocking PAR4 antibody is markedly antithrombotic in the face of a hyperreactive PAR4 variant. Blood Adv [Internet] [cited 2025 Jul 3];2(11):1283–1293. Available from: https://pubmed.ncbi.nlm.nih.gov/29884748/

Fung CYE, Cendana C, Farndale RW, Mahaut-smith MP (2007) Primary and secondary agonists can use P2X1 receptors as a major pathway to increase intracellular Ca2+ in the human platelet. J Thromb Haemost [Internet] [cited 2025 Jul 14];5(5):910–917. Available from: https://www.sciencedirect.com/science/article/pii/S153878362210437X

Gachet C (2008) P2 receptors, platelet function and pharmacological implications. Thromb Haemost [Internet] [cited 2011 Sep 6];99(3):466–472. Available from: http://www.ncbi.nlm.nih.gov/pubmed/18327393

Gibbins JM, Okuma M, Farndale R, Barnes M, Watson SP (1997) Glycoprotein VI is the collagen receptor in platelets which underlies tyrosine phosphorylation of the Fc receptor γ-chain. FEBS Lett [Internet] [cited 2025 Aug 26];413(2):255–259. Available from: https://pubmed.ncbi.nlm.nih.gov/9280292/

Gieseler F, Ungefroren H, Settmacher U, Hollenberg MD, Kaufmann R (2013) Proteinase-activated receptors (PARs) - Focus on receptor-receptor- interactions and their physiological and pathophysiological impact. Cell Commun Signal [Internet] [cited 2025 Jul 11];11(1):1–26. Available from: https://biosignaling.biomedcentral.com/articles/10.1186/1478-811X-11-86

Goggs R, Williams CM, Mellor H, Poole AW (2015) Platelet Rho GTPases–a focus on novel players, roles and relationships. Biochem J [Internet] [cited 2025 Jul 11];466(3):431–442. Available from: https://www.sciencedirect.com/org/science/article/pii/S1470872815002003

Goto S, Yamaguchi T, Ikeda Y, Kato K, Yamaguchi H, Jensen P (2010a) Safety and exploratory efficacy of the novel thrombin receptor (PAR-1) antagonist SCH530348 for non-ST-segment elevation acute coronary syndrome. J Atheroscler Thromb 17(2):156–164

Goto S, Ogawa H, Takeuchi M, Flather MD, Bhatt DL (2010b) Double-blind, placebo-controlled phase II studies of the protease-activated receptor 1 antagonist E5555 (atopaxar) in Japanese patients with acute coronary syndrome or high-risk coronary artery disease. Eur Heart J [Internet] cited 2025 Jul 3];31(21):2601–2613. Available from: https://doi.org/10.1093/eurheartj/ehq320

Gratacap MP, Herault JP, Viala C, Ragab A, Savi P, Herbert JM, et al (2000) FcγRIIA requires a Gi-dependent pathway for an efficient stimulation of phosphoinositide 3-kinase, calcium mobilization, and platelet aggregation. Blood [Internet] [cited 2025 Jul 14];96(10):3439–3446. Available from: https://www.sciencedirect.com/science/article/pii/S0006497120482825

Greenbaum AB, Grines CL, Bittl JA, Becker RC, Kereiakes DJ, Gilchrist IC, et al (2006) Initial experience with an intravenous P2Y12 platelet receptor antagonist in patients undergoing percutaneous coronary intervention: results from a 2-part, phase II, multicenter, randomized, placebo- and active-controlled trial. Am Heart J [Internet] [cited 2025 Jul 17];151(3):689.e1–689.e10. Available from: https://www.sciencedirect.com/science/article/pii/S0002870305010458?casa_token=Rpxzh9EmGY4AAAAA:z-1w56zsGUpo5aLejYN_Q1S6SCcg_ksCUaI3emaUN17uHCS6EpIwueazYXeYI72_KZGpKRFTbA

Greenbaum AB, Ohman EM, Gibson CM, Borzak S, Stebbins AL, Lu M, et al (2007) Preliminary experience with intravenous P2Y12 platelet receptor inhibition as an adjunct to reduced-dose alteplase during acute myocardial infarction: results of the safety, tolerability and effect on patency in acute myocardial infarction (STEP-AMI) angiographic trial. Am Heart J [Internet] [cited 2025 Jul 17];154(4):702–709. Available from: https://www.sciencedirect.com/science/article/abs/pii/S0002870307004929

Gresele P, Momi S (2022) Novel approaches to antiplatelet therapy. Biochem Pharmacol [Internet] [cited 2025 Aug 26];206. Available from: https://pubmed.ncbi.nlm.nih.gov/36243098/

Gryka RJ, Buckley LF, Anderson SM (2017) Vorapaxar: the current role and future directions of a novel protease-activated receptor antagonist for risk reduction in atherosclerotic disease. Drugs R D [Internet] [cited 2025 Jul 11];17(1):65. Available from: https://pmc.ncbi.nlm.nih.gov/articles/PMC5318326/

Habib A, Fitzgerald GA, Maclouf J (1999) Phosphorylation of the thromboxane receptor α, the predominant isoform expressed in human platelets. J Biol Chem [Internet] [cited 2025 Aug 26];274(5):2645–2651. Available from: https://pubmed.ncbi.nlm.nih.gov/9915793/

Hagihara K, Kazui M, Kurihara A, Iwabuchi H, Ishikawa M, Kobayashi H, et al (2010) Biotransformation of prasugrel, a novel thienopyridine antiplatelet agent, to the pharmacologically active metabolite. Drug Metab Dispos [Internet] [cited 2025 Jul 17];38(6):898–904. Available from: https://www.sciencedirect.com/science/article/abs/pii/S0090955624023730

Halkes PH, Van Gijn J, Kappelle LJ, Koudstaal PJ, Algra A (2006) Aspirin plus dipyridamole versus aspirin alone after cerebral ischaemia of arterial origin (ESPRIT): randomised controlled trial. Lancet [Internet] [cited 2025 Aug 26];367(9523):1665–1673. Available from: https://pubmed.ncbi.nlm.nih.gov/16714187/

Han X, Nieman MT (2018) PAR4 (Protease-Activated Receptor 4): PARticularly Important 4 Antiplatelet Therapy Arterioscler Thromb Vasc Biol [Internet] [cited 2025 Jul 11];38(2):287–289. Available from: /doi/pdf/10.1161/ATVBAHA.117.310550?download=true

Harrington RA, Stone GW, McNulty S, White HD, Lincoff AM, Gibson CM, et al (2009) Platelet inhibition with cangrelor in patients undergoing PCI. N Engl J Med [Internet] [cited 2025 Jul 17];361(24):2318–2329. Available from: https://www.nejm.org/doi/pdf/10.1056/NEJMoa0908628#:~:text=Efficacy End Points,also constitute evidence of ischemia

He L, Pappan LK, Grenache DG, Li Z, Tollefsen DM, Santoro SA, et al (2003) The contributions of the α2β1 integrin to vascular thrombosis in vivo. Blood [Internet] [cited 2025 Aug 26];102(10):3652–3657. Available from: https://pubmed.ncbi.nlm.nih.gov/12893751/

Hechler B, Magnenat S, Zighetti M (2005) Inhibition of platelet functions and thrombosis through selective or nonselective inhibition of the platelet P2 receptors with increasing doses of NF449 [4, 4′, 4 ″, 4 ″. J Pharmacol Exp Ther [Internet] [cited 2014 Mar 13];314(1):232–243. Available from: http://jpet.aspetjournals.org/content/314/1/232.short

Hechler B, Nonne C, Eun JR, Cattaneo M, Cazenave JP, Lanza F, et al (2006) MRS2500 [2-iodo-N6-methyl-(N)-methanocarba-2′- deoxyadenosine-3′,5′-bisphosphate], a potent, selective, and stable antagonist of the platelet P2y1 receptor with strong antithrombotic activity in mice. J Pharmacol Exp Ther [Internet] [cited 2025 Jul 10];316(2):556–563. Available from: https://jpet.aspetjournals.org/action/showFullText?pii=S0022356524324644

Heptinstall S, Espinosa DI, Manolopoulos P, Glenn JR, White AE, Johnson A, et al (2008) DG-041 inhibits the EP3 prostanoid receptor - a new target for inhibition of platelet function in atherothrombotic disease. Platelets [Internet] [cited 2025 Aug 26];19(8):605–613. Available from: https://pubmed.ncbi.nlm.nih.gov/19012178/

Hollenberg MD, Saifeddine M, Sandhu S, Houle S, Vergnolle N (2004) Proteinase-activated receptor-4: evaluation of tethered ligand-derived peptides as probes for receptor function and as inflammatory agonists in vivo. Br J Pharmacol 143(4):443–454

Hossain MM, Pan D, Arkless KL, Rahman KM, Page CP, Authi KS, et al (2025) P2Y14 receptor activation of platelets induces Ca2+ mobilization and Rho-GTPase-dependent motility that requires an interaction with P2Y1 receptors. Br J Pharmacol [Internet] [cited 2025 Jul 10];182 (13):2950–2967. Available from: https://pubmed.ncbi.nlm.nih.gov/40128640/

Hsu CC, Wu WB, Huang TF (2008) A snake venom metalloproteinase, kistomin, cleaves platelet glycoprotein VI and impairs platelet functions. J Thromb Haemost [Internet] [cited 2025 Aug 26];6(9):1578–1585. Available from: https://pubmed.ncbi.nlm.nih.gov/18624975/

Huang JS, Dong L, Kozasa T, Le Breton GC (2007) Signaling through Gα13 Switch Region I Is Essential for Protease-activated Receptor 1-mediated Human Platelet Shape Change, Aggregation, and Secretion. J Biol Chem [Internet] [cited 2025 Jul 11];282(14):10210–10222. Available from: https://www.sciencedirect.com/science/article/pii/S002192581957692X

Hung DT, Vu TKH, Nelken NA, Coughlin SR (1992) Thrombin-induced events in non-platelet cells are mediated by the unique proteolytic mechanism established for the cloned platelet thrombin receptor. J Cell Biol 116(3):827–832

Hunt SA, Baker DW, Chin MH, Cinquegrani MP, Feldman AM, Francis GS, et al (2001) ACC/AHA guidelines for the evaluation and management of chronic heart failure in the adult: executive summary. A report of the American College of Cardiology/American Heart Association task force on practice guidelines (committee to revise the 1995 guidelines for the evaluation and management of heart failure). Circulation [Internet] [cited 2025 Aug 26];104(24): 2996–3007. Available from: https://www.ahajournals.org/doi/pdf/10.1161/hc4901.102568?download=true

Husted S, Emanuelsson H, Heptinstall S, Sandset PM, Wickens M, Peters G (2006) Pharmacodynamics, pharmacokinetics, and safety of the oral reversible P2Y12 antagonist AZD6140 with aspirin in patients with atherosclerosis: a double-blind comparison to clopidogrel with aspirin. Eur Heart J [Internet] [cited 2025 Jul 17];27(9):1038–1047. Available from: https://dx.doi.org/https://doi.org/10.1093/eurheartj/ehi754

Ibanez B, James S, Agewall S, Antunes MJ, Bucciarelli-Ducci C, Bueno H, et al (2018) 2017 ESC Guidelines for the management of acute myocardial infarction in patients presenting with ST-segment elevation: The Task Force for the management of acute myocardial infarction in patients presenting with ST-segment elevation of the European Society of Cardiology (ESC). Eur Heart J [Internet] [cited 2025 Aug 26];39(2):119–177. Available from: https://doi.org/10.1093/eurheartj/ehx393

Jakubowski JA, Riesmeyer JS, Close SL, Leishman AG, Erlinge D (2012) TRITON and beyond: new insights into the profile of prasugrel. Cardiovasc Ther 30(4):e174

Jantzen HM, Milstone DS, Gousset L, Conley PB, Mortensen RM (2001) Impaired activation of murine platelets lacking Gαi2. J Clin Invest 108(3):477–483

Janus-Bell E, Mangin PH (2023) The relative importance of platelet integrins in hemostasis, thrombosis and beyond. Haematologica [Internet] [cited 2025 Aug 26];108(7):1734–1747. Available from: https://pubmed.ncbi.nlm.nih.gov/36700400/

Jin J, Kunapuli SP (1998) Coactivation of two different G protein-coupled receptors is essential for ADP-induced platelet aggregation. Proc Natl Acad Sci USA 95(14):8070–8074

Jin J, Mao Y, Thomas D, Kim S, Daniel JL, Kunapuli SP (2009) RhoA downstream of Gq and G12/13 pathways regulates protease-activated receptor-mediated dense granule release in platelets. Biochem Pharmacol [Internet] [cited 2025 Jul 14];77(5):835–844. Available from: https://www.sciencedirect.com/science/article/pii/S0006295208008289

Juif P-E, Boehler M, Dobrow M, Ufer M, Dingemanse J (2019) Clinical pharmacology of the reversible and potent P2Y 12 receptor antagonist ACT-246475 after single subcutaneous administration in healthy male subjects. Pharmacokinet J Clin Pharmacol [Internet] [cited

2025 Jul 11];2019(1):123–130. Available from: https://accp1.onlinelibrary.wiley.com/doi/10.1002/jcph.1296

Kahn ML, Nakanishi-Matsui M, Shapiro MJ, Ishihara H, Coughlin SR (1999a) Protease-activated receptors 1 and 4 mediate activation of human platelets by thrombin. J Clin Invest [Internet] [cited 2025 Jul 11];103(6):879. Available from: https://pmc.ncbi.nlm.nih.gov/articles/PMC408153/

Kahn ML, Nakanishi-Matsui M, Shapiro MJ, Ishihara H, Coughlin SR (1999b) Protease-activated receptors 1 and 4 mediate activation of human platelets by thrombin. J Clin Invest 103(6): 879–887

Kassack MU, Braun K, Ganso M, Ullmann H, Nickel P, Böing B, et al (2004) Structure-activity relationships of analogues of NF449 confirm NF449 as the most potent and selective known P2X1 receptor antagonist. Eur J Med Chem [Internet] [cited 2025 Jul 17];39(4):345–357. Available from: https://pubmed.ncbi.nlm.nih.gov/15072843/

Kim S, Foster C, Lecchi A, Quinton TM, Prosser DM, Jin J, et al (2002) Protease-activated receptors 1 and 4 do not stimulate Gi signaling pathways in the absence of secreted ADP and cause human platelet aggregation independently of Gisignaling. Blood [Internet] [cited 2025 Jul 11];99(10):3629–3636. Available from: https://www.sciencedirect.com/science/article/pii/S0006497120608412

Kim BJ, Kwon SU, Park JH, Kim YJ, Hong KS, Wong LKS, et al (2020) Cilostazol versus aspirin in ischemic stroke patients with high-risk cerebral hemorrhage: subgroup analysis of the PICASSO trial. Stroke [Internet] [cited 2025 Aug 26];51(3):931–937. Available from: https://pubmed.ncbi.nlm.nih.gov/31856691/

Koganov ES, Michelson AD, Yanachkov IB, Yanachkova MI, Wright GE, Przyklenk K, et al (2018) GLS-409, an antagonist of both P2Y1 and P2Y12, potently inhibits canine coronary artery thrombosis and reversibly inhibits human platelet activation. Sci Rep [Internet] [cited 2025 Jul 10];8(1):14529. Available from: https://pmc.ncbi.nlm.nih.gov/articles/PMC6162268/

Kogushi M, Matsuoka T, Kawata T, Kuramochi H, Kawaguchi S, Murakami K, et al (2011) The novel and orally active thrombin receptor antagonist E5555 (Atopaxar) inhibits arterial thrombosis without affecting bleeding time in Guinea pigs. Eur J Pharmacol [Internet] [cited 2025 Jul 11];657(1–3):131–137. Available from: https://pubmed.ncbi.nlm.nih.gov/21300059/

Kuijpers MJE, Pozgajova M, Cosemans JMEM, Munnix ICA, Eckes B, Nieswandt B, et al (2007) Role of murine integrin α2β1 in thrombus stabilization and embolization: contribution of thromboxane A2. Thromb Haemost [Internet] [cited 2025 Aug 26];98(5):1072–1080. Available from: http://www.thieme-connect.com/products/ejournals/html/10.1160/TH07-02-0089

Kuliopulos A, Gurbel PA, Rade JJ, Kimmelstiel CD, Turner SE, Bliden KP, et al (2020) PAR1 (protease-activated receptor 1) pepducin therapy targeting myocardial necrosis in coronary artery disease and acute coronary syndrome patients undergoing cardiac catheterization: a randomized, placebo-controlled, phase 2 study. Arterioscler Thromb Vasc Biol [Internet] [cited 2025 Jul 11];40(12):2990–3003. Available from: https://pubmed.ncbi.nlm.nih.gov/33028101/

Kumlin M, Granström E (1986) Radioimmunoassay for 11-dehydro-TXB2: a method for monitoring thromboxane production in vivo. Prostaglandins [Internet] [cited 2025 Aug 26];32(5): 741–767. Available from: https://pubmed.ncbi.nlm.nih.gov/3823488/

Larson MK, Chen H, Kahn ML, Taylor AM, Fabre JE, Mortensen RM, et al (2003) Identification of P2Y12-dependent and -independent mechanisms of glycoprotein VI–mediated Rap1 activation in platelets. Blood [Internet] [cited 2025 Jul 14];101(4):1409–1415. Available from: https://www.sciencedirect.com/science/article/pii/S0006497120574041

Léon C, Freund M, Ravanat C, Baurand A, Cazenave JP, Gachet C (2001) Key role of the P2Y1 receptor in tissue factor-induced thrombin-dependent acute thromboembolism: studies in P2Y1-knockout mice and mice treated with a P2Y1 antagonist. Circulation [Internet] [cited 2025 Aug 26];103(5):718–723. Available from: https://pubmed.ncbi.nlm.nih.gov/11156884/

Levine GN, Bates ER, Blankenship JC, Bailey SR, Bittl JA, Cercek B, et al (2011) 2011 ACCF/AHA/SCAI guideline for percutaneous coronary intervention a report of the American College of Cardiology Foundation/American Heart Association Task Force on Practice Guidelines and the Society for Cardiovascular Angiography and Interventions. Circulation [Internet] [cited 2025 Jul 17];124(23). Available from: https://pubmed.ncbi.nlm.nih.gov/22064601/

Li H, Lockyer S, Concepcion A, Gong X, Takizawa H, Guertin M, et al (2007) The fab fragment of a novel anti-GPVI monoclonal antibody, OM4, reduces in vivo thrombosis without bleeding risk in rats. Arterioscler Thromb Vasc Biol [Internet] [cited 2025 Aug 26];27(5):1199–1205. Available from: https://pubmed.ncbi.nlm.nih.gov/17322098/

Lockyer S, Okuyama K, Begum S, Le S, Sun B, Watanabe T, et al (2006) GPVI-deficient mice lack collagen responses and are protected against experimentally induced pulmonary thromboembolism. Thromb Res [Internet] [cited 2025 Aug 26];118(3):371–380. Available from: https://pubmed.ncbi.nlm.nih.gov/16139873/

Lopez J, Mark J, Duarte GJ, Shaban M, Sosa F, Mishra R, et al (2023) Role of genetic polymorphisms in clopidogrel response variability: a systematic review. Open Hear [Internet] [cited 2025 Jul 17];10(2):e002436. Available from: https://pmc.ncbi.nlm.nih.gov/articles/PMC10649851/

Lova P, Paganini S, Sinigaglia F, Balduini C, Torti M (2002) A Gi-dependent Pathway Is Required for Activation of the Small GTPase Rap1B in Human Platelets. J Biol Chem [Internet] [cited 2025 Jul 14];277(14):12009–12015. Available from: https://www.sciencedirect.com/science/article/pii/S0021925818520202

Love BB, Biller J, Gent M (1998) Adverse haematological effects of ticlopidine. Drug Saf [Internet] [cited 2025 Jul 17];19(2):89–98. Available from: https://pubmed.ncbi.nlm.nih.gov/9704247/

Mahaut-Smith MP, Jones S, Evans RJ (2011) The P2X1 receptor and platelet function. Purinergic Signal [Internet] [cited 2013 Sep 24];7(3):341–356. Available from: http://www.pubmedcentral.nih.gov/articlerender.fcgi?artid=3166991&tool=pmcentrez&rendertype=abstract

Mangin PH, Tang CJ, Bourdon C, Loyau S, Freund M, Hechler B, et al (2012) A humanized glycoprotein VI (GPVI) mouse model to assess the antithrombotic efficacies of anti-GPVI agents. J Pharmacol Exp Ther [Internet] [cited 2025 Aug 26];341(1):156–163. Available from: https://pubmed.ncbi.nlm.nih.gov/22238212/

Massberg S, Schulz C, Gawaz M (2003) Role of platelets in the pathophysiology of acute coronary syndrome. Semin Vasc Med [Internet] 3(2):147–162. Available from: https://www.ncbi.nlm.nih.gov/pubmed/15199478

Matthews JS, Jones RL (1993) Potentiation of aggregation and inhibition of adenylate cyclase in human platelets by prostaglandin E analogues. Br J Pharmacol [Internet] [cited 2025 Aug 26];108(2):363–369. Available from: https://pubmed.ncbi.nlm.nih.gov/8448586/

Mayer CL, Koeck K, Hottmann M, Redfern A, Davis M, Barth A, et al (2023) A phase 1 study in healthy participants to characterize the safety and pharmacology of inclacumab, a fully human anti-P-selectin antibody, in development for treatment of sickle cell disease. Eur J Clin Pharmacol [Internet] [cited 2025 Aug 26];79(9):1219–1228. Available from: https://pubmed.ncbi.nlm.nih.gov/37436495/

Mazharian A, Roger S, Berrou E, Adam F, Kauskot A, Nurden P, et al (2007) Protease-activating receptor-4 induces full platelet spreading on a fibrinogen matrix: involvement of ERK2 and p38 and Ca2+ mobilization. J Biol Chem [Internet] [cited 2025 Jul 11];282(8):5478–5487. Available from: https://www.sciencedirect.com/science/article/pii/S002192582068841X

Mega JL, Close SL, Wiviott SD, Shen L, Hockett RD, Brandt JT, et al (2009) Cytochrome P450 genetic polymorphisms and the response to prasugrel relationship to pharmacokinetic, pharmacodynamic, and clinical outcomes. Circulation [Internet] [cited 2025 Jul 17];119(19):2553–2560. Available from: https://pubmed.ncbi.nlm.nih.gov/19414633/

Meng D, Luo M, Liu B (2021) The role of CLEC-2 and its ligands in thromboinflammation. Front Immunol [Internet] [cited 2025 Jul 21];12:688643. Available from: www.frontiersin.org

Merali S, Wang Z, Frost C, Callejo M, Hedrick M, Hui L et al (2022) New oral protease-activated receptor 4 antagonist BMS-986120: tolerability, pharmacokinetics, pharmacodynamics, and gene variant effects in humans. Platelets 33(7):969–978

Merali S, Wang Z, Frost C, Meadows-Shropshire S, Hawthorne D, Yang J, et al (2023) First-in-human study to assess the safety, pharmacokinetics, and pharmacodynamics of BMS-986141, a novel, reversible, small-molecule, PAR4 agonist in non-Japanese and Japanese healthy participants. Platelets [Internet] [cited 2025 Jul 3];34(1). Available from: https://pubmed.ncbi.nlm.nih.gov/37394920/

Moers A, Nieswandt B, Massberg S, Wettschureck N, Grüner S, Konrad I et al (2003) G13 is an essential mediator of platelet activation in hemostasis and thrombosis. Nat Med 9(11): 1418–1422

Mohammad MA, Andell P, Koul S, James S, Scherstén F, Götberg M, et al. (2017) Cangrelor in combination with ticagrelor provides consistent and potent P2Y12-inhibition during and after primary percutaneous coronary intervention in real-world patients with ST-segment-elevation myocardial infarction. Platelets [Internet] [cited 2025 Jul 17];28(4):414–416. Available from: https://pubmed.ncbi.nlm.nih.gov/27885888/

Montalescot G, Sechtem U, Achenbach S, Andreotti F, Arden C, Budaj A, et al (2013) 2013 ESC guidelines on the management of stable coronary artery disease. Eur Heart J [Internet] [cited 2025 Jul 17];34(38):2949–3003. Available from: https://pubmed.ncbi.nlm.nih.gov/23996286/

Moore DJ, Murdock PR, Watson JM, Faull RLM, Waldvogel HJ, Szekeres PG, et al (2003) GPR105, a novel Gi/o-coupled UDP-glucose receptor expressed on brain glia and peripheral immune cells, is regulated by immunologic challenge: possible role in neuroimmune function. Mol Brain Res [Internet] [cited 2025 Jul 14];118(1–2):10–23. Available from: https://www.sciencedirect.com/science/article/pii/S0169328X03003309

Morrow DA, Braunwald E, Bonaca MP, Ameriso SF, Dalby AJ, Fish MP, et al (2012) Vorapaxar in the secondary prevention of atherothrombotic events. N Engl J Med [Internet] [cited 2025 Jul 11];366(15):1404–1413. Available from: https://pubmed.ncbi.nlm.nih.gov/22443427/

Mumaw MM, de la Fuente M, Noble DN, Nieman MT (2014) Targeting the anionic region of human protease-activated receptor 4 inhibits platelet aggregation and thrombosis without interfering with hemostasis. J Thromb Haemost [Internet] [cited 2025 Jul 14];12(8): 1331–1341. Available from: https://pubmed.ncbi.nlm.nih.gov/24888424/

Narumiya S, FitzGerald GA (2001) Genetic and pharmacological analysis of prostanoid receptor function. J Clin Invest [Internet] [cited 2025 Aug 26];108(1):25–30. Available from: https://pubmed.ncbi.nlm.nih.gov/11435452/

Neri Serneri GG, Coccheri S, Marubini E, Violi F (2004) Picotamide, a combined inhibitor of thromboxane A2 synthase and receptor, reduces 2-year mortality in diabetics with peripheral arterial disease: the DAVID study. Eur Heart J [Internet] [cited 2025 Aug 26];25(20): 1845–1852. Available from: https://pubmed.ncbi.nlm.nih.gov/15474700/

Nicolson PLR, Nock SH, Hinds J, Garcia-Quintanilla L, Smith CW, Campos J, et al (2021) Low-dose Btk inhibitors selectively block platelet activation by CLEC-2. Haematologica [Internet] [cited 2025 Jul 21];106(1):208–219. Available from: https://pubmed.ncbi.nlm.nih.gov/31949019/

Niitsu Y, Jakubowski JA, Sugidachi A, Asai F (2005) Pharmacology of CS-747 (prasugrel, LY640315), a novel, potent antiplatelet agent with in vivo P2Y12 receptor antagonist activity. Semin Thromb Hemost [Internet] [cited 2025 Jul 14];31(2):184–194. Available from: http://www.thieme-connect.de/products/ejournals/html/10.1055/s-2005-869524

Nwose EU, Yee KC (2016) Drug-disease interactions: narrative review of aspirin in gastric ulcer. Expert Opin Drug Metab Toxicol [Internet] [cited 2025 Aug 26];12(9):1081–1087. Available from: /action/showLogin?uri=%2Fdoi%2Fpdf%2F10.1080%2F17425255.2016.1201064

Nylander S, Wågberg F, Andersson M, Skärby T, Gustafsson D (2015) Exploration of efficacy and bleeding with combined phosphoinositide 3-kinase β inhibition and aspirin in man. J Thromb

Haemost [Internet] [cited 2025 Aug 26];13(8):1494–1502. Available from: https://pubmed.ncbi.nlm.nih.gov/26096765/

O'Callaghan K, Kuliopulos A, Covic L (2012) Turning receptors on and off with intracellular pepducins: New insights into G-protein-coupled receptor drug development. J Biol Chem [Internet] [cited 2025 Jul 11];287(16):12787–12796. Available from: https://pubmed.ncbi.nlm.nih.gov/22374997/

O'Gara PT, Kushner FG, Ascheim DD, Casey DE, Chung MK, De Lemos JA et al (2013) 2013 ACCF/AHA guideline for the management of st-elevation myocardial infarction: executive summary: A report of the American college of cardiology foundation/american heart association task force on practice guidelines. J Am Coll Cardiol 61(4):485–510

Offermanns S, Toombs CF, Hu Y, Simon MI (1997) Defective platelet activation in G ␣ q -deficient mice. Nature 389(September):183–186

Parodi G, Valenti R, Bellandi B, Migliorini A, Marcucci R, Comito V, et al (2013) Comparison of prasugrel and ticagrelor loading doses in ST-segment elevation myocardial infarction patients: RAPID (Rapid Activity of Platelet Inhibitor Drugs) primary PCI study. J Am Coll Cardiol [Internet] [cited 2025 Jul 17];61(15):1601–1606. Available from: https://pubmed.ncbi.nlm.nih.gov/23500251/

Patrignani P, Filabozzi P, Patrono C (1982) Selective cumulative inhibition of platelet thromboxane production by low-dose aspirin in healthy subjects. J Clin Invest [Internet] [cited 2025 Aug 26];69(6):1366–1372. Available from: https://pubmed.ncbi.nlm.nih.gov/7045161/

Patrignani P, Tacconelli S, Piazuelo E, Di Francesco L, Dovizio M, Sostres C, et al (2014) Reappraisal of the clinical pharmacology of low-dose aspirin by comparing novel direct and traditional indirect biomarkers of drug action. J Thromb Haemost [Internet] [cited 2025 Aug 26];12(8):1320–1330. Available from: https://pubmed.ncbi.nlm.nih.gov/24942808/

Patrono C, Rocca B (2017) Type 2 diabetes, obesity, and aspirin responsiveness. J Am Coll Cardiol [Internet] [cited 2025 Aug 26];69(6):613–615. Available from: https://pubmed.ncbi.nlm.nih.gov/28089179/

Patrono C, Ciabarroni G, Patrignani P, Pugliese F, Filabozzi P, Catella F, et al (1985) Clinical pharmacology of platelet cyclooxygenase inhibition. Circulation [Internet] [cited 2025 Aug 26];72(6):1177–1184. Available from: https://pubmed.ncbi.nlm.nih.gov/3933848/

Pedersen AK, FitzGerald GA (1984) Dose-related kinetics of aspirin. Presystemic acetylation of platelet cyclooxygenase. N Engl J Med [Internet] [cited 2025 Aug 26];311(19):1206–1211. Available from: https://pubmed.ncbi.nlm.nih.gov/6436696/

Perez M, Lamothe M, Maraval C, Mirabel E, Loubat C, Planty B, et al. (2009) Discovery of novel protease activated receptors 1 antagonists with potent antithrombotic activity in vivo. J Med Chem [Internet] [cited 2025 Jul 3];52(19):5826–5836. Available from: https://pubs.acs.org/doi/abs/10.1021/jm900553j

Pfefferkorn JA, Choi C, Winters T, Kennedy R, Chi L, Perrin LA, et al (2008) P2Y1 receptor antagonists as novel antithrombotic agents. Bioorg Med Chem Lett [Internet] [cited 2025 Aug 26];18(11):3338–3343. Available from: https://pubmed.ncbi.nlm.nih.gov/18445527/

Pitchford SC, Momi S, Giannini S, Casali L, Spina D, Page CP, et al (2005) Platelet P-selectin is required for pulmonary eosinophil and lymphocyte recruitment in a murine model of allergic inflammation. Blood [Internet] [cited 2012 Aug 13];105(5):2074–2081. Available from: http://www.ncbi.nlm.nih.gov/pubmed/15528309

Price MJ, Berger PB, Teirstein PS, Tanguay JF, Angiolillo DJ, Spriggs D, et al (2011) Standard- vs high-dose clopidogrel based on platelet function testing after percutaneous coronary intervention: the GRAVITAS randomized trial. JAMA [Internet] [cited 2025 Jul 17];305(11):1097–1105. Available from: https://jamanetwork.com/journals/jama/fullarticle/646144

Priestley ES, Banville J, Deon D, Dubé L, Gagnon M, Guy J, et al (2022) Discovery of two novel antiplatelet clinical candidates (BMS-986120 and BMS-986141) that antagonize protease-activated receptor 4. J Med Chem [Internet] [cited 2025 Jul 14];65(13):8843–8854. Available from: https://pubmed.ncbi.nlm.nih.gov/35729784/

Qiao JX, Wang TC, Ruel R, Thibeault C, L'Heureux A, Schumacher WA, et al (2013) Conformationally constrained ortho- Anilino diaryl ureas: discovery of 1-(2-(1′--Neopentylspiro[indoline-3,4′-piperidine]-1-yl)phenyl) -3-(4-(trifluoromethoxy)phenyl)urea, a potent, selective, and bioavailable P2Y1 antagonist. J Med Chem [Internet] [cited 2025 Aug 26];56(22):9275–9295. Available from: https://pubmed.ncbi.nlm.nih.gov/24164581/

Renda G, Tacconelli S, Capone ML, Sacchetta D, Santarelli F, Sciulli MG, et al (2006) Celecoxib, ibuprofen, and the antiplatelet effect of aspirin in patients with osteoarthritis and ischemic heart disease. Clin Pharmacol Ther [Internet] [cited 2025 Aug 26];80(3):264–274. Available from: https://pubmed.ncbi.nlm.nih.gov/16952493/

Rocca B, Patrono C (2005) Determinants of the interindividual variability in response to antiplatelet drugs. J Thromb Haemost [Internet] [cited 2025 Aug 26];3(8):1597–1602. Available from: https://pubmed.ncbi.nlm.nih.gov/16102024/

Rolf MG, Brearley CA, Mahaut-Smith MP (2001) Platelet shape change evoked by selective activation of P2X1 purinoceptors with alpha,beta-methylene ATP. Thromb Haemost [Internet]. 85(2):303–308. Available from: http://www.ncbi.nlm.nih.gov/pubmed/11246552

Rudinga GR, Khan GJ, Kong Y (2018) Protease-Activated Receptor 4 (PAR4): a promising target for antiplatelet therapy. Int J Mol Sci 19:573. [Internet]. 2018 Feb 14 [cited 2025 Jul 14];19(2): 573. Available from: https://www.mdpi.com/1422-0067/19/2/573/htm

Savcic M, Hauert J, Bachmann F, Wyld PJ, Geudelin B, Cariou R (1999) Clopidogrel loading dose regimens: kinetic profile of pharmacodynamic response in healthy subjects. Semin Thromb Hemost 25(SUPPL. 2):15–19

Savi P, Herbert JM 2005) Clopidogrel and ticlopidine: P2Y 12 adenosine diphosphate-receptor antagonists for the prevention of atherothrombosis. Semin Thromb Hemost [Internet] [cited 2025 Jul 14];31(2):174–183. Available from: http://www.thieme-connect.de/products/ejournals/html/10.1055/s-2005-869523

Scarborough RM, Kleiman NS, Phillips DR (1999) Platelet glycoprotein IIb/IIIa antagonists: what are the relevant issues concerning their pharmacology and clinical use? Circulation [Internet] [cited 2025 Aug 26];100(4):437–444. Available from: https://pubmed.ncbi.nlm.nih.gov/10421606/

Serebruany VL, Kogushi M, Dastros-Pitei D, Flather M, Bhatt DL (2009) The in-vitro effects of E5555, a protease-activated receptor (PAR)-1 antagonist, on platelet biomarkers in healthy volunteers and patients with coronary artery disease. Thromb Haemost [Internet] [cited 2025 Jul 11];102(1):111–119. Available from: https://pubmed.ncbi.nlm.nih.gov/19572075/

Shankar H, Kahner BN, Prabhakar J, Lakhani P, Kim S, Kunapuli SP (2006) G-protein-gated inwardly rectifying potassium channels regulate ADP-induced cPLA2 activity in platelets through Src family kinases. Blood [Internet] [cited 2012 Aug 13];108(9):3027–3034. Available from: http://www.pubmedcentral.nih.gov/articlerender.fcgi?artid=1895524&tool=pmcentrez&rendertype=abstract

Shapiro MJ, Weiss EJ, Faruqi TR, Coughlin SR (2000) Protease-activated receptors 1 and 4 are shut off with distinct kinetics after activation by thrombin. J Biol Chem [Internet] [cited 2025 Jul 11];275(33):25216–25221. Available from: https://www.sciencedirect.com/science/article/pii/S0021925819620788

Sinnaeve P, Fahrni G, Schelfaut D, Spirito A, Mueller C, Frenoux JM, et al (2020) Subcutaneous selatogrel inhibits platelet aggregation in patients with acute myocardial infarction. J Am Coll Cardiol [Internet] [cited 2025 Jul 17];75(20):2588–2597. Available from: https://www.sciencedirect.com/science/article/pii/S0735109720347525

Smyth SS, McEver RP, Weyrich a S, Morrell CN, Hoffman MR, Arepally GM, et al (2009) Platelet functions beyond hemostasis. J Thromb Haemost [Internet] [cited 2012 Aug 8];7(11): 1759–1766. Available from: http://www.ncbi.nlm.nih.gov/pubmed/19691483

Sostres C, Lanas A (2011) Gastrointestinal effects of aspirin. Nat Rev Gastroenterol Hepatol [Internet] [cited 2025 Aug 26];8(7):385–394. Available from: https://www.nature.com/articles/nrgastro.2011.97

Stähli BE, Gebhard C, Duchatelle V, Cournoyer D, Petroni T, Tanguay JF, et al (2016) Effects of the P-selectin antagonist Inclacumab on myocardial damage after percutaneous coronary intervention according to timing of infusion: insights from the SELECT-ACS trial. J Am Heart Assoc [Internet] [cited 2025 Aug 26];5(11). Available from: https://pubmed.ncbi.nlm.nih.gov/27852589/

Stefanini L, Roden RC, Bergmeier W (2009) CalDAG-GEFI is at the nexus of calcium-dependent platelet activation. Blood [Internet] [cited 2025 Jul 14];114(12):2506–2514. Available from: https://www.sciencedirect.com/science/article/pii/S0006497120369202

Stefanini L, Boulaftali Y, Ouellette TD, Holinstat M, Désiré L, Leblond B, et al (2012) Rap1-Rac1 circuits potentiate platelet activation. Arterioscler Thromb Vasc Biol [Internet] [cited 2012 Aug 13];32(2):434–441. Available from: http://www.pubmedcentral.nih.gov/articlerender.fcgi?artid=3262085&tool=pmcentrez&rendertype=abstract

Stone GW, Witzenbichler B, Weisz G, Rinaldi MJ, Neumann FJ, Metzger DC, et al (2013) Platelet reactivity and clinical outcomes after coronary artery implantation of drug-eluting stents (ADAPT-DES): a prospective multicentre registry study. Lancet [Internet] [cited 2025 Jul 17];382(9892):614–623. Available from: https://www.thelancet.com/action/showFullText?pii=S0140673613611708

Storey RF, Gurbel PA, Berg J ten, Bernaud C, Dangas GD, Frenoux JM, et al (2020) Pharmacodynamics, pharmacokinetics, and safety of single-dose subcutaneous administration of selatogrel, a novel P2Y12 receptor antagonist, in patients with chronic coronary syndromes. Eur Heart J [Internet] [cited 2025 Jul 17];41(33):3132–3140. Available from: https://pubmed.ncbi.nlm.nih.gov/31994703/

Tantry US, Bonello L, Aradi D, Price MJ, Jeong YH, Angiolillo DJ, et al (2013) Consensus and update on the definition of on-treatment platelet reactivity to adenosine diphosphate associated with ischemia and bleeding. J Am Coll Cardiol [Internet] [cited 2025 Jul 17];62(24):2261–2273. Available from: /doi/pdf/10.1016/j.jacc.2013.07.101?download=true

Tardif J-C, Tanguay J-F, Wright SR, Duchatelle V, Petroni T, Grégoire JC et al (2013) Effects of the P-selectin antagonist inclacumab on myocardial damage after percutaneous coronary intervention for non–ST-segment elevation myocardial infarction results of the SELECT-ACS trial. J Am Coll Cardiol 61:2048–2055

Tilly P, Charles AL, Ludwig S, Slimani F, Gross S, Meilhac O, et al (2014) Blocking the EP3 receptor for PGE2 with DG-041 decreases thrombosis without impairing haemostatic competence. Cardiovasc Res [Internet] [cited 2025 Aug 26];101(3):482–491. Available from: https://doi.org/10.1093/cvr/cvt276

Toyoda K, Uchiyama S, Yamaguchi T, Easton JD, Kimura K, Hoshino H, et al (2019) Dual antiplatelet therapy using cilostazol for secondary prevention in patients with high-risk ischaemic stroke in Japan: a multicentre, open-label, randomised controlled trial. Lancet Neurol [Internet] [cited 2025 Aug 26];18(6):539–548. Available from: https://pubmed.ncbi.nlm.nih.gov/31122494/

Tricoci P, Huang Z, Held C, Moliterno DJ, Armstrong PW, Van de Werf F, et al (2012) Thrombin-Receptor Antagonist Vorapaxar in Acute Coronary Syndromes. N Engl J Med [Internet] [cited 2025 Jul 11];366(1):20–33. Available from: https://www.nejm.org/doi/pdf/10.1056/NEJMoa1109719

Tullemans BME, Karel MFA, Léopold V, ten Brink MS, Baaten CCFMJ, Maas SL, et al (2021) Comparison of inhibitory effects of irreversible and reversible Btk inhibitors on platelet function. EJHaem [Internet] [cited 2025 Jul 21];2(4):685–699. Available from: https://pubmed.ncbi.nlm.nih.gov/35845214/

Tyler HM, Saxton CAPD, Parry MJ (1981) Administration to man of UK-37,248-01, a selective inhibitor of thromboxane synthetase. Lancet [Internet] [cited 2025 Aug 26];317(8221):629–632. Available from: https://pubmed.ncbi.nlm.nih.gov/6110861/

Uphaus T, Richards T, Weimar C, Neugebauer H, Poli S, Weissenborn K, et al (2022) Revacept, an inhibitor of platelet adhesion in symptomatic carotid stenosis: a multicenter randomized phase II trial. Stroke [Internet] [cited 2025 Aug 26];53(9):2718–2729. Available from: https://pubmed.ncbi.nlm.nih.gov/35695006/

van der Wicken LR, Simoons ML, Laarman GJ, van den Brand M, Nijssen KM, Dellborg M, et al (1995) Ridogrel as an adjunct to thrombolysis in acute myocardial infarction. Int J Cardiol [Internet] [cited 2025 Aug 26];52(2):125–134. Available from: https://pubmed.ncbi.nlm.nih.gov/8749872/

Vane JR (1971) Inhibition of prostaglandin synthesis as a mechanism of action for aspirin-like drugs. Nat New Biol [Internet] [cited 2025 Aug 26];231(25):232–235. Available from: https://www.nature.com/articles/newbio231232a0

Voors-Pette C, Lebozec K, Dogterom P, Jullien L, Billiald P, Ferlan P, et al (2019) Safety and tolerability, pharmacokinetics, and pharmacodynamics of ACT017, an antiplatelet GPVI (Glycoprotein VI) Fab: first-in-human healthy volunteer trial. Arterioscler Thromb Vasc Biol [Internet] [cited 2025 Aug 26];39(5):956–964. Available from: https://pubmed.ncbi.nlm.nih.gov/31017822/

Voss B, McLaughlin JN, Holinstat M, Zent R, Hamm HE (2007) PAR1, but Not PAR4, activates human platelets through a Gi/o/Phosphoinositide-3 kinase signaling Axis. Mol Pharmacol [Internet] [cited 2025 Jul 11];71(5):1399–1406. Available from: https://www.sciencedirect.com/science/article/pii/S0026895X24044419

Vretenbrant K, Ramström S, Bjerke M, Lindahl TL (2007) Platelet activation via PAR4 is involved in the initiation of thrombin generation and in clot elasticity development. Thromb Haemost 97(3):417–424

Vu TKH, Hung DT, Wheaton VI, Coughlin SR (1991) Molecular cloning of a functional thrombin receptor reveals a novel proteolytic mechanism of receptor activation. Cell [Internet] [cited 2025 Jul 14];64(6):1057–1068. Available from: https://www.sciencedirect.com/science/article/pii/009286749190261V

Wagner B, Smieško M, Jakob RP, Mühlethaler T, Cramer J, Maier T, et al (2024) Analogues of the pan-selectin antagonist rivipansel (GMI-1070). Eur J Med Chem [Internet] [cited 2025 Aug 26];272. Available from: https://pubmed.ncbi.nlm.nih.gov/38728868/

Wallentin L, Becker RC, Budaj A, Cannon CP, Emanuelsson H, Held C, et al (2009) Ticagrelor versus clopidogrel in patients with acute coronary syndromes. N Engl J Med [Internet] [cited 2025 Jul 17];361(11):1045–1057. Available from: https://www.nejm.org/doi/pdf/10.1056/NEJMoa0904327

Wielders SJH, Bennaghmouch A, Reutelingsperger CPM, Bevers EM, Lindhout T (2007) Anticoagulant and antithrombotic properties of intracellular protease-activated receptor antagonists. J Thromb Haemost [Internet] [cited 2025 Jul 11];5(3):571–576. Available from: https://pubmed.ncbi.nlm.nih.gov/17166251/

Wilson SJ, Ismat FA, Wang Z, Cerra M, Narayan H, Raftis J, et al (2018) PAR4 (Protease-Activated Receptor 4) antagonism with BMS-986120 inhibits human ex vivo thrombus formation. Arterioscler Thromb Vasc Biol [Internet] [cited 2025 Jul 14];38(2):448–456. Available from: /doi/pdf/10.1161/ATVBAHA.117.310104?download=true

Wiviott SD (2007) Prasugrel versus Clopidogrel in Patients with Acute Coronary Syndromes. N Engl J Med [Internet] [cited 2014 Jan 21];357(20):2001–2015. Available from: http://scholar.google.com/scholar?hl=en&btnG=Search&q=intitle:new+england+journal#2

Wolska N, Rozalski M (2019) Blood platelet adenosine receptors as potential targets for anti-platelet therapy. Int J Mol Sci [Internet] [cited 2025 Aug 26];20(21). Available from: https://pubmed.ncbi.nlm.nih.gov/31684173/

Wong PC, Seiffert D, Bird JE, Watson CA, Bostwick JS, Giancarli M, et al (2017) Blockade of protease-activated receptor- 4(PAR4) provides robust antithrombotic activity with low bleeding. Sci Transl Med [Internet] [cited 2025 Jul 3];9(371). Available from: /doi/pdf/10.1126/scitranslmed.aaf5294?download=true

Woulfe D, Jiang H, Mortensen R, Yang J, Brass LF (2002) Activation of Rap1B by Gi family members in platelets. J Biol Chem [Internet] [cited 2025 Jul 14];277(26):23382–23390. Available from: https://www.sciencedirect.com/science/article/pii/S0021925819667116

Xu H, Tilley DG (2022) Pepducin-mediated G protein-coupled receptor signaling in the cardiovascular system. J Cardiovasc Pharmacol [Internet] [cited 2025 Jul 3];80(3):378–385. Available from: https://pubmed.ncbi.nlm.nih.gov/35170495/

Xu WF, Andersen H, Whitmore TE, Presnell SR, Yee DP, Ching A, et al (1998) Cloning and characterization of human protease-activated receptor 4. Proc Natl Acad Sci USA [Internet] [cited 2025 Jul 11];95(12):6642–6646. Available from: https://www.pnas.org/doi/pdf/10.1073/pnas.95.12.6642

Xu H, Bonaca MP, Goodrich E, Scirica BM, Morrow DA (2021) Efficacy and safety of vorapaxar for secondary prevention in low body weight in patients with atherosclerosis: analyses from the TRA 2°P-TIMI 50 trial. Eur Heart J Acute Cardiovasc Care [Internet] [cited 2025 Jul 11];10(2):190–199. Available from: https://pubmed.ncbi.nlm.nih.gov/31642690/

Yang J, Wu J, Jiang H, Mortensen R, Austin S, Manning DR, et al (2002) Signaling through Gi Family Members in Platelets: redundancy and specificity in the regulation of adenylyl cyclase and other effectors. J Biol Chem [Internet] [cited 2025 Jul 14];277(48):46035–46042. Available from: https://www.sciencedirect.com/science/article/pii/S002192581933203X

Zhang C, Srinivasan Y, Arlow DH, Fung JJ, Palmer D, Zheng Y, et al (2012a) High-resolution crystal structure of human protease-activated receptor 1 bound to the antagonist vorapaxar. Nature [Internet] [cited 2025 Jul 11];492(7429):387. Available from: https://pmc.ncbi.nlm.nih.gov/articles/PMC3531875/

Zhang P, Gruber A, Kasuda S, Kimmelstiel C, O'Callaghan K, Cox DH et al (2012b) Suppression of arterial thrombosis without affecting hemostatic parameters with a cell-penetrating PAR1 pepducin. Circulation 26(1):83–91

Zheng SL, Roddick AJ (2019) Association of aspirin use for primary prevention with cardiovascular events and bleeding events: a systematic review and meta-analysis. JAMA - J Am Med Assoc [Internet] [cited 2025 Aug 26];321(3):277–287. Available from: https://pubmed.ncbi.nlm.nih.gov/30667501/

Zheng B, Li J, Jiang J, Xiang D, Chen Y, Yu Z, et al (2021) Safety and efficacy of a platelet glycoprotein Ib inhibitor for patients with non-ST segment elevation myocardial infarction: a phase Ib/IIa study. Pharmacotherapy [Internet] [cited 2025 Aug 26];41(10):828–836. Available from: https://pubmed.ncbi.nlm.nih.gov/34478577/

Platelet Function Tests and Monitoring Antiplatelet Therapies

Simon Davidson

Contents

Abstract

In the late 1990s, the antiplatelet agent clopidogrel, a P2Y12 inhibitor, was introduced into clinical practice. Concurrently, several new methods for assessing platelet function emerged, such as the PFA-100 in 1995, marking the beginning of a sustained expansion in platelet function testing. It soon became apparent that patient responses to clopidogrel varied significantly, with some individuals exhibiting high on-treatment platelet reactivity. This variability prompted

S. Davidson (✉)
Faculty of Medical Science, Division of Medicine, University College London, London, UK
e-mail: simon.davidson@ucl.ac.uk

E. Gray, J. Hogwood (eds.), *Antithrombotic and Antiplatelet Agents*, Handbook of Experimental Pharmacology 291, https://doi.org/10.1007/164_2025_788

discussions around the utility of platelet function testing to tailor antiplatelet therapy. Additionally, such testing was proposed for patients preparing for cardiac surgery to better manage the balance between thrombotic risk before surgery and bleeding risk during the perioperative period. This chapter explores widely used platelet function tests in these contexts, particularly those considered point-of-care (POC) or requiring minimal laboratory processing. It also reviews recent guidelines and clinical trial evidence, building on a previously published chapter, regarding the role and effectiveness of platelet function testing in these clinical scenarios.

Keywords

Antiplatelet monitoring · Aspirin · Multiplate · P2Y12 inhibitors · PFA · Rotem · TEG · VerifyNow

1 Introduction

The greater use of thienopyridine antiplatelet agents such as clopidogrel or dual antiplatelet therapy, in which aspirin is added alongside the thienopyridine, occurred in clinical practice at the same time as several new platelet function devices were being developed and launched into the diagnostic market during the mid-1990s. This subsequently led to some publications suggesting platelet function testing should be performed to tailor therapy for patients to ascertain both bleeding and thrombotic risk and drug regimen efficacy (Orban and Sibbing 2013; Lordkipanidzé et al. 2016; Kong et al. 2015). Other published platelet function testing work was based on studies performed in the acute setting with 6- to 24-month follow-up showing the benefit of platelet function monitoring and antiplatelet drug dose adjustment on long-term outcomes (Geisler et al. 2015; Price et al. 2008; Sibbing 2017).

Clopidogrel carries a 30% risk of patient non-responsiveness due primarily to genetic factors of converting it to a prodrug. Other P2Y12 inhibitors have come to market in the past decade that have faster onset offset activity but may present more bleeding challenges. These drugs include prasugrel (also metabolised to a prodrug via the liver enzyme cytochrome P450) and ticagrelor (a direct and reversible P2Y12 inhibitor), both of which are currently included in the treatment recommendations in acute coronary syndromes (along with the front-line antiplatelet agents clopidogrel and aspirin) in the European Cardiology guidelines (Collet 2020). There remains an interest in platelet function testing to detect those patients with a 'high-on-treatment' platelet reactivity and subsequent thrombotic risk, or conversely their bleeding risk while on antithrombotic antiplatelet therapy and requiring surgery or interventions.

There is limited data on using platelet function tests to monitor antiplatelet therapy in the paediatric population. A review from 2019 showed most data were from light transmission aggregometry, PFA-100, VerifyNow and TEG-platelet mapping. The results were inconsistent, and outcomes were variable, with there being a need for more trials to be performed (Huang et al. 2019). A recent publication looking at aspirin dosing in children <2 years with congenital heart disease using TEG-platelet mapping demonstrated this younger cohort required high doses of aspirin based on the TEG results. Concluding platelet function testing would be beneficial in these children to reduce under and overdosing of aspirin (Regan et al. 2024).

This chapter, an update on the previous chapter published in 2023 (Davidson 2023), will discuss the commonly used platelet function tests, focusing on adults and point-of-care assays or those with minimal required laboratory sample handling, to discuss the ease of using the test and the clinical relevance of the test at the current time. Genetic testing for clopidogrel polymorphisms in the CYP2C19 enzyme will not be discussed; however, there is a useful update on genetic testing in percutaneous coronary interventions, an international consensus by the American College of Cardiology Foundation (Angiolillo et al. 2024).

2 Antiplatelet Drugs

The antiplatelet drugs currently employed are aspirin, clopidogrel, prasugrel and ticagrelor. Other antiplatelet drugs that are available include the P2Y12 inhibitor Cangrelor (Kengreal, FDA approved 2015), which has a rapid onset and offset action of 3–6 min and is given intravenously (Feng and Mahaffey 2020), and the PAR-1 receptor antagonist Vorapaxar (Zontivity, FDA approved 2014) (Tantry et al. 2020).

The platelet glycoprotein (GP) receptor (GP IIb/IIIa) for fibrinogen has attracted interest since the 1970s, resulting in the production of GPIIb/IIIa inhibitors such as Reopro (Abciximab), Integrilin and Tirofiban. These antiplatelet agents are not usually monitored as they are used in the acute setting of percutaneous coronary intervention and stenting patients with recent cardiac arrest. Previous studies have shown some patients to display variability in their response to these drugs, possibly increasing their thrombotic risk post procedure (Mahtta and Bavry 2019). The VerifyNow device did have a GpIIb/IIIa cartridge, but this has been withdrawn from the market.

3 Mode of Action of Antiplatelet Drugs

Aspirin's mode of action is through the inactivation of the platelets' cyclooxygenase pathway. The isoenzymes COX-1 and 2 catalyse the conversion of arachidonic acid to prostaglandin H2, this being the precursor to a number of prostanoids, one of which is thromboxane A2. It is thromboxane A2 that induces platelet aggregation and vasoconstriction. When thromboxane A2 is released from platelets, it amplifies the local platelet activation signal and recruits additional platelets, and via a specific G-protein-coupled transmembrane receptor, it facilitates dense granule secretion and integrin GpIIb/IIIa activation. Aspirin is a relatively weak inhibitor of platelet function, and platelet activation can still be achieved, with the effect of aspirin circumvented by a number of other stimulants, including ADP, thrombin and shear stress (Patrono and Rocca 2012).

Adenosine diphosphate (ADP) is a platelet agonist that induces shape change and reversible aggregation; however, it is its potentiating action during aggregation that is key. When released from platelet-dense granules, ADP amplifies the platelets' response to other agonists, permitting stabilisation of platelet aggregates and the mobilisation and increase in intracellular calcium. Platelets have two G-coupled receptors for ADP, the $P2Y_1$ and P2Y12. The $P2Y_1$ receptor is responsible for the increase in cytoplasmic calcium, reversible aggregation and platelet shape change. The P2Y12 receptor inhibits adenylyl cyclase (cyclic AMP) and amplifies the aggregation response. The P2Y12 antagonist clopidogrel is a prodrug that undergoes biotransformation via a two-step process in the liver via the P450 cytochrome, which includes an initial oxidative step to produce 2-hydoxy thiophene, the isomerised 2-oxo thiophene ring that is then hydrolysed to give the active metabolite. Clopidogrel irreversibly inhibits ADP-induced platelet aggregation by 30–60% and ADP-induced inhibition of adenylyl cyclase by selective binding and antagonism of the P2Y12 receptor (Cattaneo 2019). Prasugrel is also a prodrug and is metabolised via the liver and the P450 cytochrome to generate the metabolite that irreversibly inhibits the P2Y12 receptor. The formation of the active metabolite of prasugrel is more efficient than that of clopidogrel due to a single esterification process that is less reliant upon the CYP enzymes, which are the cause of clopidogrel resistance or drug failure (Cattaneo 2019). The mechanism of action of ticagrelor is different from that of clopidogrel and prasugrel. Ticagrelor is a direct acting reversible P2Y12 receptor inhibitor. Ticagrelor prevents ADP from binding to the receptor in a non-competitive manner and achieves quicker onset/offset action and more consistent platelet inhibition (Cattaneo 2004, 2010). Cangrelor also has a rapid onset platelet inhibition, 2 min, and offset, 60 min. Cangrelor is used as a i.v. infusion and is given to patients previously P2Y12 naïve undergoing PCI to reduce the thrombotic risk (Feng and Mahaffey 2020).

Vorapaxar is a PAR-1 inhibitor given orally on as a daily dose for patients with peripheral artery disease and previous myocardial infarction (Tantry et al. 2020). Treatment failure with vorapaxar has to date not been reported. In the Thrombin Receptor Antagonist for Clinical Event Reduction in Acute Coronary Syndrome (TRACER study) using LTA with TRAP as an agonist, it showed potent PAR-1 inhibition (Storey et al. 2014). In this study, the VerfiyNow GpIIb/IIIa assay was used, as it contains a TRAP isoform.

The GpIIb/IIIa inhibitors (Abciximab, Eptifibatide and Tirofiban) are platelet glycoprotein inhibitors that work in slightly different ways. Abciximab is a monoclonal antibody c7E3 that irreversibly inhibits the GPIIb/IIIa receptor on platelets preventing the binding of von Willebrand factor and fibrinogen and subsequent platelet activation. Eptifibatide is a small peptide Barbourin from the pygmy rattlesnake (*Sistrurus miliarius barbouri*). It binds reversibly to the GpIIa/IIIb receptor exclusively preventing binding of fibrinogen to the glycoprotein. Tirofiban is a competitive, reversible exosite inhibitor of GpIIa/IIIb, preventing binding of fibrinogen (Gelbenegger and Jilma 2022).

4 Clinical Use and Cessation of Antiplatelet Drugs Before Surgical Procedures

Antiplatelet medications are mostly used in patients with cardiovascular disease, including thrombotic stroke, and for reducing the risk of venous thromboembolism in hospitalised patients. For example, use of cangrelor in patients at high risk of thrombosis when having to stop their standard P2Y12 medication as they await cardiac surgery. Efficacy of antiplatelet therapy, reducing bleeding risk and recovery of platelet function after stopping antiplatelet medication are areas where platelet function testing is of potential benefit to the patient.

In patients with acute coronary syndrome undergoing percutaneous coronary intervention (PCI), the P2Y12 inhibitors ticagrelor and prasugrel are preferred over clopidogrel due to faster onset of antiplatelet effect with reduced ischaemic events. However, ticagrelor and prasugrel have a high bleeding rates when compared to clopidogrel. In patients with chronic coronary syndromes undergoing PCI, clopidogrel is the preferred antiplatelet. It has been shown that up to 30% of patients given clopidogrel have residual high platelet reactivity (HPR). In patients treated with ticagrelor or prasugrel, HRP is 5%. This in turn is implicated in the increased post PCI thrombotic events who are treated with clopidogrel. A low platelet reactivity with all three compounds has been associated with an increased bleeding risk in these patients. Clopidogrel is affected by polymorphisms of the CYP2C19 enzyme with loss-of-function alleles involved in its conversion to its active metabolite, which increase the risk of thrombosis. Whereas prasugrel and ticagrelor are not (Angiolillo et al. 2024).

The use of platelet function with these three P2Y12 compounds can be in the following scenarios: patients on clopidogrel with HRP and therefore increased thrombotic risk can be switched to prasugrel or ticagrelor. Or de-escalation from patients on prasugrel or ticagrelor where there is increased bleeding or risk thereof to clopidogrel if this is deemed effective by platelet function.

For patients that need to stop their antiplatelet medication for a medical procedure, this can be guided by platelet function testing to ensure platelet reactivity has sufficiently recovered for the procedure. With aspirin, this can vary depending on the bleeding risk of the procedure; low risk continues and high risk (cardiac surgery) stops (Swan et al. 2024). See Table 1 for a list of drugs and suggested times to stop therapy pre-procedure.

5 Methods Available to Monitor Platelet Function?

The assays available to monitor platelet function are summarised in Table 2. The considered gold standard (although not very well standardised) laboratory method for assessing platelet function has been light transmission aggregometry (LTA). Other methods that can be classed as POC include Multiplate (MEA), VerifyNow, TEG platelet mapping, ROTEM, PFA-100/−200 (Innovance) and Plateletworks. The most common methods used for assessing antiplatelet therapy are Multiplate,

Table 1 Antiplatelet drugs – mode of action – half-life, when to stop for surgical intervention with increased risk of bleeding, time for recovery of platelet function

Antiplatelet drug	Mode of inhibition	Half-life	Time to stop before surgical intervention	Time for platelet function to recover
Abciximab	GpIIb/IIIa	10–15 min	12 h	12 h
Aspirin	COX-1	15–20 min	5–10 days	2 days
Cangrelor	P2Y12	3–6 min	1 h	5 min
Clopidogrel	P2Y12	7 h	5–7 days	3 days
Prasugrel	P2Y12	7 h	7 days	2–3 days
Ticagrelor	P2Y12	8 h	5 days	1 day
Tirofiban	GpIIa/IIIb	2 h	3 h	3 h
Vorapraxar	PAR-1	5–13 days	3 days	4–8 weeks

Gp Glycoprotein, *COX* cyclo-oxygenase, *PAR* protease activated receptor

VerfiyNow, TEG and Rotem. It will be these methods that will be the focus of this chapter; other methods will be discussed briefly. The flow cytometric method VASP is dependent on the degree of P2Y12 activation and therefore a good marker of efficacy of P2Y12 inhibitors. This method will not be discussed as this is not widely available and needs some degree of sample pretreatment, a flow cytometer and specialised staff to perform the test (Mallouk et al. 2018).

The questions for the different assays are (1) can they predict the risk of thrombotic and bleeding events? (2) Are they sufficiently sensitive to show when the effects of antiplatelet therapy have worn off? (3) What is the cutoff level to segregate responders from non-responders? (4) Does a change in therapy (based on the results of these assays) improve clinical outcome? (5) Concordance of results and interpretation between the assays.

6 Monitoring Antiplatelet Therapy

6.1 Light Transmission Aggregometry (LTA) (Gold Standard as Comparator for the Point of Care Devices)

LTA was developed in the 1960s and essentially uses a spectrophotometer which measures changes in increasing light transmission through a suspension of stirred platelet-rich plasma (PRP) (Born 1962) that develops when platelets aggregate in response to agonists such as ADP, collagen, thrombin, arachidonic acid, epinephrine, ristocetin (Born 1962), thrombin receptor-activating peptide (TRAP), calcium ionophore A23187 and the thromboxane receptor agonist U46619. Blood is collected into citrate, neutralising not only any plasma calcium but also intracellular calcium which can impact on the assay. PRP is harvested from whole blood by room

Table 2 Tests of platelet function used for antiplatelet drug monitoring

Platelet function assay	Agonist	Detection end point	Advantages	Disadvantages
LTA	ADP 3–10 μM AA 0.5 mM	Light transmission	Reference method	Sample preparation, poorly standardised
Multiplate MEA	ADP 6.5 μM AA 0.5 mM TRAP 32 μM	Impedance	No sample manipulation, disposable cuvettes	Skilled laboratory user operator required or trained health care professional, 30-min wait time until testing after sample taken
VerifyNow	ADP 20 μM AA NI	Light transmission	No sample manipulation, easy to use	Drug interference between different test cartridges
PFA-100/200 innovance	ADP 46 μM (coated cartridge)	High shear platelet aggregation	No sample manipulation, easy to use	Low dose P2Y12 inhibitors lacks sensitivity
Plateletworks	ADP 20 μM AA 0.4 μM	Platelet count	Very simple test, small blood sample	None direct test of platelet aggregation, poor correlation with other assays
TEG platelet mapping TEG6	ADP 2 μM AA 1 mM NI	Viscoelastic Platelet count Viscoelastic resonance	Whole blood test Whole blood	Relatively long time to generate result Limited clinical data
Rotem delta platelet module	ADP 10 μM AA 0.42 mM TRAP 36 μM	Electrode impedance	Technology similar to MEA	Lack of clinical data

LTA light transmission aggregometry, *MEA* Multiple electrode platelet aggregation, *NI* no information available, *ADP* adenosine diphosphate, *AA* arachidonic acid, *TRAP* thrombin receptor activating peptide, *RUO* research use only

temperature (15° to 28°C) centrifugation at low speeds (e.g. 150× *g* for 10 min). After separation and aliquoting into a secondary tube, the PRP must be capped before use to avoid changes in pH. PRP should be tested within 3–4 h of collection as recommended by reagent manufacturer instructions for use. The aggregometer is attached to a computer from which interrogation of the aggregation traces can occur. The lag time, slope and amplitude of the curves are used to assess platelet function and can most simply be expressed as % aggregation. This method is traditionally used to assess inherited disorders of platelet function. Samples with reduced platelet counts may require a modified panel of agonists.

LTA may not be the optimal method available for testing platelet responsiveness to aspirin or thienopyridines for several reasons. By comparison to other methods, a large sample volume is required. LTA is also time-consuming (about two hours to prepare samples and perform testing using specialised trained personnel), and it is often only available in larger, more specialised clinical laboratories. There are numerous pre-analytical and analytical variables that affect the results including PRP preparation and final concentration of agonists used. Even when all the variables are controlled, the accuracy and reproducibility of the method are relatively poor. An international survey of assessment of platelet function by LTA was conducted by the platelet physiology subcommittee of the scientific and standardisation committee of the International Society on Thrombosis and Haemostasis (ISTH) and the findings published in 2013 (Cattaneo et al. 2013). There was marked variation in practice worldwide, as highlighted by users and quality assurance organisations. This has driven the ISTH to develop a methodological guideline for LTA. Recommendations include addressing pre-analytical variables such as sample collection and the exposure of other platelet-function-interacting drugs that should be omitted before tests are performed. Additional guidance includes the optimal sample required anticoagulant, preparation of PRP, LTA as the preferred testing method, select agonist concentrations and result reporting (Hayward et al. 2008).

The LTA agonist results obtained within one laboratory may not directly compare to another testing laboratory. Reference intervals or normal response to agonists may be locally determined or derived from reagent manufacturer. This means that attempting to define cut-off values of platelet aggregation to identify non-responders to antiplatelet therapy would be extremely difficult. However, despite numeric differences that may exist between LTA testing sites, the overall LTA interpretation should demonstrate equivalence and efforts for assuring interpretation accuracy is monitoring using external quality assurance programs (http://nascola.com/PlateletEQA).

It remains questionable whether the pharmacological effects of aspirin in relation to any platelet function assays should be measured at all as there is sufficient evidence to show that true 'aspirin resistance' is a rare entity (Michelson et al. 2005; Cattaneo 2004). It has also been suggested that noncompliance is in the main responsible for this variation in platelet function as well as variability in laboratory assays to measure the antiplatelet effect of aspirin and poor design of trails (Gasparyan et al. 2008; Weber et al. 2002). In stable coronary artery disease, aspirin resistance was relatively low when LTA was used (Lordkipanidzé et al. 2007). However, in recent meta-analyses, the incidence of aspirin resistance has been quoted as 23% in patients given aspirin for ischaemic stroke (Van Oosterom et al. 2022). The inadequacy of LTA for measuring the effect of aspirin was demonstrated in a 2006 study by the fact that although platelet COX-1 activity was uniformly inhibited in all studied patients via collagen-induced thromboxane B_2 production, LTA studies, however, showed marked inter-individual differences (Ohmori et al. 2006). Therefore, this technique may overestimate the incidence of drug resistance, including assays using ADP to monitor thienopyridines due to its aggregating inducing effect on the P2Y1 receptor (Cattaneo 2011). However, LTA when used to assess aspirin resistance does compare well with clinical outcomes in some studies (Van Oosterom et al. 2022).

The problem may lie in that aspirin 'resistance' may vary in different patient groups due to numerous factors including genetic polymorphisms, increased platelet turnover, drug interactions (e.g. nonsteroidal anti-inflammatories that compete for the COX-1 receptor and proton pump inhibitors) and other inflammatory conditions.

6.2 Multiple Electrode Platelet Aggregation (MEA) (Roche Diagnostics, Switzerland)

The MEA or multiplate aggregometer is based on impedance aggregation in whole blood (Cardinal and Flower 1980). The principle of impedance aggregation is based on resting non-activated platelets are not thrombogenic. When activated, the platelet glycoprotein receptors allow them to attach to surfaces, which they do to artificial surfaces as well as within the vasculature. The MEA device has disposable single-use-only cuvettes with sensor wires, and as activated platelets bind to these, they increase the electrical resistance between the two wires, which can be measured. The MEA cuvettes contain two copper wire sensors silver coated, and when the impedance measurements are collated, the analyser software calculates the area under the curve and reaction velocity (Würtz et al. 2014).

The MEA has two reagents that allow assessment of platelet function while on antiplatelet treatment. The Aspirin (ASPI) test uses arachidonic acid as the agonist, which is the substrate for cyclooxygenase, which through the COX pathway produces thromboxane A2, the potent platelet agonist. Aspirin inhibits the COX pathway and MEA results of <30 AU show an aspirin antiplatelet effect. The ADP (P2Y12) reagent uses a final concentration of 6.5 μM ADP (lower than the 20 μM ADP employed in the VerifyNow P2Y12 test cartridge). A suggested range of 0–45 AU has been proposed as the P2Y12 therapeutic range, although care should be taken when reviewing the literature as the range currently does vary slightly between researchers. For example, a cut-off of >47 AU was suggested by Meen et al. (2012) and > 49 AU Kruger et al. (2014).

A cut-off of 35 AU pre-surgery test has recently been proposed for patients on clopidogrel undergoing cardiac surgery and predicting the potential need for platelet transfusion (Baryshnikova et al. 2022).

There has also been a consensus publication to predict the need for platelet transfusion in the perioperative period for patients undergoing cardiac surgery who have been taking P2Y12 antagonists and to help determine an individualised waiting period after cessation of P2Y12 antagonists before cardiac surgery (Kong et al. 2015).

The recommendations were that if ADP AUC >50, no platelet transfusion is required, and post-operatively the bleeding is unlikely due to platelet dysfunction. This included all P2Y12 inhibitors – clopidogrel, prasugrel and ticagrelor – and was based on clinical experience and expert opinion. An ADP AUC 30–50 has platelets reserved, and if there is significant bleeding post-operatively, then give/transfuse platelets. If the ADP AUC <30, there remains considerable inhibited platelet function; consider delaying procedure or transfuse platelets post-operatively (Kong et al. 2015). These are broadly similar to another study that looked at blood product usage after cardiac surgery using the Multiplate (Schimmer et al. 2013).

Other cut-offs have been suggested for bleeding complications, which have also been reported as an ADP AUC of <30 (Sibbing et al. 2010; Siller-Matula et al. 2016). However, these were not in patients undergoing cardiac surgery.

The initial preferred sample collection tube was one containing Hirudin, thereby retaining the platelets intracellular calcium stores. However, the original hirudin blood collection tubes have been discontinued in some countries, and alternate supplies may be difficult to source. Hirudin monovette tubes are still available from Sarstedt. Alternatively, blood collected in tubes containing Benzylsulfonyl-D-Arg-Pro-4-amidinobenzylamide (BAPA) may be suitable as well as blood collected in other anticoagulants, including citrate and heparin. Consistency in blood collection tubes is necessary to assure consistent result reporting.

Platelet counts normally should be greater than 100×10^9/L to perform the test and obtain reliable quantitative results; however, samples with platelet counts $<100 \times 10^9$/L can be used to qualitatively assess platelet function with some caution. We have found platelet counts as low as 70×10^9/L will give reliable results if the platelet function is normal (unpublished data S.Davidson) post-cardiac surgery.

TRAP reagent is also available and can be used as a comparator as normal result would be expected. If the TRAP result is abnormally low then another cause of platelet dysfunction should be suspected including thrombocytopenia (Kong et al. 2015).

The multiplate has also been shown to be beneficial in guiding antiplatelet therapy in patients having had carotid stenting following acute ischaemic stroke. These patients are at high risk of intercranial haemorrhage (ICH) and stent thrombosis. A study of 105 acute stroke patients where carotid stenting was performed and dual antiplatelet therapy was given: aspirin and clopidogrel. When antiplatelet therapy was monitored using the multiplate, 27% of patients were found to be clopidogrel non-responders <50% platelet inhibition, according to their cut-off. These patients were then switched to ticagrelor. A more favourable outcome was found in those patients on ticagrelor, and ICH was lower than in the clopidogrel treated patients. This study showed personalised antiplatelet therapy via testing platelet response to clopidogrel gave better outcomes when non-responders were switched to ticagrelor using the multiplate (Kreiberg et al. 2024).

6.3 VerifyNow (Accriva Diagnostics, San Diego, CA)

The VerifyNow device was originally developed as a point-of-care test (POCT) device (Ultegra rapid platelet function analyser) to detect adequate antiplatelet response to GPIIb/IIIa inhibitors such as Abciximab (Reopro (Eli Lilly, Indianapolis, IN) (Smith et al. 1999). The GpIIb/IIIa is no longer marketed. The antiplatelet test repertoire now includes individual disposable P2Y12 Platelet Reactivity Test, Aspirin Platelet Reactivity, and PRUTest Platelet Reactivity cartridges. The device uses a modified optical platelet aggregometry method of measurement. The device contains a light source and optical detectors and magnets to move steel balls in each of the four reaction chambers of the disposable cartridge allowing mixing of the blood and reagents. The assay is based on the ability of activated platelets to agglutinate fibrinogen-coated beads. Each test uses different agonists in the different chambers to increase the sensitivity and specificity of the assay. For instance, the P2Y12 cartridge ADP and prostaglandin E1 (PGE1) are used in the test channel to activate the platelets. The PGE1 is a suppressor of intracellular calcium, reducing the contribution of ADP binding to other receptors (e.g. P2Y1) and initiating platelet aggregation. The contribution of prostaglandin is to increase intracellular adenosine monophosphate thereby optimising the sensitivity and specificity of the test for ADP-induced activation of platelets via P2Y12.

Two other agonists, iso-TRAP (Thrombin Receptor Activating Peptide) and PAR-4-AP (PAR4-Activating Peptide), are included in another channel; with the fibrinogen-coated beads, they activate the platelets and measure the baseline platelet activity from which the percentage of platelet inhibition can be calculated using the ADP channel. The test is initiated by automatic addition of citrated blood to each channel, which reconstitutes the reagents (Lordkipanidzé et al. 2019).

Agglutination of the fibrinogen-coated beads by platelets is quantified by the use of a microprocessor algorithm that considers both the rate and extent of agglutination. The data are reported as a rate of platelet function or platelet reaction units (PRU) in millivolts per 10 s (mV/10 s). In the P2Y12 cartridge, this can also be expressed as % inhibition which for POCT users is sometimes easier to understand and translate into clinical practice. Although most studies report PRU using PRU cut-offs for clinical efficacy of drugs, there appears to be good agreement between the % inhibition and PRU, as the % inhibition is automatically calculated using the following equation $\% \text{ Inhibition} = [1-(PRU_{ON\text{-}TREATMENT} / PRU_{BASELINE})] \times 100\%$ (Liu et al. 2020; Luddington 2005).

Although the VerifyNow has been reported to correlate moderately with LTA platelet aggregation and MEA multiplate aggregation, there are differences in results from some samples and generally a wide spread of data across patients treated with clopidogrel (Paniccia et al. 2010). It has been suggested that the variation in results is due to the inclusion of PGE_1 in the VerifyNow ADP channel making it specific for the P2Y12 receptor and acting to suppress any additional ADP receptor contribution from P2Y1, unlike LTA / MEA methods of platelet aggregation that will include some additional influence between ADP receptors P2Y1 (Paniccia et al. 2010).

If the clopidogrel response is high in the VerifyNow P2Y12 Reactivity test indicating, significant platelet inhibition, then interference in the VerifyNow Aspirin Reactivity cartridge can also be seen. However, the interference does not affect the classification of aspirin treated patients (VerifyNow Aspirin package insert). The cartridges will currently only accept Greiner Bio-One citrate tubes.

Haematocrit levels between 33 and 52 and platelet counts between 119 and $502 \times 10^{9/L}$ have shown no effect on the test. Other drugs include the glycoprotein

IIb/IIIa inhibitors, cilostazol and potentially other platelet function-interfering drugs may adversely affect the test.

6.4 Thromboelastography (TEG Platelet Mapping/TEG 6) (Haemonectics, Boston, USA)

Thromboelastography measures the viscoelastic changes that occur as blood clots under low shear stress. Native (nonanticoagulated) blood is added to a warmed cuvette (37°C) containing an activator (kaolin). A suspended pin is lowered into the blood and rotates through a 4.5° arc back and forth. As fibrin develops, the strands interact with the cuvette, pin and activated platelets. The resistance of the pin movement as the fibrin clot forms is relayed to a computer where the classical TEG traces are visualised. These traces are plotted over time, and there are several parameters that are reported. The main parameters used in the clinical setting giving the user information on the patient's coagulation status are the clot time, which relates to clotting factor levels (r time), the angle of clot formation (relating to fibrinogen contribution; α angle), strength of the clot (which relates to platelet involvement of clot formation; MA, maximum amplitude) and clot lysis at times of 30 and 60 min (Ly30 and Ly60) (Luddington 2005).

The traditional TEG used in the surgical setting has been modified to allow measurement of the effect of antiplatelet therapy (TEG Platelet Mapping, TEGPM). Testing is normally performed in heparinised blood and should be analysed after a 30-min rest period at room temperature. TEGPM uses reptilase and factor XIIIa to clot the sample without thrombin generation. Reptilase cleaves fibrinogen to form fibrin in a similar way to thrombin and factor XIIIa stabilises the clot allowing measurement of the maximum amplitude. Two tests are performed simultaneously, one with only reptilase and factor XIIIa and one with reptilase, factor XIIIa and platelet agonist to either arachidonic acid or ADP. The MA of these tracings is sensitive to certain platelet antagonists, and a response to drug is regarded as 50% inhibition of the MA compared to the test performed without platelet agonist present. A partial response to antiplatelet drug is deemed 30–50% inhibition, and less than 30% inhibition is no drug response (Agarwal et al. 2006). A study comparing LTA, PFA and TEGPM showed the TEGPM to have good agreement with LTA when similar concentrations of agonists were used in both assay systems (Agarwal et al. 2006). Two studies have evaluated the use of the modified TEG in the surgical setting and use of antiplatelet drugs. In a small study, one group looked at bleeding in coronary surgery post-operatively in those patients that had received clopidogrel and aspirin. In one study, TEGPM had a sensitivity of 78% and specificity of 84% in discriminating between those patients where bleeding was attributed to the continued influence of clopidogrels antiplatelet effect. Aspirin platelet dysfunction as measured with the TEGPM did not appear to influence post-operative bleeding in this small study of 59 patients (Preisman et al. 2010). A second group investigated the use of the TEGPM in the pre-operative setting of the predictive value of using this test to assess bleeding risk in patients taking clopidogrel and aspirin compared to a control group. They found that although the TEGPM could identify significant platelet inhibition following antiplatelet therapy, the overlap of results between the control group and the antiplatelet groups was so great that the use of this test was limited clinically (Collyer et al. 2009).

TEG 6 uses a cartridge-based system to analyse the same parameters by visco-elastic blood coagulation using a resonance method. The signal from this is converted to the standard TEG readout. The TEG6 offers an ADP/AA cartridge for platelet mapping; the sample type required for this is heparinised whole blood. There are also cartridges available for Koalin, Koalin Heparinase, Rapid TEG and Functional Fibrinogen, sample type: citrated whole blood [website http://www.teg.haemonetics.com last accessed 15 Oct 2022]. There is limited data on the use of TEG6 and antiplatelet monitoring (Olechowski et al. 2018; Kirmani et al. 2017).

6.5 Rotem (IL Werfen, Barcelona, Spain)

The Rotem platelet module is an add-on to the Rotem Delta. As well as the four channels used to monitor viscoelastic haemostasis, there are two channels that perform impedance platelet aggregometry, similar to the Multiplate. There are three agonists available. The ADP (ADPTEM) final concentration 10 μM, arachidonic acid (ARATEM) final concentration is 0.42 mM and thrombin activating peptide (TRAPTEM) final concentration is 36 μM. Initial studies have shown the Rotem platelet able to detect patients taking aspirin; however, the detection of clopidogrel was less clear (Schultz-Lebahn et al. 2022). The timing of sampling may have been a factor in this study, as samples were taken 1–1.5 h after taking clopidogrel. Effects are not normally seen until 4–8 h (Feng and Mahaffey 2020).

One study from 2019 looked at normal patients receiving aspirin or dual aspirin and clopidogrel. The receiver operating curves (ROC) showed r0.99 for aspirin and r0.8 for dual antiplatelet therapy, distinguishing well between treated and untreated patients. However, there was only moderate correlation with other assays (Polzin et al. 2019).

Further studies are needed using the Rotem platelet to fully elucidate the effects of antiplatelet therapy in different clinical settings.

When standard Rotem parameters have been investigated for their usefulness to detect antiplatelet drugs, they have shown a lack of sensitivity (INTEM, EXTEM and FIBTEM), although prolonged showing significant overlap with controls (Hulshof et al. 2021).

6.6 PFA-100/-200 (Siemens Healthcare Diagnostics, Marburg, Germany)

The platelet function analyser (PFA)-100/−200 is designed to measure high shear whole blood aggregation that is based on a cartridge system whereby activated platelets occlude an aperture in a membrane that has been treated with collagen and epinephrine (CEPI) or collagen and ADP (CADP). The time for the blood to stop flowing across the membrane under a standard negative pressure (40 mm mercury equivalent) is recorded as the closure time (CT) with results available in approximately 5 min. A relatively small volume of citrated blood (800 μL) is required per cartridge. This method was introduced in the mid-to-late 1990s and was seen as a replacement for the bleeding time (Harrison 2005). The CT was shown to be sensitive to aspirin treatment, although not all patients taking aspirin had a prolonged CEPI closure time. It is also sensitive to most forms of von Willebrand disease and useful as a screen for primary haemostatic defects both inherited and acquired (Harrison 2005).

The standard CADP cartridge is insensitive to clopidogrel antiplatelet therapy, and this led to the development of the Innovance PFA P2Y test cartridge. This cartridge has a membrane coated with 20 μg ADP, 5 ng prostaglandin E1 and 459 μg calcium chloride. The cartridge has been shown to be sensitive to clopidogrel (in vitro spiking evaluation) and comparable to other methods for monitoring clopidogrel therapy (Edwards et al. 2012; Tsantes et al. 2012). Although the sensitivity of the cartridge is high, it does tend to show an 'all or nothing' effect with many results being >300 s (maximum CT) and does not allow any stratification of results. It is unknown whether this is clinically important, but patients with a raised bleeding risk may benefit from a reduced level of platelet inhibition, and it is unclear with the currently published data that this test would help in this scenario.

6.7 Plateletworks (Helena Biosciences, Boston, USA)

Plateletworks is a screening assay for the determination of percentage platelet aggregation or inhibition in a whole blood method of platelet counting. The method is adapted from LTA and is relatively cheap and easy to perform assuming there is access to a Haematology cell counter that can accurately measure platelet numbers. Plateletworks is a two-step method, where a baseline platelet count is performed, and then a second platelet count is performed following the exposure of the platelets to a platelet agonist. The agonist stimulates platelets to aggregate, and those that form platelet clumps will not be counted by the analyser (Campbell et al. 2008). The difference in platelet counts at baseline and following agonist activation gives a measure of platelet function by the following formula:

$$\frac{\text{Baseline platelet count–Agonist platelet count}}{\text{Baseline platelet count}} \times 100 = \%\text{Aggregation}$$

The vacutainers available are a 0.024 mL EDTA tube for baseline and a 1 mL tube of either ADP 20 μM in 3.2% sodium citrate or Collagen 10 μM in 3.2% sodium citrate. Once the sample has been taken into the agonist tube, it must be tested within 10 min. This may restrict its use in certain hospital or clinic settings.

Obviously, all those interfering aspects that can cause spurious platelet counting on automated haematology analysers will affect this test. Thrombocytopenia, whether genuine or pseudo forms caused by EDTA dependent agglutination, will invalidate the test as will the presence of giant platelets, microcytic red cells or cellular fragments.

In the POPULAR study (Do platelet function assays predict clinical outcomes in clopidogrel pretreated patients undergoing elective PCI), which looked at on-treatment platelet activity as measured by LTA, Plateletworks, Impact-R, VerifyNow P2Y12, PFA-100 (Innovance ADP/Collagen cartridge) and cut-off values derived from receiver operating curves for each assay, the Plateletworks method was as good as LTA and the VerifyNow methods when associated with the primary endpoint (Breet et al. 2010). This endpoint being all cause death, non-fatal myocardial infarction, stent thrombosis and ischaemic stroke, along with the safety endpoints of major and minor bleeding. All these tests' predictive value in this study were, however, only modest (Breet et al. 2010).

7 Discussion

The current evidence published by 2017, level B IIb, states platelet function testing may be considered to guide the decision on the timing of cardiac surgery in patients who have recently received P2Y12 inhibitors or who have ongoing DAPT. Although platelet function testing to adjust the dose before or after elective stenting is not recommended, level A III.

(Level A data is derived from multiple randomised clinical trials or meta-analyses and class III evidence or general agreement that the given treatment or procedure is not useful/effective. Level B evidence is from a single randomised control trial or a large non-randomised study, and IIb signifies the usefulness/efficacy is less well established by evidence/opinion and may be considered) (Valgimigli 2017).

In patients with myocardial revascularisation de-escalation from prasugrel to clopidogrel in patients with a normal clopidogrel response guided by platelet function testing can be considered (Neumann 2019). The American Heart Association (AHA) and American College of Cardiology (ACC) also agree on no platelet function testing for patients dose adjustment pre- or post-stenting and also agree with the ESC/ECAT de-escalation from prasugrel to clopidogrel guided by platelet function. Levels of evidence COB IIb LOE B (COR IIb benefit/risk case by case, may or might be considered although usefulness is unclear/unknown/not well established. LOE B: moderate quality of evidence (>1 RCT, well designed and executed nonrandomised studies, observational studies and registries) (Capodanno et al. 2018). The latter recommendation is based on the TROPICAL study (see below). The AHA/ACC also gives a similar level of evidence for platelet function testing of patients undergoing cardiopulmonary bypass on antiplatelet therapy as the EC/ECAT, COB IIb/LOE B.

The TROPICAL ACS study investigated guided de-escalation of antiplatelet treatment in patients with acute coronary syndrome undergoing PCI. The authors concluded that guided de-escalation of antiplatelet treatment was non-inferior to standard treatment with prasugrel at 1 year after PCI in terms of net clinical benefit (Sibbing 2017). This was a multicentre study that used the Multiplate. The APACS study investigated high platelet reactivity in patients with acute coronary syndromes undergoing PCI and was a randomised controlled trial comparing prasugrel and clopidogrel. The authors found that routine platelet function testing identifies patients with high residual platelet reactivity ('poor responders') on clopidogrel (Geisler et al. 2015). A strategy of prasugrel rather than clopidogrel reloading results in earlier and more sustained suppression of platelet reactivity. This was also conducted using the multiplate analyser (Geisler et al. 2015; Sibbing 2017).

The VerifyNow P2Y12 assay and the Multiplate are the most widely used in clinical practice for assessing antiplatelet therapy. As shown by the published clinical trials and small cohort studies, laboratory staff should be aware that the inter-assay correlation is modest; therefore, the results are not readily interchangeable. The questions of clinical utility and cost effectiveness still need to be answered. It should also be noted that due to platelet circadian rhythm, the timing of platelet function testing is also a laboratory preanalytical variable that will affect the results of any platelet function tests. The timing of these tests should therefore be standardised as much as possible (Cattaneo 2019; Dalby et al. 2000).

True 'aspirin resistance' or treatment failure of aspirin is rare, and reported 'aspirin resistance' appears to be caused by non-compliance in most cases. Although this varies among patient groups, particularly cardiac, low prevalence and ischaemic stroke patients, where the prevalence appears higher. The wide range of aspirin responses in published studies has been ascribed to differences in study design, different assays used, dosing regimens and compliance (Lordkipanidzé et al. 2007). The circulating platelet pool is dynamic with 10% being replenished daily. The half-life of aspirin is also short, approximately 20 min, which means that the timing of the platelet function test can expose differences in the degree of platelet inhibition. In contrast, studies that used specific P2Y12 tests to measure the pharmacological efficacy of clopidogrel showed broad variability of response, with in the order of 30% of treated patients categorised as poor responders. Inter-individual difference in the extent of metabolism of clopidogrel to its active metabolite by liver cytochrome P450 isoforms has been proposed as the commonest cause of the observed variability in platelet inhibition, except that it has been shown that the CYP2C10*2 mutation accounts for only 5–10% of this variation. The sensitivity of the assays for genotyping the CYP2C19 is approximately only 40%. It is currently proposed that genetic testing not be performed (Cattaneo 2012).

Platelet function testing in the acute phase, like myocardial infarction or acute coronary syndrome, will often show little or no antiplatelet effect if the patient is loaded with clopidogrel. This is due to the underlying inflammatory response and the platelets' role in the humoral immune defence mechanism. The release of younger more active platelets aided by interleukin-6 and thrombopoietin gives the patient a 'high-on-treatment' platelet reactivity. Another possible cause of this clopidogrel 'resistance' may be due to down regulation of some of the liver CYP isoenzymes required for clopidogrel metabolism during inflammation (Bernlochner et al. 2010; Bongiovanni et al. 2022).

The predictive value of P2Y12-directed platelet function testing has shown that high on-treatment platelet reactivity was associated with higher risk for ischaemic events, including stent thrombosis (Chau et al. 2021). In contrast, randomised trials (TRIGGER and GRAVITAS) in stable patients that have investigated the value of altering an individual's treatment based on test results (both studies used the Verifynow device) have shown negative findings and do not support routine P2Y12 testing (Trenk et al. 2012; Price et al. 2011). It should be noted that the TRIGGER study was stopped due to the low rate of adverse events, and therefore the clinical utility of platelet function testing could not be demonstrated. The GRAVITAS study also showed a similar constraint in patient selection, and only low-risk patients were enrolled into the study. The ARCTIC study of high-on-treatment PCI patients also showed no benefit from point-of-care testing using the VerifyNow device and dose escalation or changing treatment (Collet 2012). The ARCTIC study cohort did include high-risk patients with significantly higher mortality rates at 1 year than generally encountered in this population. Again, a point to stress here is that different cut-offs for the same test were used in the ARTIC and GRAVITAS studies.

The TRIGGER-PCI was a high-on-treatment study switching from clopidogrel to prasugrel in high-risk patients following PCI. It showed effective inhibition by switching to prasugrel; however, due to low rates of ischaemic events, clinical utility could not be shown. The ANTARCTIC study used older patients, >75 years and higher-risk of ischaemia and bleeding, than ARTIC and showed no benefit. Both studies used the VerifyNow for platelet function testing (Trenk et al. 2012; Cayla et al. 2016).

However as mentioned above, the TROPICAL-ACS and APACS studies using the Multiplate analyser did show non-inferiority or benefit in changing individual antiplatelet treatment using platelet function testing (Sibbing 2017; Geisler et al. 2015).

In summary, both European and American cardiology societies support the use of platelet function testing to guide antiplatelet de-escalation from prasugrel to clopidogrel. They also support the use of platelet function testing pre-cardiac surgery for patients on P2Y12 inhibitors to guide the timing of surgery. All of these studies supporting these recommendations have used VerfiyNow or Multiplate.

For a summary of the platelet function tests, agonists and concentrations, where appropriate, and advantages and disadvantages, see Table 2.

References

Agarwal S, Coakley M, Reddy K, Riddell A, Mallett S (2006) Quantifying the effect of antiplatelet therapy: a comparison of the platelet function analyzer (PFA-100) and modified thromboelastography (mTEG) with light transmission platelet aggregometry. Anesthesiology 105:676–683. https://doi.org/10.1097/00000542-200610000-00011

Angiolillo DJ, Galli M, Alexopoulos D, Aradi D, Bhatt DL, Bonello L, Capodanno D, Cavallari LH, Collet JP, Cuisset T, Ferreiro JL, Franchi F, Geisler T, Gibson CM, Gorog DA, Gurbel PA, Jeong YH, Marcucci R, Siller-Matula JM, Mehran R, Neumann FJ, Pereira NL, Rizas KD, Rollini F, So DYF, Stone GW, Storey RF, Tantry US, Berg JT, Trenk D, Valgimigli M, Waksman R, Sibbing D (2024) International consensus statement on platelet function and genetic testing in percutaneous coronary intervention: 2024 update. JACC Cardiovasc Interv 17(22):2639–2663. https://doi.org/10.1016/j.jcin.2024.08.027

Baryshnikova E, Di Dedda U, Ranucci M (2022) A comparative study of multiple electrode aggregometry technologies in cardiac surgery: different values, same clinical relevance. J Cardiothorac Vasc Anesth 36:1927–1933. https://doi.org/10.1053/j.jvca.2021.11.030

Bernlochner I, Steinhubl S, Braun S, Morath T, Jaitner J, Stegherr J, Mehilli J, von Beckerath N, Schömig A, Kastrati A, Sibbing D (2010) Association between inflammatory biomarkers and platelet aggregation in patients under chronic clopidogrel treatment. Thromb Haemost 104: 1193–1200. https://doi.org/10.1160/TH10-05-0266

Bongiovanni D, Han J, Klug M, Kirmes K, Viggiani G, von Scheidt M, Schreiner N, Condorelli G, Laugwitz KL, Bernlochner I (2022) Role of reticulated platelets in cardiovascular disease. Arterioscler Thromb Vasc Biol 42:527–539. https://doi.org/10.1161/ATVBAHA.121.316244

Born GVR (1962) Aggregation of blood platelets by adenosine diphosphate and its reversal. Nature 194:927–929. https://doi.org/10.1038/194927b0

Breet NJ, van Werkum JW, Bouman HJ, Kelder JC, Ruven HJ, Bal ET, Deneer VH, Harmsze AM, van der Heyden JA, Rensing BJ, Suttorp MJ, Hackeng CM, ten Berg JM (2010) Comparison of platelet function tests in predicting clinical outcome in patients undergoing coronary stent implantation. JAMA 303:754–762. https://doi.org/10.1001/jama.2010.181

Campbell J, Ridgway H, Carville D (2008) Plateletworks: a novel point of care platelet function screen. Mol Diagn Ther 12:253–258. https://doi.org/10.1007/BF03256290

Capodanno D, Alfonso F, Levine GN, Valgimigli M, Angiolillo DJ (2018) ACC/AHA versus ESC guidelines on dual antiplatelet therapy: JACC guideline comparison. J Am Coll Cardiol 72: 2915–2931. https://doi.org/10.1016/j.jacc.2018.09.057

Cardinal DC, Flower RJ (1980) The electronic aggregometer: a novel device for assessing platelet behavior in blood. J Pharmacol Methods 3:135–358. https://doi.org/10.1016/0160-5402(80)90024-8

Cattaneo M (2004) Aspirin and clopidogrel: efficacy, safety, and the issue of drug resistance. Arterioscler Thromb Vasc Biol 24:1980–1987. https://doi.org/10.1161/01.ATV.0000145980.39477.a9

Cattaneo M (2010) New P2Y12 inhibitors. Circulation 121:171–179. https://doi.org/10.1161/CIRCULATIONAHA.109.853069

Cattaneo M (2011) The platelet P2Y12 receptor for adenosine diphosphate: congenital and drug-induced defects. Blood 117:2102–2112. https://doi.org/10.1182/blood-2010-08-263111

Cattaneo M (2012) The role of laboratory monitoring in antiplatelet therapy. In: Gresele P, Born GVR, Patrono C, Page CP (eds) Handbook of experimental pharmacology vol 210. Antiplatelet agents, 1st edn. Springer, pp 474–491

Cattaneo M (2019) P2Y12 Antagonists. In: Michelson A (ed) Platelets, 4th edn. Elsevier Inc., pp 937–956

Cattaneo M, Cerletti C, Harrison P, Hayward CP, Kenny D, Nugent D, Nurden P, Rao AK, Schmaier AH, Watson SP, Lussana F, Pugliano MT, Michelson AD (2013) Recommendations for the standardization of light transmission aggregometry: a consensus of the working party from the platelet physiology subcommittee of SSC/ISTH. J Thromb Haemost 11:1183–1189. https://doi.org/10.1111/jth.12231

Cayla G, Cuisset T, Silvain J, Leclercq F, Manzo-Silberman S, Saint-Etienne C, Delarche N, Bellemain-Appaix A, Range G, El Mahmoud R, Carrié D, Belle L, Souteyrand G, Aubry P, Sabouret P, du Fretay XH, Beygui F, Bonnet JL, Lattuca B, Pouillot C, Varenne O, Boueri Z, Van Belle E, Henry P, Motreff P, Elhadad S, Salem JE, Abtan J, Rousseau H, Collet JP, Vicaut E, Montalescot G, ANTARCTIC investigators. (2016) Platelet function monitoring to adjust antiplatelet therapy in elderly patients stented for an acute coronary syndrome (ANT-ARCTIC): an open-label, blinded-endpoint, randomised controlled superiority trial. Lancet 388: 2015–2022. https://doi.org/10.1016/S0140-6736(16)31323-X

Chau KH, Kirtane AJ, Easterwood RM, Redfors B, Zhang Z, Witzenbichler B, Weisz G, Stuckey TD, Brodie BR, Rinaldi MJ, Neumann FJ, Metzger DC, Henry TD, Cox DA, Duffy PL, Mazzaferri EL Jr, Mehran R, Stone GW (2021) Stent thrombosis risk over time on the basis of clinical presentation and platelet reactivity: analysis from ADAPT-DES. JACC Cardiovasc Interv 14:417–427. https://doi.org/10.1016/j.jcin.2020.12.005

Collet JP, Cuisset T, Rangé G, Cayla G, Elhadad S, Pouillot C, Henry P, Motreff P, Carrié D, Boueri Z, Belle L, Van Belle E, Rousseau H, Aubry P, Monségu J, Sabouret P, O'Connor SA, Abtan J, Kerneis M, Saint-Etienne C, Barthélémy O, Beygui F, Silvain J, Vicaut E, Montalescot G, ARCTIC Investigators (2012) Bedside monitoring to adjust antiplatelet therapy for coronary stenting. N Engl J Med 367:2100–2109. https://doi.org/10.1056/NEJMoa1209979

Collet JP, Thiele H, Barbato E, Barthélémy O, Bauersachs J, Bhatt DL, Dendale P, Dorobantu M, Edvardsen T, Folliguet T, Gale CP, Gilard M, Jobs A, Jüni P, Lambrinou E, Lewis BS, Mehilli J, Meliga E, Merkely B, Mueller C, Roffi M, Rutten FH, Sibbing D, Siontis GCM, ESC Scientific Document Group (2020) ESC guidelines for the management of acute coronary syndromes in patients presenting without persistent ST-segment elevation. Eur Heart J 42:1289–1367

Collyer TC, Gray DJ, Sandhu R, Berridge J, Lyons G (2009) Assessment of platelet inhibition secondary to clopidogrel and aspirin therapy in preoperative acute surgical patients measured by Thrombelastography Platelet Mapping. Br J Anaesth 102:492–498. https://doi.org/10.1093/bja/aep039

Dalby MC, Davidson SJ, Burman JF, Davies SW (2000) Diurnal variation in platelet aggregation with the PFA-100 platelet function analyser. Platelets 11:320–324. https://doi.org/10.1080/09537100050144731

Davidson SJ (2023) Monitoring of antiplatelet therapy. Methods Mol Biol 2663:381–402. https://doi.org/10.1007/978-1-0716-3175-1_25

Edwards A, Jakubowski JA, Rechner AR, Sugidachi A, Harrison P (2012) Evaluation of the INNOVANCE PFA P2Y test cartridge: sensitivity to P2Y(12) blockade and influence of anticoagulant. Platelets 23:106–115. https://doi.org/10.3109/09537104.2011.601361

Feng KY, Mahaffey KW (2020) Cangrelor in clinical use. Futur Cardiol 16:89–102. https://doi.org/10.2217/fca-2019-0095c1

Gasparyan AY, Watson T, Lip GY (2008) The role of aspirin in cardiovascular prevention: implications of aspirin resistance. J Am Coll Cardiol 51:1829–1843. https://doi.org/10.1016/j.jacc.2007.11.080

Geisler T, Booth J, Tavlaki E, Karathanos A, Müller K, Droppa M, Gawaz M, Yanez-Lopez M, Davidson SJ, Stables RH, Banya W, Zaman A, Flather M, Dalby M (2015) High platelet reactivity in patients with acute coronary syndromes undergoing percutaneous coronary intervention: randomised controlled trial comparing prasugrel and clopidogrel. PLoS One 10: e0135037. https://doi.org/10.1371/journal.pone.0135037

Gelbenegger G, Jilma B (2022) Clinical pharmacology of antiplatelet drugs. Expert Rev Clin Pharmacol 15(10):1177–1197. https://doi.org/10.1080/17512433.2022.2121702

Harrison P (2005) The role of PFA-100 testing in the investigation and management of haemostatic defects in children and adults. Br J Haematol 130:3–10. https://doi.org/10.1111/j.1365-2141.2005.05511.x

Hayward CP, Moffat KA, Pai M, Liu Y, Seecharan J, McKay H, Webert KE, Cook RJ, Heddle NM (2008) An evaluation of methods for determining reference intervals for light transmission platelet aggregation tests on samples with normal or reduced platelet counts. Thromb Haemost 100:134–145

Huang JY, Soeharto DA, Damara I, Ignjatovic V, Linden MD, Monagle P (2019) Antiplatelet therapy monitoring in neonates and children. Semin Thromb Hemost 45(1):73–85. https://doi.org/10.1055/s-0038-1676375

Hulshof AM, Olie RH, Vries MJA, Verhezen PWM, van der Meijden PEJ, Ten Cate H, Henskens YMC (2021) Rotational thromboelastometry in high-risk patients on dual antithrombotic therapy after percutaneous coronary intervention. Front Cardiovasc Med 8:788137. https://doi.org/10.3389/fcvm.2021.788137

Kirmani BH, Johnson RI, Agarwal S (2017) Platelet function testing in cardiac surgery: a comparative study of electrical impedance aggregometry and thromboelastography. Platelets 28:550–554. https://doi.org/10.1080/09537104.2016.1237626

Kong R, Trimmings A, Hutchinson N, Gill R, Agarwal S, Davidson S, Arcari M (2015) Consensus recommendations for using the Multiplate(®) for platelet function monitoring before cardiac surgery. Int J Lab Hematol 37:143–147. https://doi.org/10.1111/ijlh.12279

Kreiberg MPB, Laugesen NG, Brandt AH, Stavngaard T, Højgaard J, Truelsen T (2024) Platelet-function-monitoring-guided therapy after emergent carotid artery stenting. J Clin Med 13(22): 6690. https://doi.org/10.3390/jcm13226690

Krüger JC, Meves SH, Kara K, Mügge A, Neubauer H (2014) Monitoring ASA and P2Y12-specific platelet inhibition--comparison of conventional (single) and multiple electrode aggregometry. Scand J Clin Lab Invest 74:568–574. https://doi.org/10.3109/00365513.2014.913305

Liu Z, Tian R, Wang Y, Chen Q, Li J, Xu L, Zhang S (2020) Platelet inhibition with ticagrelor versus clopidogrel in diabetic patients after percutaneous coronary intervention for chronic coronary syndromes. Thromb Haemost 120:1221–1229. https://doi.org/10.1055/s-0040-1713375

Lordkipanidzé M, Pharand C, Schampaert E, Turgeon J, Palisaitis DA, Diodati JG (2007) A comparison of six major platelet function tests to determine the prevalence of aspirin resistance in patients with stable coronary artery disease. Eur Heart J 28:1702–1708. https://doi.org/10.1093/eurheartj/ehm226

Lordkipanidzé M, So D, Tanguay JF (2016) Platelet function testing as a biomarker for efficacy of antiplatelet drugs. Biomark Med 10:903–918. https://doi.org/10.2217/bmm-2016-0070

Lordkipanidzé M, Hvas AM, Harrison P (2019) Clinical Tests of platelet function. In: Michelson A (ed) Platelets, 4th edn. Elsevier Inc, pp 593–608

Luddington RJ (2005) Thromboelastography / Thromboelastometry. Clin Lab Haematol 27:81–90. https://doi.org/10.1111/j.1365-2257.2005.00681.x

Mahtta D, Bavry A (2019) αIIbβ3 (GPIIb-IIIa) antagonists. In: Michelson A (ed) Platelets, 4th edn. Elsevier Inc., pp 957–971

Mallouk N, Varvat J, Berger A, Epinat M, Accassat S, Garcin A, Montmartin A, Li G, Garnier P, Mismetti P, Lambert C (2018) Assessment of a flow cytometry technique for studying signaling pathways in platelets: monitoring of VASP phosphorylation in clinical samples. Pract Lab Med 11:10–18. https://doi.org/10.1016/j.plabm.2018.02.002

Meen O, Brosstad F, Liestøl K, Kunszt G, Bendz B, Wettergreen M, Schjelderup NM, Andreassen T, Erikssen G (2012) Sequential ADP-stimulated light transmission and multiple electrode aggregometry in patients taking aspirin and clopidogrel after non ST-elevation myocardial infarction. Scand J Clin Lab Invest 72:318–325. https://doi.org/10.3109/00365513.2012.666565

Michelson AD, Cattaneo M, Eikelboom JW, Gurbel P, Kottke-Marchant K, Kunicki TJ, Pulcinelli FM, Cerletti C, Rao AK (2005) Aspirin resistance: position paper of the Working Group on Aspirin Resistance. J Thromb Haemost 3:1309–1311. https://doi.org/10.1111/j.1538-7836.2005.01351.x

Neumann FJ, Sousa-Uva M, Ahlsson A, Alfonso F, Banning AP, Benedetto U, Byrne RA, Collet JP, Falk V, Head SJ, Jüni P, Kastrati A, Koller A, Kristensen SD, Niebauer J, Richter DJ, Seferovic PM, Sibbing D, Stefanini GG, Windecker S, Yadav R, Zembala MO, ESC Scientific Document Group (2019) ESC/EACTS Guidelines on myocardial revascularization. Eur Heart J 40(2):87–165. https://doi.org/10.1093/eurheartj/ehy394

Ohmori T, Yatomi Y, Nonaka T, Kobayashi Y, Madoiwa S, Mimuro J, Ozaki Y, Sakata Y (2006) Aspirin resistance detected with aggregometry cannot be explained by cyclooxygenase activity:

involvement of other signaling pathway(s) in cardiovascular events of aspirin-treated patients. J Thromb Haemost 4:1271–1278. https://doi.org/10.1111/j.1538-7836.2006.01958.x

Olechowski B, Dalton RT, Khanna V, Ashby A, Vavyla M, Mariathas M, Harris S, Nicholas Z, Mahmoudi M, Curzen N (2018) Detection of individual responses to clopidogrel: validation of a novel, rapid analysis using thrombelastography 6s. Cardiovasc Ther 36:e12433. https://doi.org/10.1111/1755-5922.12433

Orban M, Sibbing D (2013) Platelet function testing in patients with acute coronary syndrome. J Cardiovasc Transl Res 6:371–377. https://doi.org/10.1007/s12265-013-9450-7

Paniccia R, Antonucci E, Maggini N, Miranda M, Gori AM, Marcucci R, Giusti B, Balzi D, Prisco D, Abbate R (2010) Comparison of methods for monitoring residual platelet reactivity after clopidogrel by point-of-care tests on whole blood in high-risk patients. Thromb Haemost 104:287–292. https://doi.org/10.1160/TH09-12-0832

Patrono C, Rocca B (2012) Aspirin and other COX-1 inhibitors. In: Gresele P, Born GVR, Patrono C, Page CP (eds) Handbook of experimental pharmacology vol 210. Antiplatelet agents, 1st edn. Springer, pp 137–164

Polzin A, Helten C, Dannenberg L, Mourikis P, Naguib D, Achilles A, Knoop B, Zako S, Rehder S, Görlinger K, Levkau B, Zeus T, Kelm M, Hohlfeld T, Hoffmann T (2019) Platelet reactivity in patients on aspirin and clopidogrel therapy measured by a new bedside whole-blood assay. J Cardiovasc Pharmacol 73:40–47. https://doi.org/10.1097/FJC.0000000000000631

Preisman S, Kogan A, Itzkovsky K, Leikin G, Raanani E (2010) Modified thromboelastography evaluation of platelet dysfunction in patients undergoing coronary artery surgery. Eur J Cardiothorac Surg 37:1367–1374. https://doi.org/10.1016/j.ejcts.2009.12.044

Price MJ, Endemann S, Gollapudi RR, Valencia R, Stinis CT, Levisay JP, Ernst A, Sawhney NS, Schatz RA, Teirstein PS (2008) Prognostic significance of post-clopidogrel platelet reactivity assessed by a point-of-care assay on thrombotic events after drug-eluting stent implantation. Eur Heart J 29:992–1000. https://doi.org/10.1093/eurheartj/ehn046

Price MJ, Angiolillo DJ, Teirstein PS, Lillie E, Manoukian SV, Berger PB, Tanguay JF, Cannon CP, Topol EJ (2011) Platelet reactivity and cardiovascular outcomes after percutaneous coronary intervention: a time-dependent analysis of the gauging responsiveness with a VerifyNow P2Y12 assay: impact on thrombosis and safety (GRAVITAS) trial. Circulation 124:1132–1137. https://doi.org/10.1161/CIRCULATIONAHA.111.029165

Regan IE, Cox D, Kelleher ST, McMahon CJ (2024) The effects of aspirin dose in children with congenital and acquired heart disease. Results from the Paediatric Study of Aspirin Efficacy using Diagnostic and Monitoring Tools (PAED-M). Pediatr Cardiol. Ahead of print. https://doi.org/10.1007/s00246-024-03509-6

Schimmer C, Hamouda K, Sommer SP, Özkur M, Hain J, Leyh R (2013) The predictive value of multiple electrode platelet aggregometry (multiplate) in adult cardiac surgery. Thorac Cardiovasc Surg 61:733–743. https://doi.org/10.1055/s-0033-1333659

Schultz-Lebahn A, Nissen PH, Pedersen TF, Tang M, Hvas AM (2022) Platelet function assessed by ROTEM®*platelet* in patients receiving antiplatelet therapy during cardiac and vascular surgery. Scand J Clin Lab Invest 82(1):18–27. https://doi.org/10.1080/00365513.2021.2012820

Sibbing D, Schulz S, Braun S, Morath T, Stegherr J, Mehilli J, Schomig A, von Beckerath N, Kastrati A (2010) Antiplatelet effects of clopidogrel and bleeding in patients under- going coronary stent placement. J Thromb Haemost 8:250–256. https://doi.org/10.1111/j.1538-7836.2009.03709.x

Sibbing D, Aradi D, Jacobshagen C, Gross L, Trenk D, Geisler T, Orban M, Hadamitzky M, Merkely B, Kiss RG, Komócsi A, Dézsi CA, Holdt L, Felix SB, Parma R, Klopotowski M, Schwinger RHG, Rieber J, Huber K, Neumann FJ, Koltowski L, Mehilli J, Huczek Z, Massberg S, TROPICAL-ACS Investigators (2017) Guided de-escalation of antiplatelet treatment in patients with acute coronary syndrome undergoing percutaneous coronary intervention (TROPICAL-ACS): a randomised, open-label, multicentre trial. Lancet 390:1747–1757. https://doi.org/10.1016/S0140-6736(17)32155-4

Siller-Matula JM, Hintermeier A, Kastner J, Kreiner G, Maurer G, Kratochwil C, Lang IM, Delle-Karth G (2016) Distribution of clinical events across platelet aggregation values in all-comers treated with prasugrel and ticagrelor. Vasc Pharmacol 79:6–10. https://doi.org/10.1016/j.vph.2016.01.003

Smith JW, Steinhubl SR, Lincoff AM, Coleman JC, Lee TT, Hillman RS, Coller BS (1999) Rapid platelet-function assay: an automated and quantitative cartridge-based method. Circulation 99: 620–625. https://doi.org/10.1161/01.cir.99.5.620

Storey RF, Kotha J, Smyth SS, Moliterno DJ, Rorick TL, Moccetti T, Valgimigli M, Dery JP, Cornel JH, Thomas GS, Huber K, Harrington RA, Hord E, Judge HM, Chen E, Strony J, Mahaffey KW, Tricoci P, Becker RC, Jennings LK (2014) Effects of vorapaxar on platelet reactivity and biomarker expression in non-ST-elevation acute coronary syndromes. The TRACER Pharmacodynamic Substudy. Thromb Haemost 111(5):883–891. https://doi.org/10.1160/TH13-07-0624

Swan D, Turner R, Douketis J, Thachil J (2024) How to undertake procedures while on antiplatelet agents: a hematologist's view. Res Pract Thromb Haemost 8(6):102539. https://doi.org/10.1016/j.rpth.2024.102539

Tantry US, Bliden KP, Chaudhary R, Novakovic M, Rout A, Gurbel PA (2020) Vorapaxar in the treatment of cardiovascular diseases. Futur Cardiol 16:373–384. https://doi.org/10.2217/fca-2019-0090

Trenk D, Stone GW, Gawaz M, Kastrati A, Angiolillo DJ, Müller U, Richardt G, Jakubowski JA, Neumann FJ (2012) A randomized trial of prasugrel versus clopidogrel in patients with high platelet reactivity on clopidogrel after elective percutaneous coronary intervention with implantation of drug-eluting stents: results of the TRIGGER-PCI (testing platelet reactivity in patients undergoing elective stent placement on clopidogrel to guide alternative therapy with prasugrel) study. J Am Coll Cardiol:2159–2164. https://doi.org/10.1016/j.jacc.2012.02.026

Tsantes A, Ikonomidis I, Papadakis I, Kottaridi C, Tsante A, Kalamara E, Kardoulaki A, Kopterides P, Kapsimali V, Karakitsos P, Lekakis J, Travlou A (2012) Evaluation of the role of the new INNOVANCE PFA P2Y test cartridge in detection of clopidogrel resistance. Platelets 23:481–489. https://doi.org/10.3109/09537104.2012.689037

Valgimigli M, Bueno H, Byrne RA, Collet JP, Costa F, Jeppsson A, Jüni P, Kastrati A, Kolh P, Mauri L, Montalescot G, Neumann FJ, Petricevic M, Roffi M, Steg PG, Windecker S, Zamorano JL, Levine GN, ESC Scientific Document Group; ESC Committee for Practice Guidelines (CPG); ESC National Cardiac Societies (2017) ESC focused update on dual antiplatelet therapy in coronary artery disease developed in collaboration with EACTS: the task force for dual antiplatelet therapy in coronary artery disease of the European Society of Cardiology (ESC) and of the European Association for Cardio-Thoracic Surgery (EACTS). Eur Heart J 39:213–260. https://doi.org/10.1093/eurheartj/ehx419.d

Van Oosterom N, Barras M, Cottrell N, Bird R (2022) Platelet function assays for the diagnosis of aspirin resistance. Platelets 33:329–338. https://doi.org/10.1080/09537104.2021.1942816

Weber AA, Przytulski B, Schanz A, Hohlfeld T, Schrör K (2002) Towards a definition of aspirin resistance: a typological approach. Platelets 13:37–40. https://doi.org/10.1080/09537100120104890

Würtz M, Hvas AM, Christensen KH, Rubak P, Kristensen SD, Grove EL (2014) Rapid evaluation of platelet function using the Multiplate® Analyzer. Platelets 25:628–633. https://doi.org/10.3109/09537104.2013.849804

MIX
Papier aus verantwortungsvollen Quellen
Paper from responsible sources
FSC® C105338

If you have any concerns about our products,
you can contact us on
ProductSafety@springernature.com

In case Publisher is established outside the EU,
the EU authorized representative is:
Springer Nature Customer Service Center GmbH
Europaplatz 3, 69115 Heidelberg, Germany

Printed by Libri Plureos GmbH
in Hamburg, Germany